Color Atlas of Immunology

Gerd-Rüdiger Burmester, M.D.

Professor of Medicine
Charité University Hospital
Humboldt University of Berlin
Berlin, Germany

Antonio Pezzutto, M.D.

Professor of Hematology and Oncology
Charité University Hospital
Humboldt University of Berlin
Berlin, Germany

With contributions by
Timo Ulrichs and Alexandra Aicher

131 color plates by Jürgen Wirth
13 tables

Thieme
Stuttgart · New York

Library of Congress Cataloging-in-Publication Data is available from the publisher

Contributors:
Timo Ulrichs, M.D.
Max-Planck-Institute
for Infection Biology
and Institute of Infection Medicine
Free University of Berlin
Berlin, Germany

Alexandra Aicher, M.D.
Molecular Cardiology
Department of Internal Medicine IV
University of Frankfurt
Frankfurt, Germany

Jürgen Wirth
Professor of Visual Communication
University of Applied Sciences
Darmstadt, Germany

This book is an authorized and updated translation of the German edition published and copyrighted 1998 by Georg Thieme Verlag, Stuttgart, Germany.
Title of the German edition:
Taschenatlas der Immunologie.
Grundlagen, Labor, Klinik
Translated by
Suzyon O'Neal Wandrey, Berlin, Germany

© 2003 Georg Thieme Verlag,
Rüdigerstrasse 14, D-70469 Stuttgart, Germany
http://www.thieme.de

Thieme New York, 333 Seventh Avenue,
New York, NY 10001, U.S.A.
http://www.thieme.com

Cover design: Cyclus, Stuttgart
Typesetting by Mitterweger & Partner
Kommunikationsgesellschaft mbH, Plankstadt

Printed in Germany by Grammlich, Pliezhausen
ISBN 3-13-126741-0 (GTV)
ISBN 0-86577-964-3 (TNY)   1 2 3 4 5

Important Note: Medicine is an ever-changing science undergoing continual development. Research and clinical experience are continually expanding our knowledge, in particular our knowledge of proper treatment and drug therapy. Insofar as this book mentions any dosage or application, readers may rest assured that the authors, editors, and publishers have made every effort to ensure that such references are in accordance with **the state of knowledge at the time of production of the book.**

Nevertheless, this does not involve, imply, or express any guarantee or responsibility on the part of the publishers in respect to any dosage instructions and forms of application stated in the book. **Every user is requested to examine carefully** the manufacturer's leaflets accompanying each drug and to check, if necessary in consultation with a physician or specialist, whether the dosage schedules mentioned therein or the contraindications stated by the manufacturers differ from the statements made in the present book. Such examination is particularly important with drugs that are either rarely used or have been newly released on the market. Every dosage schedule or every form of application used is entirely at the user's own risk and responsibility. The authors and publishers request every user to report to the publishers any discrepancies or inaccuracies noticed.

About the Authors

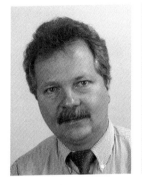 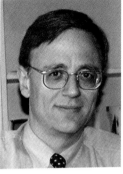 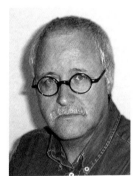

Gerd-Rüdiger Burmester *Antonio Pezzutto* *Jürgen Wirth*

Gerd-Rüdiger Burmester was born in Hanover, Germany in 1953. He studied medicine at the University of Hanover Medical School from 1972 to 1978 and did his doctoral research under the aegis of Professor Joachim R. Kalden in Hanover. His active interest in clinical immunology and rheumatology began during medical school and intensified after his studies as a Postdoctoral Fellow in the laboratories of Professors Henry Kunkel and Robert Winchester at the Rockefeller University in New York on a scholarship from the Deutsche Forschungsgemeinschaft. Dr. Burmester subsequently took up a teaching position at the University of Erlangen Medical School. He completed his additional research requirements for a *Habilitation* (German qualification for professorship) in 1989 and was appointed Associate Professor in 1990. He later accepted a chair at the Department of Rheumatology and Clinical Immunology, Charité Hospital, Humboldt University in Berlin. Professor Burmester is engaged in clinical and experimental rheumatology and clinical immunology. Other interests include medical didactics on both the undergraduate and postgraduate levels. Professor Burmester has a wife and two children.

This pocket atlas was made with substantial help from **Timo Ulrichs**, MD at the Department of Microbiology, Free University of Berlin, and lecturer at the Department of Rheumatology, Charité Hospital. Dr. Ulrichs studied in Marburg and did his doctoral research in immunology. He is currently engaged in studies of immunological infectology in tuberculosis and vaccine development.

Antonio Pezzutto was born in Mirano near Venice in 1953. He studied medicine at the University of Padua from 1972 to 1978 and did his doctoral research in tumor immunology and was subsequently licensed as a specialist for clinical hematology and laboratory hematology. In 1983 he transferred to the University of Heidelberg's Medical Clinic and Policlinic, where he was influenced for 10 years by the exceptional professional competence and personality of Professor Werner Hunstein. Dr. Pezzutto did his *Habilitation* in hematology and clinical immunology. He has served as a professor at the Department of Hematology, Oncology, and Tumor Immunology, Charité Hospital, Humboldt University in Berlin since 1994. He heads the Work Group "Molecular Immunotherapy" at the Max-Delbrück-Center for Molecular Medicine in the Berlin district of Buch. His work mainly focuses on tumor immunology. Professor Pezzutto's wife is a scientist from Great Britain; they have two children.

Alexandra Aicher was essential in compiling the illustrations and texts. She obtained her M.D. at the University of Ulm in 1995 and received post-doctoral training at the Max-Delbrück-Center/Robert-Rössle-Clinic, Berlin until 1997. After 2 years as post-doctoral fellow in immunology and micro-biology at the University of Washington in Seattle, USA, she now works in molecular cardiology at the University of Frankfurt, Germany, focusing on dendritic cells and macrophages in atherosclerosis as well as on hematopoietic stem cells in neovascularization.

Jürgen Wirth began his studies in graphic design at the Offenbach School of Working Arts. He later transferred to the University of Graphic Arts in Berlin, where he majored in free graphics and illustration. He later completed his undergraduate degree at the Offenbach College of Design. Jürgen Wirth developed innovative exhibition concepts as a member of the exhibition design team during the renovation of the Senckenberg Museum in Frankfurt/Main. By that time, he was also working as a freelance graphic designer for several publishing companies, designing the illustrations for a number of school textbooks, nonfiction books, and scientific publications. Jürgen Wirth has received several awards for outstanding book graphics and design. In 1978, he was appointed professor at the School of Design in Schwäbisch Gmünd. Professor Wirth has taught foundation studies, design, and visualization at the Faculty of Design at the University of Applied Sciences in Darmstadt since 1986.

Preface

Immunology is a dynamic discipline with rapid research developments unparalleled by those of any other field except, perhaps, the neurosciences. This research has provided valuable new data for medicine and biology. Immunology, including its fundamental principles and clinical applications, is a very exciting field in which to specialize.

Nowadays, we still live to a ripe old age despite hostile attacks by myriads of pathogenic organisms. Immunological mechanisms have become highly sensitive and specific in the process. This color atlas graphically depicts these mechanisms. Its main goal is to explain the diverse interactions between the fundamental principles and the laboratory and clinical applications of immunology so as to create a vivid mental picture. The book's main target group includes medical students, biology students, and students in other branches of the biosciences. However, it also targets physicians and biologists who are active in their respective fields.

By definition, an atlas must focus on the graphic presentation of subject matter, the explanation of which is limited to brief text segments. Especially in immunology, a graphic presentation of the subject matter must depict certain processes and their progression through time and different phases as well as the interactions between a number of different substances and elements. In order to present an unmistakable picture of these "protagonists," the graphic designers must create archetypal models and skillfully use colors to ensure a clear understanding of the subject matter. We have mainly concentrated on harmonization of the color plates for different topics. The goal was to ensure that the visual elements were not overloaded with internal structures and to have the individual pieces combine to form a mosaic whole. This was sometimes achieved at the expense of aesthetics, and there is inevitably a certain loss of anatomical detail.

Due to space limitations and the emphasis on human medicine, the book mainly focuses on human immunology; space does not permit us to present all areas of the immense field of immunology in their entirety. A number of excellent textbooks of immunology are already on the market. Some of our colleagues may prefer a more comprehensive presentation of the subject matter. We must also remember the enormous developments in immunological research, the constant discovery of new information and processes that are still unclear today, but will soon be well understood. A constant exchange of paradigms is taking place, especially on the subject of tolerance and autoimmunity. The current edition cannot provide full coverage of this new information. We naturally hope that there will be many future editions that will allow us to revise the contents of the book to keep abreast of the latest advances. We would greatly appreciate any suggestions, additions, and corrections proposed by the readers of this color atlas.

Spring 2003

Gerd-Rüdiger Burmester, Berlin
Antonio Pezzutto, Berlin
Jürgen Wirth, Darmstadt

Introduction

This book targets students of medicine and biosciences as well as physicians and bioscientists. As was mentioned in the preface, the book mainly focuses on human immunology. This information will be conveyed in 131 color plates accompanied by explanatory texts on the facing pages.

The atlas is broken down into three main segments. The fundamental principles of human immunology are presented in the opening segment, the essential laboratory tests used in immunology are described in the second section, and the clinical aspects of immunological diseases are presented in the final section. The appendix contains a glossary of important immunological terms and tables including CD nomenclature for immunologically relevant molecules, criteria for classification of rheumatic diseases, an overview of the most important cytokines and growth factors, and important reference values for immunology. Besides providing an introduction to all relevant aspects of modern immunology, this color atlas also serves as an important source of reference for important questions in clinical medicine and laboratory practice.

The **fundamental principles** section begins with the organs of the immune system, followed by a description of the relevant cells of the immune system and the mechanisms by which T and B lymphocytes acquire high levels of specificity. Surface molecules are described in detail in deference to the enormous emphasis placed on them in most immunological publications. A description of accessory cells and natural killer cells follows. Next, the human lymphocyte antigen system is analyzed, followed by the principles of antigen processing and hypersensitivity reactions. Autoimmunity and tolerance are described in the last part of the section.

The **laboratory applications** section describes the most important test systems in immunology. "Conventional" methods such as precipitation, agglutination, and complement-binding reactions are presented along with newer methods such as immunoblotting, molecular biology tests, and a number of test systems for the detection of expressed genes.

The **clinical immunology** section describes immunodeficiencies and the essential immunological features of a number of immune diseases. The main focus is on rheumatology and hematology.

Uniform symbols are used to represent the various cell systems as well as their receptors and products. The symbols are explained on the inside front and inside back covers.

Contents

Fundamental Principles

Laboratory Applications

Clinical Immunology

Appendix

Acknowledgments

The authors thank Professor Falk Hiepe, Dr. Susanne Priem, Dr. Bruno Stuhlmüller, and Dr. Bernhard Thiele, Department of Medicine, Rheumatology and Clinical Immunology, Charité Hospital, for their help in preparing the laboratory section. Our special thanks go to Professor Hans-Eberhard Völker and Professor Herrmann Krastel, Department of Ophthalmology, University of Heidelberg, for their helpful suggestions and for supplying slides on immunological diseases of the eye, and to Professor Wolfgang Schneider, Head of the Pathological Institute, Krankenhaus Berlin Buch, for his constructive comments and a number of photographs on immunological diseases of the kidney.

Valuable photographs and slides were also provided by Dr. Andreas Breitbart, Department of Hematology, University of Ulm, Dr. Uwe Pleyer, Department of Ophthalmology, Charité Hospital, Professor Heidrun Moll, Center for Infection Research, University of Würzburg, Professor Peter Möller, Director of the Institute of Pathology, University of Ulm, Professor Michael Hüfner, Medical Department and Policlinic, University of Göttingen, Professor Herwart Otto, Director of the Institute of Pathology, University of Heidelberg, Dr. Hans R. Gelderblom, Robert Koch Institute, Berlin, Professor Hans-Michael Meinck, Department of Neurology, University of Heidelberg, and Dr. Thomas Wolfensberger, Hôpital Jules Gonin, Lausanne.

List of Abbreviations

AA	amino acid	DT	diphtheria, tetanus (vaccination)
Ab	antibody	DTH	delayed-type hypersensitivity
ACE	angiotensin-converting enzyme	EAE	experimental autoimmune encephalitis
ACh	acetylcholine	EAU	experimental autoimmune uveoretinitis
ADCC	antibody-dependent cell-mediated cytotoxicity	EBV	Epstein–Barr virus
		EC	endothelial cell
Ag	antigen	ECP	eosinophil cationic protein
AIDS	acquired immunodeficiency syndrome	EGF	epithelial growth factor
AIHA	autoimmune hemolytic anemia	ELISA	enzyme-linked immunosorbent assay
AILD	angioimmunoblastic lymphadenopathy with dysproteinemia	EMA	epithelial membrane antigen
		ENA	extractable nuclear antigen
ALCL	anaplastic large-cell lymphoma	ER	endoplasmic reticulum
ALL	acute lymphoblastic leukemia	ESR	erythrocyte sedimentation rate
ALT	alanine aminotransferase	FACS	fluorescence-activating cell sorter
AMA	antimitochondrial antibody	Fc$(\gamma-\varepsilon)$R	Fc receptors for γ, α, δ, μ, and ε immunoglobulins
AML	acute myeloid leukemia		
ANA	antinuclear antibody	FDC	follicular dendritic cell
ANCA	antineutrophil cytoplasmic antibody	FGH	fibroblast growth factor
AP	alkaline phosphatase	FISH	fluorescence in situ hybridization
APC	antigen-presenting cell	FITC	fluorescein isothiocyanate
ARC	AIDS-related complex	GAD	glutamate decarboxylase
AST	aspartate aminotransferase	GALT	gut-associated lymphoid tissue
BAL	bronchoalveolar lavage	GBM	glomerular basal membrane
BALT	bronchus-associated lymphoid tissue	GCDC	germinal center dendritic cell
BCG	bacillus Calmette–Guérin	G-CSF	granulocyte colony-stimulating factor
BCR	B-cell receptor	GM-CSF	granulocyte-macrophage colony-stimulating factor
Cn	complement factor n		
CALLA	common acute lymphoblastic leukemia-associated antigen	GN	glomerulonephritis
		GPI	glycosylated phosphatidylinositol
CBR	complement-binding reaction	GVHD	graft-versus-host disease
CD	cluster of differentiation	GVL	graft-versus-leukemia (effect)
CDR	complementarity-determining region	HAMA	human antimurine antibody
CFU	colony-forming unit	HCV	hepatitis C virus
CLL	chronic lymphatic leukemia	HD	Hodgkin's disease
CMV	cytomegalovirus	HEV	high endothelial venules
COX	cyclooxygenase	HIV	human immunodeficiency virus
CR	complement receptor	HLA	human leukocyte antigen
CRP	C-reactive protein	hsp	heat-shock protein
CSF	colony-stimulating factor	HSV	herpes simplex virus
CTL	cytotoxic T lymphocyte	HTLV	human T-lymphotropic virus
CVID	common variable immune deficiency	IC	immune complex
cyt	intracytoplasmic	ICAM	intercellular adhesion molecule
Da	dalton	ICE	interleukin-1β-converting enzyme
DAF	decay-accelerating factor	IDC	interdigitating cell
DC	dendritic cell	IDDM	insulin-dependent diabetes mellitus
del	chromosomal deletion	IFN	interferon
DPT	diphtheria, pertussis, tetanus	Ig	immunoglobulin

IL	interleukin
ILT	Ig-like transcript
inv	chromosomal inversion
IRAK	IL-1 receptor-associated kinase
IRBP	interphotoreceptor retinoid-binding protein
ITAM	immunoreceptor tyrosine-based activation motif
ITIM	immunoreceptor tyrosine-based inhibiting motif
ITP	idiopathic thrombocytopenic purpura
IVIG	intravenous immunoglobulin therapy
JCA	juvenile chronic arthritis
JRA	juvenile rheumatoid arthritis
kDa	kilodalton
KIR	killer cell Ig-like receptor
L	ligand
LAM	lipoarabinomannane
LBL	lymphoblastic lymphoma
LC	Langerhans cell
LCF	lymphocyte chemotactic factor
LFA	lymphocyte function-associated antigen
LGL	large granular lymphocyte
LIR	leukocyte Ig-like receptor
LKM	liver-kidney microsomal antibody
LPS	lipopolysaccharide
LTR	long terminal repeats
MAb	monoclonal antibody
MAG	myelin-associated glycoprotein
MALT	mucosa-associated lymphoid tissue
MASP	mannan-binding lectin-associated serine protease
MBP	major basic protein
MCP	monocyte chemoattractant protein
M-CSF	monocyte colony-stimulating factor
MCTD	mixed connective tissue disease
MGUS	monoclonal gammopathy of unknown significance
MHC	major histocompatibility complex
MIF	migration inhibition factor
MIRL	membrane inhibitor of reactive lysis
MOG	myelin oligodendrocyte glycoprotein
MPGN	membranoproliferative glomerulonephritis
MPO	myeloperoxidase
MPS	mononuclear phagocytic system
NF	nuclear factor
NFAT	nuclear factor-activated T cell
NGF	nerve growth factor
NHL	non-Hodgkin's lymphoma
NK	natural killer (cell)

NPM-ALK	nucleophospamine anaplastic lymphoma kinase
NSAID	nonsteroidal anti-inflammatory drugs
PAF	platelet-activating factor
PALS	periarteriolar lymphocyte sheath
PAMP	pathogen-associated molecular pattern
PBC	primary biliary cirrhosis
PCR	polymerase chain reaction
PDGF	platelet-derived growth factor
PE	phycoerythrin
PEG	polyethylene glycol
PFC	plaque-forming cell
PIBF	progesterone-induced blocking factor
PLP	proteolipid protein
PMN	polymorphonuclear neutrophil granulocyte
PMR	polymyalgia rheumatica
poly-IgR	polymeric immunoglobulin receptor
POX	peroxidase
PRR	pattern recognition receptors
PSC	primary sclerosing cholangitis
RA	rheumatoid arthritis
REAL	revised European-American lymphoma classification
RF	rheumatoid factor
Rh	rhesus
RID	radial immunodiffusion
RPGN	rapidly progressive glomerulonephritis
RR	relative risk
RS	Reed–Sternberg
S	Svedberg unit
SAA	serum amyloid A
SAP	serum amyloid P
SCID	severe combined immune deficiency
SLE	systemic lupus erythematosus
t (n:n)	chromosomal translocation from chromosome n to n
TAP	transporter associated with presentation
TBII	TSH-binding inhibiting immunoglobulin
TCR	T-cell receptor
TdT	terminal desoxyribonucleotransferase
TG	thyroglobulin
TGF	transforming growth factor
TIL	tumor-infiltrating lymphocyte
TNF	tumor necrosis factor
TPO	thyroidal peroxidase
TSBI	thyroid stimulation-blocking immunoglobulin
TSH	thyroid-stimulating hormone
TSI	thyroid-stimulating immunoglobulin
VCAM	vascular cell adhesion molecule

The Immune System

It took more than 400 million years of evolution for our immune system to develop into the highly complex and adaptable defense mechanism that it is today. Its primary task is to protect us from foreign and harmful substances, microorganisms, toxins, and malignant cells. Only through the continuous development of the immune system was it possible to protect living organisms against constant attacks from both the external and internal environments. In the process, the immune system has learned to inactivate destructive responses to endogenous substances and to prevent irreparable damage to the surrounding tissue. Most immunological responses are of limited duration and are restricted by regulatory mechanisms to prevent overreactions.

An essential task of the immune system is to distinguish dangerous from harmless. Infiltration with microorganisms or bacterial toxins, for example, is a dangerous attack on an organism, whereas the inhalation of pollen or the infiltration of food antigens from the stomach into the blood system is harmless. The destruction of malignant cells or foreign cell material is desirable (e.g., in parasite infestation), but direct attacks against the host tissue are undesirable (e.g., in autoimmune disease). The processes by which the immune system avoids the development of destructive self-reactivity are collectively referred to as *tolerance*. The large majority of lymphocytes directed against self-antigens present throughout the primary lymphoid organs are destroyed in a process known as *central tolerance*. *Peripheral tolerance* is still another mechanism that occurs in less common endogenous structures or in those present only in certain regions of the body.

Nonspecific Immune System

The historically older congenital defense mechanisms are defined as nonspecific because they become active independently of the invading pathogen. They are also called *nonclonal defense mechanisms* because no individual cell clone is required for their specific development. Some examples include the acid layer of the skin, the intact epidermis, the complement system, antimicrobial enzyme systems, and nonspecific mediators such as interferons and interleukins. Examples on the cellular level include granulocytes, the monocyte–macrophage system, and natural killer (NK) cells. The latter represent an interface between the specific and nonspecific immune systems.

The inflammatory response permits an on-the-site concentration of defensive forces via the complex interplay of soluble and cellular components; this is an important nonspecific defense mechanism. The first step in this process is the release of mediators that dilate the blood vessels and make the capillary walls more permeable. The site of infection is then penetrated by granulocytes, which are replaced by macrophages in the later course of the reaction. The granulocytes carry out the "first line of defense" in which the majority of invading pathogens are destroyed. The remaining pathogenic organisms and waste products of this first-line defense are phagocytosed by macrophages.

Specific Immune System

The process of such an immune response paves the way for the specific immune response. In a specific cytokine environment, the body can decide whether to proceed to a more humoral line of defense or a more cellular line of defense. The migration of antigen-presenting cells (APC) to the lymphoid organs first triggers a systemic immune response, then a *memory response*. The specific immune system consisting of T and B lymphocytes is responsible for this. These cell systems can produce highly specific reactions to their respective antigens and undergo clonal expansion, thus achieving a highly effective response to and memory for those antigens.

Fundamental Principles

A. Origin of Cells of the Immune System

All components of the blood, including the cells of the immune system, originate from pluripotent hematopoietic stem cells of the bone marrow. With the aid of soluble mediators (cytokines) and contact signals emitted by stromal cells, these highly undifferentiated progenitor cells can give rise to the different blood cells (A). These cells are among the few body cells capable of self-renewal. Hence, they can divide without differentiating, thereby producing an unlimited supply of blood cells. The bone marrow produces 1.75×10^{11} erythrocytes (red blood cells) and 7×10^{10} leukocytes (white blood cells) each day and has the capacity to increase this production up to severalfold if needed. In vitro, these so-called progenitor cells can form colonies of differentiated cells. Myeloid progenitor cells can differentiate into the following types of cells: *megakaryocytes*, very large multinucleated cells that break up into small particles which constitute the platelets (thrombocytes) of the blood; *erythroblasts*, which further multiply and differentiate into circulating erythrocytes (red blood cells); *myeloblasts*, which can differentiate into neutrophils, eosinophils, and basophils (they all have a segmented nucleus and are therefore called polymorphonuclear leukocytes in order to distinguish them from the other mononuclear cells); *monoblasts* (monocyte precursors); and *dendritic cells*. Granulocytes, monocytes, and dendritic cells have the ability to ingest particles, microorganisms and fluids and are therefore called *phagocytes* (from the Greek word "phago" = "eat").

In response to soluble mediators called *chemokines*, the leukocytes migrate from the blood into the tissue, where they repair damaged tissue and remove bacteria, parasites, and dead cells that induce inflammation. After migration into the tissue, the blood monocytes differentiate into macrophages.

The most important cells of the immune system are the lymphocytes, which originate from a common progenitor cell in the bone marrow. Two types of lymphocytes can be distinguished: T lymphocytes, which are responsible for the cellular immune reponse, and B lymphocytes, which produce antibodies (humoral immune response). Cells of a third type, the natural killer cells, are also part of the lymphatic system. These cells are related to T lymphocytes, but their origin is still a matter of debate since they also express some features of myeloid cells.

B. Defense Mechanisms against Infections

The primary function of the immune system is the protection of the organism against infection. *Innate immunity* is a more ancient line of defense, which is highly conserved between the different species. It consists mainly of phagocytic cells, blood proteins, and natural killer cells. All of its strategies are based on the recognition of typical molecular structures that are shared among different pathogens. The mechanisms of innate immunity are deployed shortly after the body has been invaded by a pathogen—usually within hours.

Phagocytosis is the main mechanisms of innate immunity. In this process, the microorganism is coated with blood components such as complement, which induces lysis of the invader or the release of cytotoxic lytic enzymes from killer cells.

Adaptive immunity, the phylogenetically modern mechanism, is based on the presence of receptors that are highly specific for certain regions (epitopes) of the pathogens. These receptors are either cell-bound (T lymphocytes and some B lymphocytes) or secreted (antibodies produced by B lymphocytes). A single T or B lymphocyte proliferates and produces large quantities of identical daughter cells (clonal expansion). This specific response process takes days to weeks.

C. Plasticity of Stem Cells

When present in specialized tissue, hematopoietic progenitor cells can differentiate into various different blood cells or tissue-specific cells, such as hepatocytes, neurons, muscle cells, or endothelial cells. The signals that regulate their differentiation into specialized cells are still largely unknown. Hematopoietic stem cells circulate in small numbers in the peripheral blood. They are morphologically indistinguishable from small lymphocytes.

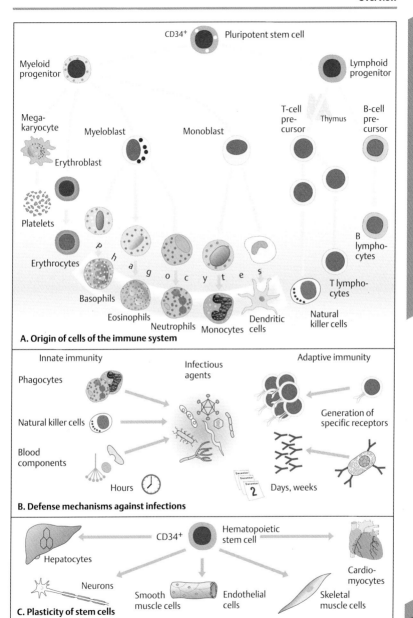

CD34⁺ Pluripotent stem cell

Myeloid progenitor

Lymphoid progenitor

Mega-karyocyte

Myeloblast

Monoblast

T-cell pre-cursor

Thymus

B-cell pre-cursor

Erythroblast

Platelets

Erythrocytes

p h a g o c y t e s

B lympho-cytes

T lympho-cytes

Basophils

Eosinophils

Neutrophils

Monocytes

Dendritic cells

Natural killer cells

A. Origin of cells of the immune system

Innate immunity

Infectious agents

Adaptive immunity

Phagocytes

Natural killer cells

Blood components

Generation of specific receptors

Hours

December 2

Days, weeks

B. Defense mechanisms against infections

Hepatocytes

CD34⁺

Hematopoietic stem cell

Neurons

Smooth muscle cells

Endothelial cells

Cardio-myocytes

Skeletal muscle cells

C. Plasticity of stem cells

Fundamental Principles

3

A. Structure of the Lymphatic System

All blood cells develop from common, pluripotent bone marrow stem cells. They can be detected in the fetal liver, which has hematopoietic properties, from the 8th week of gestation until shortly before birth. The stem cells give rise to the precursor cells of the lymphatic and myelopoietic systems. Erythrocytes, granulocytes, and thrombocytes have common precursor stages (progenitor cells), whereas lymphatic cells develop early into separate cell lines. Starting from the 13th week of gestation, some stem cells migrate to the thymus and bone marrow, which are referred to as the *primary lymphoid organs*. There, the cells continue to proliferate and differentiate. **T** lymphocytes require passage through the **t**hymus to complete their maturation, whereas **B** lymphocytes complete their maturation in the bone marrow (equivalent to the **b**ursa of Fabricius in birds).

Specialized receptors are located on the surface of T and B lymphocytes (antigen receptors made of two glycoprotein chains). The structure of the receptors varies from one cell to another. Each receptor recognizes and binds with only one specific antigen ("lock-and-key" principle). Unlike T lymphocytes, B lymphocytes can mature into plasma cells, produce large quantities of receptors in modified form, and enter the bloodstream as circulating antibodies.

Immature T lymphocytes make contact with specialized epithelial cells, dendritic cells, and macrophages in the thymus, which provides an opportunity for the selection and differentiation of T cells useful to the immune system. Cytokines (soluble regulatory factors or "messengers" for the immune system), such as interleukins 1, 2, 6, and 7, also play an important role. A large number of lymphocytes, especially those which recognize self-components of the body, are destroyed during this process of selection.

B lymphocytes start to develop from stem cells in the bone marrow around the 14th week of gestation. Contact with stromal cells of the bone marrow and cytokines is important for the differentiation of B cells. Interleukins 1, 6, and 7 are the most important cytokines in this process. The bone marrow is the lifetime production site of B lymphocytes.

Mature T and B lymphocytes leave their differentiation sites and migrate to peripheral or *secondary lymphoid organs* (e.g., spleen, lymph nodes, and mucosa-associated lymphoid tissue).

Mucosa-associated lymphoid tissue (MALT) is a collection of lymphatic cells in the submucosal tissue of the gastrointestinal (GI) tract, bronchial tract, urinary tract, and lacrimal glands. Organized lymphoid tissue (e.g., tonsils or Peyer's patches) and a large number of lymphatic cells loosely distributed throughout the pericapillary and periendothelial tissue can be found there.

B. Lymphatic Recirculation

The cells of the lymphatic system circulate continuously and reach all parts of the body with a few exceptions (e.g., vitreous body, brain, testicles). They reach the lymph nodes, skin, and intestine via a specialized endothelium of postcapillary venules, the so-called **h**igh **e**ndothelial **v**enules (**HEV**). The cells of this endothelium are much higher than normal endothelial cells. They express high levels of adhesion molecules that serve as homing receptors for lymphocytes. In response to certain chemotactic factors, lymphocytes migrate to the underlying tissue (diapedesis). The lymphatic cells reenter the circulation through efferent lymph vessels that merge into the thoracic duct. The lymphocytes enter the spleen via arterioles and sinusoids and exit the organ via the splenic vein.

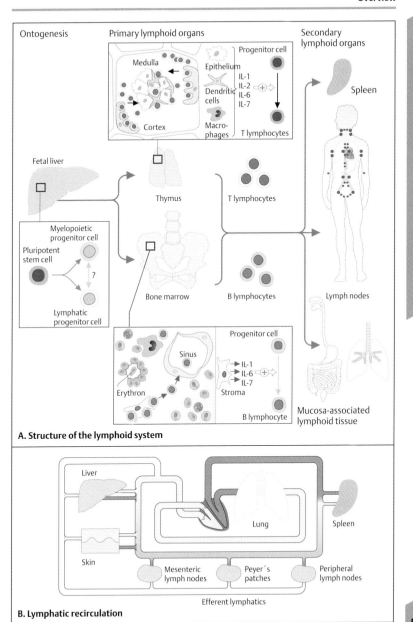

A. Structure of the lymphoid system

Ontogenesis — Primary lymphoid organs — Secondary lymphoid organs

Medulla

Epithelium
Dendritic cells
Macrophages

Cortex

Progenitor cell

IL-1
IL-2
IL-6
IL-7

T lymphocytes

Fetal liver

Thymus

T lymphocytes

Spleen

Myelopoietic progenitor cell

Pluripotent stem cell

?

Lymphatic progenitor cell

Bone marrow

B lymphocytes

Lymph nodes

Sinus

Erythron

Stroma

Progenitor cell

IL-1
IL-6
IL-7

B lymphocyte

Mucosa-associated lymphoid tissue

B. Lymphatic recirculation

Liver

Lung

Spleen

Skin

Mesenteric lymph nodes

Peyer's patches

Peripheral lymph nodes

Efferent lymphatics

Fundamental Principles

5

The thymus is the central organ for the differentiation and functional maturation of T lymphocytes. Like the bone marrow and bursa of Fabricius (in birds), it is one of the primary lymphoid organs and is distinguished from secondary lymphoid organs, such as the spleen, lymph nodes, and mucosa-associated lymphoid tissue.

A. Anatomy and Development of the Thymus

1 In the ontogenic sense, the thymus develops as an outgrowth of the third branchial pouch and later migrates through the anterior mediastinum to its final destination between the sternum and the major vessel trunks. It consists of two lobes that unite cranially to form the horns of the thymus, which sometimes extend to the thyroid gland.

2 The size of the thymus is age-dependent. It reaches a maximum weight of around 40 g around the 10th year of life and then undergoes a continuous process of involution. As a result, the parenchyma of the thymus consists almost entirely of fat and fibrous tissue in old age. Only a few clusters of parenchyma and lymphocytes remain intact (see also paragraphs **3** and **4**). In many cases, it is not possible to reliably differentiate between the involuted organ and the surrounding mediastinal fat by macroscopic means.

3, 4 Each lobe of the thymus is subdivided by fibrous septa (trabeculae) into smaller lobes, each of which consists of an outer layer (cortex) and an inner layer (medulla). The cortex contains a dense cluster of lymphocytes; the abundance of mitoses is indicative of extensive proliferation. The medulla, on the other hand, has a much smaller population of lymphatic cells. It also contains structures known as Hassall's bodies that are made of densely packed cell layers. These structures may be the remnants of degenerated epithelial cells. An intrathymic barrier similar to the blood–brain barrier divides the cortex from the circulating blood. No such barrier exists for the marrow.

The lymphocytes that mature into T cells in the thymus are often called *thymocytes* for functional and anatomical reasons. The specific combination of important surface markers permits immunophenotypic differentiation between thymocytes and mature T cells. Thymocytes are extremely cortisone-sensitive in the early stages of development (important for maturation studies), but as the process of differentiation continues, they become more and more cortisone-resistant. The cortisone-sensitive, immature thymocytes are located mainly in the cortex, and the cortisone-insensitive ones are mainly localized in the medulla.

5 Apart from lymphocytes and Hassall's bodies, the thymus also contains epithelial cells with a large cytoplasm and dendritic cells and macrophages (the latter cell groups are not shown in the illustration). Moreover, the thymus contains a large number of blood vessels and efferent lymphoid tissues that drain into the mediastinal lymph nodes.

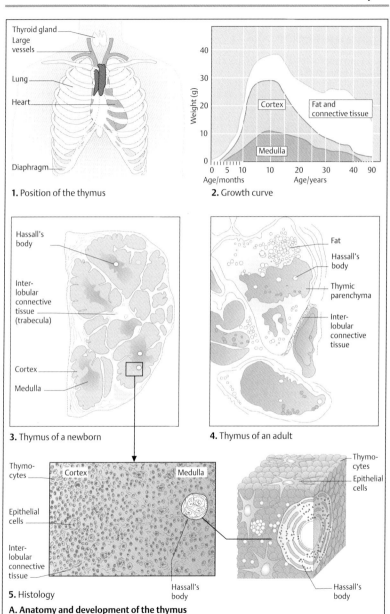

1. Position of the thymus

2. Growth curve

3. Thymus of a newborn

4. Thymus of an adult

5. Histology

A. Anatomy and development of the thymus

A. Structure of the Spleen

The spleen is the largest lymphoid organ (size about 12×7×4 cm, weight about 200 g). It consists of two types of tissue: red pulp and white pulp. The *white pulp* consists of lymphocytes. The *red pulp* resembles a sponge made of erythrocytes; it is the site of elimination of old and/or damaged erythrocytes. The spleen is surrounded by a capsule of collagen fibers. Collagen septa (trabeculae) accompanied by arterioles radiate from the capsule into the splenic parenchyma, where the white pulp is located. T lymphocytes are mainly located in the periarteriolar region, thus forming the periarteriolar lymphocyte sheath (PALS). They are surrounded by B lymphocytes that form the so-called *marginal zone*. Small clusters of B lymphocytes (*primary follicles*) can always be found in the marginal zone of the PALS. During an immune response, the primary follicles develop into true follicles (*secondary follicles*) with a germinal center and follicular cortex.

B cells escape from the bloodstream into the T-cell-rich periarteriolar region and continue on to the follicle. They then pass the marginal zone and venous sinusoidal vessels in the region of the white pulp, where they ultimately reenter the circulation (B-cell recirculation; see also pp. 22 and 24).

B. Structure of the Lymph Nodes

Lymph nodes are situated along the lymphatic vessels; they form a complex network that drains the skin and the internal organs. Like the spleen, the lymph nodes are invested in a capsule of collagen fibers. Normal lymph nodes are round to kidney-shaped structures that are 1–15 mm in diameter. The lymphatics penetrate the capsule and form the *marginal sinuses* in the subcapsular region and the *interfollicular sinuses* in the deeper zones down to the center of the lymph node. At the center of the node, the sinuses merge to form central *medullary sinuses*. Lymph leaves the lymph node via a single efferent lymphatic which runs along the blood vessels.

The external cortex of the lymph node contains mainly B lymphocytes, whereas the T lymphocytes are mainly localized in the underlying paracortical region. After antigen stimulation, loose clusters of B cells in the cortex (*primary follicles*) give rise to the so-called *secondary follicles*, which contain a germinal center made of blastic elements (centrocytes and centroblasts) and a mantle zone made of small lymphocytes.

C. Mucosa-associated Lymphoid Tissue (MALT)

Loosely organized lymphoid tissues with small aggregates of T cells, B cells, and plasma cells (mainly of the IgA type) are located in the submucosa of the gastrointestinal tract, respiratory tract, lacrimal glands, and urinary tract.

The gastrointestinal tract also contains complex structures, such as the tonsils and Peyer's patches. The tonsillar architecture is similar to that of lymph nodes.

In the terminal ileum, Peyer's patches consist of follicles with germinal centers and mantle zones. A large number of antigen-presenting cells can be found in the region between the follicle and the follicle-associated intestinal epithelium ("dome region"). The dome epithelium is characterized by the presence of so-called *microfold cells* (M cells), which have numerous microfolds (not microvilli) on the epithelial side and are specialized transporters of antigens. The apical surface of these cells therefore contains specific oligosaccharides instead of the usual glycocalyces. M cells can also bring in lymphocytes and monocytes, which can pick up antigens even within the M cells.

T lymphocytes are mainly loosely distributed throughout the interfollicular tissue: some are also found in the intraepithelial region. The number of intraepithelial lymphocytes and plasma cells increases dramatically when inflammation occurs.

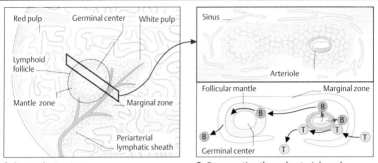

1. Anatomic structure

2. Cross-section through arteriole and follicle; lymphocyte circulation

A. Structure of the spleen

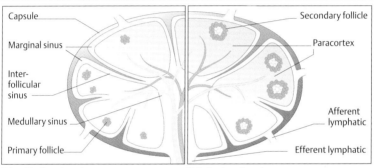

1. Inactive lymph node

2. Active lymph node

B. Structure of the lymph node

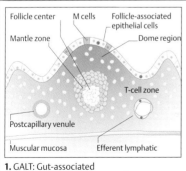

1. GALT: Gut-associated lymphoid tissue; Peyer's patch

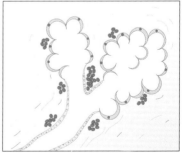

2. BALT: Bronchus-associated lymphoid tissue

C. Mucosa-associated lymphoid tissue

Fundamental Principles

9

A. Maturation of T cells

Pre-thymocytes are precursors of the T cells (T lymphocytes); they mature in the bone marrow and fetal liver. In the embryonal stages, the thymus arises from the 3rd branchial pouch and incoming precursor cells; the branchial pouch thereby forms the epithelial component and the precursor cells the lymphatic component of the thymus. The thymic epithelial cells provide hormones important for the development of the pre-thymocytes. In the thymus the precursor cells mature into thymocytes and are ultimately released as mature T cells into the circulation.

B. Phases of Thymocyte Development

Pre-thymocyte development takes place in the fetal liver and bone marrow, where the rearrangement of T-cell receptors (TCR) and the change in genetic information required for gamma chains also occur. These precursor cells are characterized by the presence of terminal deoxynucleotidyl transferase (TdT) enzyme. Once they enter the thymus, the cells differentiate into early thymocytes distinguished by surface expression of CD2 and CD7 antigens (stage 1 of T-cell differentiation). Transcription of the T-cell receptor's gamma chain and rearrangement of the beta chain also occurs in the thymus. These cells are described as double negative since they contain neither the CD4 nor the CD8 antigen.

In the next stage of maturation (stage 2), the common thymocyte contains characteristic CD1 antigens as well as CD4 and CD8 surface antigens (double positive). Expression of the TCR on the cell surface occurs in conjunction with the formation of alpha and beta chains. Molecules of the CD3 antigen receptor complex also appear on the cell surface.

A decisive step toward the maturation of the actual T cells now occurs (stage 3). The CD1 antigen is lost, and the cells divide to form two T-cell populations that bear either the CD4 antigen or the CD8 antigen. The CD4 antigen is characteristic of the T-helper (T_H) cell population, and the CD8 antigen is characteristic of the cytotoxic T cell population (T_C, CTL). The cells are now said to be single positive. Over 99% of all mature T cells bear TCRα/β on the surface; the rest have TCRγ/δ. The T-cell receptors are distinguished functionally in their ability to recognize antigens.

C. Development of Mature T Cells

After being released into the circulation, the mature T cells undergo further differentiation in the blood and lymphatic system. These *naive T cells* circulate until antigen contact has been established outside the lymphoid organs. They bear the CD45RA surface antigen. This antigen contact leads to the development of memory T cells that are characterized by the presence of the CD45RO and CD29 antigens. CD45RO is a variant of common leukocyte antigen (see also p. 17), a cell surface phosphatase. CD29, on the other hand, is a fibronectin receptor important for the adhesion of T cells and for their migration in tissue.

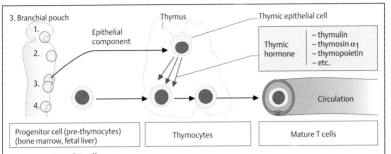

A. Maturation of T cells

Location	Fetal liver Bone marrow	Thymus		
Cell	Pre-thymocytes	Early thymocyte	General thymocyte	Mature thymocyte
TCR	Rearrangement of TCRγ	Transcription of TCRγ rearrangement of TCRβ	Cell surface expression of TCRγ, α, β	Mainly expression of TCRα, β
Marker	TdT enzyme	TdT, CD2, CD7 (CD1) Double negative	TdT, CD1, CD2, CD3, CD5, CD4 and CD8 Double positive	T_H: CD2, CD5, CD7, CD3, CD4 T_C: CD2, CD5, CD7, CD3, CD8 Single positive

B. Phases of thymocyte development

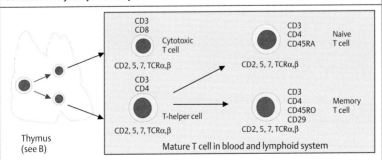

C. Development of mature T cells

Fundamental Principles

The thymus ensures that most T cells that are released into the circulation function in conjunction with the corresponding *major histocompatibility complex* (MHC) genes of the body's immune system but do not identify endogenous substances as foreign material.

A. Mechanisms of T-Cell Selection in the Thymus

After pre-thymocytes migrate to the thymus, they come into contact with thymic epithelial cells. T-cell receptors then develop and interact with MHC molecules on epithelial cells. One of the following events may occur in the process.

The thymocytes may be unable to bind with MHC molecules via the T-cell receptor (case A). This is necessary, however, for destruction of virus-infected cells that present the viral antigen to T cells on the corresponding MHC molecules. If the "partner" of the infected cell were a T cell incapable of forming such a bond, the T cell would not be able to recognize the antigen. As a result, the infected cell would not be destroyed. Such "misprogrammed" T cells are of no use to the immune system and are eliminated right away. This is not done by actively killing the cells, but by an endogenous "suicide program" referred to as *programmed cell death* or *apoptosis*. These cells do not receive a positive, life-saving signal to terminate the process of programmed cell death; see also p. 65.

The T cells may be able to cooperate with the correctly matching MHC molecule. The T-cell receptor is able to form a bond with a thymus epithelial cell via the MHC molecule, and the T cell receives a signal to abort the suicide program, thus saving its life. The cell is allowed to continue to mature and may ultimately be released into the circulation. Another important protective mechanism determines whether this occurs. If the bond between the T-cell receptor and the MHC molecule is too strong, a cytotoxic response to the body's own antigen-presenting cells may later occur. In this case also, the T cell will be destroyed (case B).

In some cases, the T-cell receptor and the MHC antigen may match but the receptor recognizes an endogenous antigen. Responses by such "autoimmune" T cells could ultimately destroy the organism. Hence, this type of cell is also "sorted out" in a process that is probably mediated by dendritic cells that migrate to the thymus. Dendritic cells possess most, but not all, surface autoantigens known to exist (see also p. 59A). T cells that react with one of these autoantigens will not receive a life-saving signal and will be destroyed (case C).

Only those cells that recognize the matching MHC molecule, form a moderately strong bond with it, and are not directed against any autoantigens will be allowed to fully mature and pass as fully functional T cells into the circulation (case D).

Considering this strict process of selection, 90% of the thymocytes that migrate into the thymus will perish. Apart from these selective mechanisms, certain peripheral safety mechanisms also work to suppress autoaggressive T cells. This provides an additional degree of safety when the autoaggressive cells are not eliminated in the first process of selection (see also p. 59**B**).

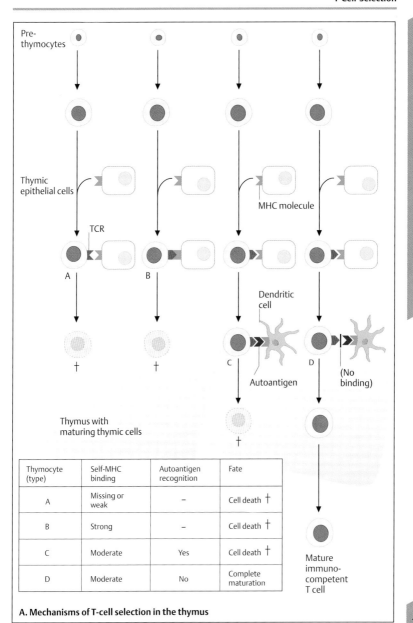

A. Mechanisms of T-cell selection in the thymus

A. T-Cell Receptor Gene Families

Alpha (α) and beta (β) chains are the most commonly expressed TCR genes. TCRγ/δ is expressed on immature T cells and on a minority of T cells in the peripheral blood. Alpha and beta chains are located on chromosome 14, whereas delta and gamma chains are situated on chromosome 7. Similarly to the immunoglobulins, the variable regions of the T-cell receptor are located on various exons, which are ultimately linked with the constant regions of the receptor by splicing. This ensures a very high degree of receptor variability, which is further enhanced by the variable selection of J elements (α and β chains) and D segments (β chains).

B. T-Cell Receptor Rearrangement

The recombination process that occurs while the information needed for the T-cell receptor chain formation is being organized results in *gene rearrangement*, a process in which a particular gene element or elements may be deleted or altered in an unbalanced chromosome exchange. *Inversion* is a process characterized by the formation of loops, subsequent chromosome cleavage, and reconnection to inversions. In other words, the transcription order of the original genetic information is reversed.

C. Configuration of the T-Cell Receptor

The α chain of the T-cell receptor is a 40–60 kDa glycoprotein, whereas the β chain has a molecular weight of 40–50 kDa. Like the immunoglobulins, T-cell receptor chains have *variable regions* and *constant regions*. In the β chain, the C-terminal ends of the V region (link between the V and C regions) are encoded by J and D genes. The V regions of the α and β chains have 102–119 amino acids and contain two cysteine compounds that permit the formation of a disulfide bridge.

The C regions of the α and β chains contain 138–179 amino acids and have four functional domains, which are normally encoded by different exons.

The amino-terminal C domain contains two cysteine compounds with disulfide bridges within the chain; hence, the tertiary structure presumably corresponds to that of the constant region of the immunoglobulin molecule. The transmembrane domain comprises 20–24 primarily hydrophobic amino acids.

In contrast to the α and β chains, the γ and δ chains are located only on T cells that express CD3 but not α/β receptors. The structure of γ and δ chains is similar to that of the α and β chains. The amino acid sequence of the γ chain very closely resembles that of the β chain, and the sequence of the δ chain corresponds to that of the α chain.

D. T-Cell Receptor Combination Potential

As in the immunoglobulins, the different possibilities for combining V, D, and J genes and other mechanisms create an enormous diversity resulting in a combination potential of 10^{15} for T-cell receptors.

E. Distribution of α/β and γ/δ T Cells

The large majority of mature T cells in the blood (and, presumably, also those in tissue) express TCRα/β. This includes the ca. 66% CD4-positive and ca. 33% CD8-positive T-cells (average figures). TCRα/β cells are seldom double negative or double positive (see p. 9**B**). In contrast, the majority of γ/δ T cells are double negative. Some are double positive, and only a few express the CD4 antigen.

The function of the TCRγ/δ-positive cells is still unknown. They are thought to play an important role in the defense against mycobacteria and in their response to superantigens.

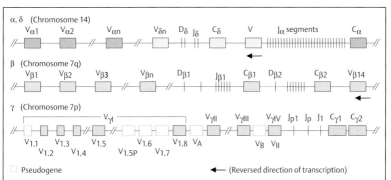

A. T-cell receptor gene families

□ Pseudogene   ◀── (Reversed direction of transcription)

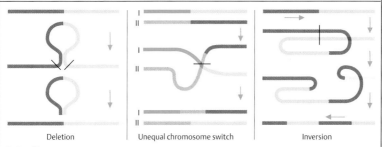

Deletion   Unequal chromosome switch   Inversion

B. T-cell receptor rearrangement

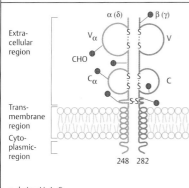

α chain = V - J - C
β chain = V - D - J - C
δ chain = V - D - J - C
γ chain = V - J - C

C. Configuration of the T-cell receptor

Gene segments	α-chain	β-chain
V	100	100
D	0	2
J	100	13
V×D×J-combinations	10^4	$2×10^3$
N-sequences	10^4	10^4
Total number of α/β combinations		10^{15}

D. Possible combinations of the T-cell receptor (α/β)

	$\frac{α/β}{95\%}$	$\frac{γ/δ}{5\%}$	
Total:			

Marker:	CD4$^+$	CD8$^-$	66%	<1%	
	CD4$^-$	CD8$^+$	33%	25%	Weak
	CD4$^-$	CD8$^-$	<1%	70%	
	CD4$^+$	CD8$^+$	<1%	<12%	

E. Distribution of α/β and γ/δ T cells

Fundamental Principles

15

In addition to the T-cell receptor, numerous helper molecules are also needed for the development, differentiation, activation, and antigen recognition of T cells. These molecules play an important role in the binding of T cells with antigen-presenting cells (accessory molecules). Some of these molecules, such as the CD3 antigens, occur exclusively on cells of the T-cell line, whereas others occur on B cells and accessory cells. These molecules can be recognized and analyzed with the help of monoclonal antibodies. This method has not only greatly increased the understanding of lymphatic cell function, but it is also one of the most important advances in immunological diagnostics. It is the method used to determine the immune status and the type category of malignant lymphatic tumors. At consensus conferences, antigens identified using monoclonal antibodies have been (and will continue to be) given internationally valid designations starting with "CD" (cluster of differentiation) and a corresponding number.

A. Human T-Cell Differentiation Molecules

The CD1 antigen has five isoforms (a, b, c, d, e) and is expressed on cortical thymocytes and dendritic cells. CD1 molecules are structurally similar to class I major histocompatibility antigens. Like the MHC antigens, they form complexes with β_2-microglobulin. CD1 antigens are thought to be involved in the presentation of lipid-containing antigens to T cells. Mycobacterial lipidic antigens are also presented by CD1.

The CD2 molecule serves as a receptor for the CD58 antigen, e.g., the lymphocyte functional antigen (LFA)-1. CD2 is an important factor in alternative T-cell activation. It is an early T-cell marker that is encoded by all T lymphocytes and natural killer (NK) cells.

The CD3 cluster consists of a number of important membrane-based molecules that are closely associated with T-cell receptors. These molecules, especially their zeta (ζ) and eta (η) chains, are required for signal transduction once contact with MHC molecules has been established. MHC molecules are directly responsible for T-cell activation. An exact description of how these molecules function can be found on p. 17.

The CD4 molecule is characteristic of T-helper cells. Apart from immature thymocytes, it is also expressed by accessory cells and eosinophilic granulocytes. It plays an important role in class II MHC molecule binding and interacts with p56[lck] tyrosine kinase. It also serves as the binding protein for the human immunodeficiency virus (HIV). The CD4 antigen corresponds to the CD8 molecule, which consists of two chains and is characteristic of cytotoxic T cells. It is also located on immature thymocytes and is weakly characteristic of natural killer cells. It is responsible for binding to class I MHC molecules and interacts with p56[lck] tyrosine kinase.

The CD5 antigen and CD7 antigen are also characteristic of T cells. CD5 is involved in signal transduction and cell-to-cell interactions. The CD7 antigen can be described as the earliest T-cell marker; its mode of action is still largely unknown. The CD5 antigen is also expressed in a subpopulation of B lymphocytes.

CD28 and CD152 (CTLA-4) molecules interact with CD80 and CD86 molecules on antigen-presenting cells. Interaction between CD28 and CD80/CD86 generates an important co-stimulatory signal for T-cell activation and proliferation. The binding of CTLA-4 to this molecule, on the other hand, represents a negative signal for the T cell.

Molecule	Molecular weight (kDa)	Gene locus	Cell expression	Function
α β2m CD1a b,c,d,e	43 – 49	1q22-23	Thymocytes, dendritic cells, few B cells (CD1c)	Antigen-presentation (glycolipids)
CD2	50	1p13	Thymocytes, all T cells, NK cells	Receptor for CD58 (LFA-1), T-cell activation
γ δ ζ/η α(δ) β(γ) ε CD3/TCR	CD3g 25 CD3d 20 CD3e 20 ζ-chain 16 η-chain 22	11q23 11q23 11q23 1q22 1q22	Maturing thymocytes, T cells	Signal-transduction after MHC-TCR contact
CD4	55	12p12	Thymocytes, T-helper cells, monocytes/macrophages, dendritic cells, eosinophilic granulocytes	Binding to MHC class II MHC
CD5	67	11q13	Thymocytes, all maturing T cells, few B cells	Signal transduction
CD7	40	17q25	All cells of T-cell lineage	Not known
α β CD8	CD8α 33 CD8β 33	2p12 2p1	Thymocytes, cytotoxic T-cells, NK cells (weak, CD8a)	Binding to class I MHC molecules
CD154 (CD40L)	33	Xq26.3-27.1	CD4+ T cells (after activation), CD8+ T cells (subpopulation), basophils	Binds to CD40, activates B cells and dendritic cells
CD28	40	2q33	Thymocytes CD4+ T cells, CD8+ T cells, (subpopulation)	Ligand for CD80, CD86 ("co-stimulatory signal")
CD152 (CTLA-4)	33	2q33	Activated T cells	Ligand for CD80, CD86 (negative regulator of T-cell activation)

A. Human T-cell differentiation molecules

A. T-Cell Activation and Signal Transduction

Once it has been bound by MHC α and β molecules (see p. 51), the antigenic peptide is presented to the specific T cell, which first forms a bond with α and β chains to form a trimolecular complex (see p. 35). The bond is stabilized by the CD4/CD8 molecule. The actual signal transduction process finally takes place mainly via the ζ and η molecules of the CD3 complex. CD4 and CD8 (α chain) cells are involved in signal transduction via p56^{lck} tyrosine kinase, but the CD45 antigen plays a very important role. The latter occurs in several isomeric forms and exhibits intracellular tyrosine phosphatase activity. Hence, phosphorylation activity mediated by phosphotyrosine kinase is the first step toward T-cell activation after the ligand binds to the TCR molecule. This process permits other proteins with specific tyrosine-binding properties to combine with phosphorylated proteins. These structurally preserved binding motifs are referred to as *Src-homology-2 domains* (SH2 domains) because they were first identified in the Src protein.

Phosphorylation of tyrosine amino acids on the cytoplasmic part of a membrane-based protein leads to the binding of SH2-containing proteins at this binding site. Besides CD45, p59^{fyn}, and p56^{lck}, zeta-associated protein (70 kDa) and zeta-associated protein kinases (ZAP kinase) also play an important role.

Phosphatidylinositol phospholipase (PIP) enzyme is stimulated during the activation process. This triggers other processes that ultimately lead to an increase in the concentrations of inositol trisphosphate (IP$_3$) and diacylglycerol (DAG) in cytoplasm. This, in turn, causes a considerable increase in cellular calcium levels due to the mobilization of membrane-based intracellular calcium deposits. This influx of DAG and calcium first activates protein kinase C (PKC), a serine/threonine phosphokinase, then the proto-oncogene product Ras. This initiates a specific signal transduction cascade that leads to the activation of transcription activators, such as AP/1 (see below). Calmodulin and calcineurin are also involved in this activity.

These events ultimately lead to gene activation and the regulation of gene transcription. The initiation of interleukin-2 (IL-2) gene transcription is a key factor in T-cell activation. The transformation of the nuclear factor of activated T cells (NFAT) from the preexisting form to the active form by way of phosphorylation plays a decisive role in the process. NFAT migrates to the nucleus, binds to the specific IL-2 promoter region, and cooperates with another nuclear binding factor (AP-1 complex) in starting IL-2 gene transcription via RNA polymerase II.

B. T-Cell Activation: The Time Course of Gene Expression

A distinction is made between immediate, early, and late T-cell activation processes. Proto-oncogenes (c-*fos* and c-*myc*), nuclear binding proteins (see section **A**), and cytokine genes become involved in this order of succession. The increased expression of MHC determinants (on certain cell systems) and adhesion molecules occurs only several days later.

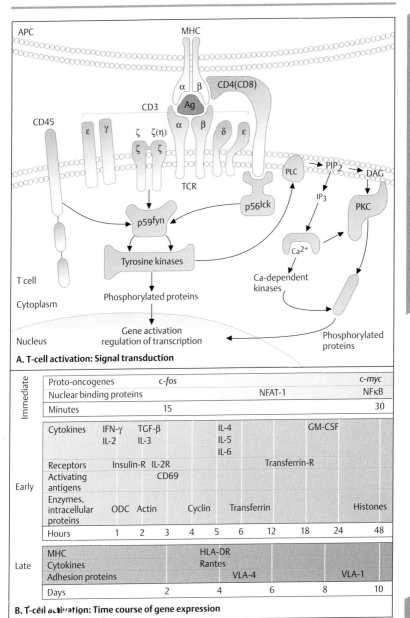

A. T-cell activation: Signal transduction

Immediate	Proto-oncogenes		c-*fos*						c-*myc*
	Nuclear binding proteins						NFAT-1		NFκB
	Minutes			15					30

Early	Cytokines	IFN-γ IL-2	TGF-β IL-3			IL-4 IL-5 IL-6			GM-CSF		
	Receptors	Insulin-R	IL-2R				Transferrin-R				
	Activating antigens		CD69								
	Enzymes, intracellular proteins	ODC	Actin		Cyclin		Transferrin				Histones
	Hours	1	2	3	4	5	6	12	18	24	48

Late	MHC		HLA-DR			
	Cytokines		Rantes			
	Adhesion proteins			VLA-4		VLA-1
	Days	2	4	6	8	10

B. T-cell activation: Time course of gene expression

Fundamental Principles

Fundamental Principles

A. Differentiation into T_H1 and T_H2 cells

Peripheral T cells can differentiate into naive T cells and memory T cells (see page 9C). After further antigen contact, they form two distinct subpopulations known as the T_H1 and T_H2 subgroups.

After the initial contact with various antigens (e.g., bacteria, fungi, protozoans, grass pollens), most T_H cells encounter elements of the nonspecific immune system, especially macrophages, natural killer cells, and mast cells. The establishment of such contact and the corresponding antigen response are subject to the genetic susceptibility (predisposition) of the host, which is determined by MHC components, T-cell receptors, and other still unknown factors.

Antigen processing by nonspecific defense cells produces a cytokine milieu that has a decisive effect on the further course of the immune response. Interleukin (IL)-12, which is secreted by macrophages, also plays an important role. Further antigen presentation is carried out by "professional" antigen-presenting cells (mainly dendritic cells). The trimolecular TCR–antigenic peptide–MHC complex and the bond between the B7/1 (CD80) and CD28 molecules are also important. Due to the predominantly cytokine milieu and the different manners of antigen presentation, the originally undetermined T-helper null cell (T_H0) transforms into either a T_H1 or T_H2 cell.

T_H1 T cells mainly secrete IL-2, IFN-γ, TNF-β, and GM-CSF. They lead via macrophage activation to extensive inflammatory processes that also enable the killing of intracellular pathogens.

T_H2 cells mainly form IL-4 and IL-5 (and also IL-3, IL-6, IL-7, IL-8, IL-9, IL-10, and IL-14) and activate B cells for production of antibodies.

The nature of these processes in *Leishmania* infection has been studied in an exemplary fashion. Different mouse strains react differently to the infection depending on the cytokine pattern. A T_H1 cytokine pattern ensures the survival of the laboratory animals after contact with the pathogen, whereas the predominance of T_H2 cells leads to a lethal course of infection.

Both T-helper cell groups are able to inhibit the activation of the other group using their own cytokines. Hence, IFN-γ leads to inhibition of T_H2 cells, whereas IL-10 impedes macrophage activation and leads to marked immuno-suppression. The characteristic cytokines, on the other hand, have a positive, intensifying effect on the respective subpopulation. IL-2, for example, acts on T_H1 cells and IL-4 on T_H2 cells. We must stress, however, that there are often no strict lines between the subpopulations in the human defense system. On the contrary, it is possible to have smooth, pathogen-dependent transitions between the subpopulations.

B. Regulation of IgE Production

The T_H2 cell plays an essential role in the regulation of IgE production. Activation of the B cell takes place mainly via the CD40/CD40 ligand system. There occurs a release of IL-4, IL-13 and/or soluble receptors of IL-4 (IL-4-R) that also contribute to IgE production. IL-4 leads to the differentiation of B cells in IgG1 and IgE-producing plasma cells, whereas IL-13 induces the formation of IgG4 and IgGE antibodies.

C. Regulatory T cells

Regulatory T cells have a suppressor function. They represent a minority of CD4$^+$ T cells that co-express CD25 even in the absence of activation. CD4$^+$ CD25$^+$ regulatory T cells have been shown to present autoimmunity, as their depletion promotes development of various autoimmune diseases in mice. They also seem to play a role in preventing effective immunosurveillance in patients with cancer (see p. 152).

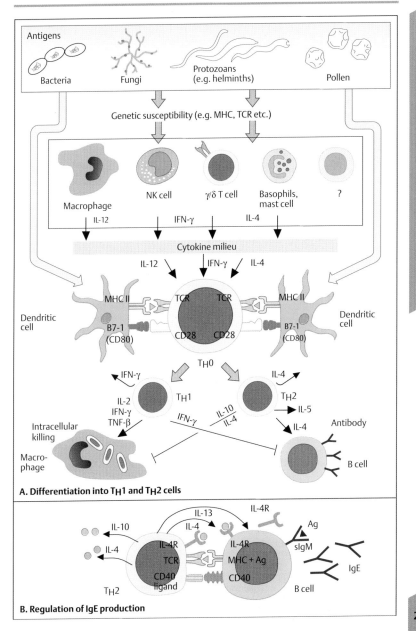

A. Differentiation into T$_H$1 and T$_H$2 cells

B. Regulation of IgE production

A. Development of B Lymphocytes

B lymphocytes develop in the bone marrow from pluripotent stem cells in reaction to signals from stromal cells (soluble cytokines; cell–cell contact).

The progenitor B cell (pro-B cell) is the first recognizable stage of B-cell development. Pro-B cells are self-replenishing cells that express stem cell-associated antigens (CD34 and CD117) and B-cell line-specific antigens CD19 and CD22 (the latter is expressed only in cytoplasm).

Immunoglobulin synthesis begins in the further stage of development. Heavy chains of the IgM immunoglobulins (μ chains) can be detected in the cytoplasm of pre-B cells. The next stage of differentiation is called the "virgin B cell" because the cells have not yet come into contact with foreign antigens. Complete IgM immunoglobulins are expressed on the surface of the virgin cells. The further course of differentiation is antigen-guided. The immature B cells are killed by apoptosis if their immunoglobulins are bound by autoantigens presumably presented to them by stromal cells in the bone marrow (clonal deletion/clonal anergy). The others leave the bone marrow at this stage of maturation and then migrate to the T-cell-rich zones of the peripheral lymphoid organs, where a process of selection occurs once more. All cells that have not received a "survival signal" from the T cells die due to apoptosis. The remaining B cells migrate to the lymphatic follicles. On the surface, they express IgD immunoglobulins and the cell differentiation antigens CD21, CD22, CD23, and CD37. As circulating follicular B cells, they continuously recirculate between the bone marrow and the secondary lymphoid organs until they meet a matching antigen. This usually takes place the in T-cell-rich zone of the lymph nodes or in mucosa-associated lymphoid tissue, where the B cells develop into IgM-producing plasma cells (primary B-cell response). These IgM antibodies have only a low affinity for the antigen. To produce "better" antibodies, the B cells undergo a special process of development in the lymphatic follicles (germinal center reaction; see p. 24) when they encounter immune complexes bound to follicular dendritic cells. The germinal center reaction allows the B cells to develop the ability to produce antibodies of other classes (immunoglobulin switch) and of higher affinity. Terminal maturation of B cells into plasma cells then occurs in the bone marrow or in the mucosa of the gastrointestinal tract.

Some of the antigen-stimulated B cells migrate to the marginal zone of the peripheral organs and differentiate into IgD-negative, CD23-negative, and CD39-positive cells (extrafollicular B cells). In contrast to most other B cells, these cells can also react to carbohydrate antigens (T-cell-independent response), but only generate IgM antibodies of low affinity.

B. CD5⁺ B Cells

A small fraction of B cells is distinguished by the expression of the T-cell-associated differentiation antigen CD5 (Ly1 antigen in the mouse). These B cells (B1+ B-cell fraction) are believed to belong to a subpopulation that diverges from the normal B-cell line early on in the course of ontogenesis and colonizes the pleural and peritoneal cavities. However, the existence of this B-cell population has only been confirmed in the mouse. CD5⁺ B cells are long-lived, self-replenishing, and secrete low-affinity, polyreactive autoantibodies of the IgM class. Their differentiation in the pleural and peritoneal cavities might explain the autoreactivity of these cells (absence of clonal deletion due to contact with stromal cells of the bone marrow).

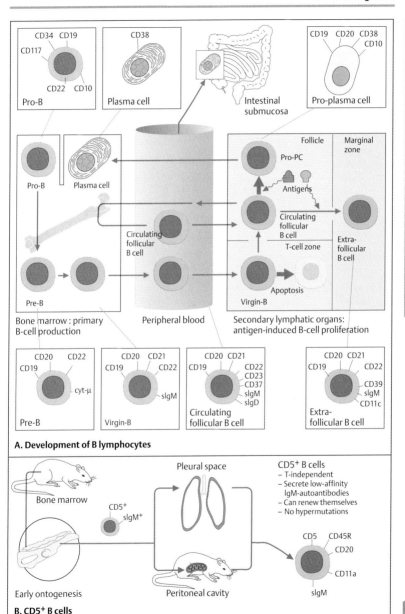

A. Development of B lymphocytes

Pro-B
- CD34 CD19
- CD117
- CD22 CD10

Plasma cell
- CD38

Intestinal submucosa

Pro-plasma cell
- CD19 CD20 CD38
- CD10

Follicle — Marginal zone

Pro-PC
Antigens
Circulating follicular B cell
Extra-follicular B cell
T-cell zone

Virgin-B
Apoptosis

Bone marrow : primary B-cell production

Peripheral blood

Secondary lymphatic organs: antigen-induced B-cell proliferation

Pre-B
- CD20 CD22
- CD19
- cyt-μ

Virgin-B
- CD20 CD21
- CD19 CD22
- sIgM

Circulating follicular B cell
- CD20 CD21
- CD19 CD22
- CD23
- CD37
- sIgM
- sIgD

Extra-follicular B cell
- CD20 CD21
- CD19 CD22
- CD39
- sIgM
- CD11c

B. CD5+ B cells

Bone marrow

CD5+ sIgM+

Pleural space

Peritoneal cavity

CD5+ B cells
- T-independent
- Secrete low-affinity IgM-autoantibodies
- Can renew themselves
- No hypermutations

CD5 CD45R
CD20
CD11a
sIgM

Early ontogenesis

Fundamental Principles

23

A. B-Cell Activation and the Germinal Center Reaction

Unstimulated resting lymphatic follicles such as those in fetal lymph nodes consist of a network of follicular dendritic cells (FDCs) in loose contact with small follicular B cells that exhibit surface expression of IgM and IgD. Once antigen contact takes place, secondary lymphoid follicles with prominent germinal centers develop. The exponential growth of B cells takes place in the germinal center of the follicle only 3–4 days after the initial antigen contact. The B cells first develop into large cells with large amounts of cytoplasm (primary B blasts) and small, "resting" cells along the follicular margin. A few days later, the blasts are concentrated primarily in the basal region of the follicle (*dark zone* of the germinal center), where the branching cytoplasmic processes of the FDCs form a fine, loose network. The blasts (centroblasts) have a doubling time of around seven hours. Nonetheless, they do not increase in number since they quickly transform into small cells with lobular nuclei (centrocytes) that migrate away from the dark zone. These centrocytes then form the so-called *light zone* of the germinal center, where they come into close contact with a very dense network of dendritic cells. A large fraction of centrocytes die due to apoptosis, especially near the boundary between the light and dark zones, where numerous macrophages with phagocytosed apoptotic nuclei (*tingible bodies*) are located. The germinal center reaction lasts for about three weeks. Only a few B-cell blasts (secondary B-blasts) can be found in the center of a "burnt-out" follicle after 2–3 months.

B. B-Cell Antigen Profile During the Germinal Center Reaction

Centroblasts and centrocytes have a high level of CD38 antigen expression. In contrast to follicular and extrafollicular B cells, they have lost the CD23 and CD39 antigens. Centroblasts also express a high density of CD77.

Because the transcription of immunoglobulin genes is temporarily halted while "somatic hypermutation" takes place in centroblasts, the centroblasts are Ig-negative. Centrocytes have renewed expression of immunoglobulin, which permits them to react with antigen presented by FDCs. They may differentiate again into centroblasts, but may also transform into memory B cells or plasmablasts, which then differentiate into plasma cells in the bone marrow or in the mucosal lining of the gastrointestinal tract.

C. Selection of High-Affinity Antibodies by Hypermutation in the Germinal Center

Centroblasts achieve an extremely high mutation rate in immunoglobulin genes (somatic hypermutation) in order to generate antibodies of different affinity. As centrocytes, they migrate to the light zone of the germinal center. Once there, only strong binding to antigen-presenting follicular dendritic cells can prevent them from undergoing apoptosis. The centrocytes receive a further survival signal via CD40 from CD40 ligand-positive T lymphocyzes in the light zone. They then migrate back to the dark zone and begin a new process of cell division as centroblasts. The affinity of the surface immunoglobulins for the antigen can increase due to point mutation. Substitution of a single amino acid, for example, can increase the affinity of the immunoglobulin tenfold. This mechanism helps to select B cells that produce high-affinity antigen-adapted antibodies. The "demand" for these antibodies determines whether a B cell will be able to survive and produce antibodies of the desired affinity and specificity.

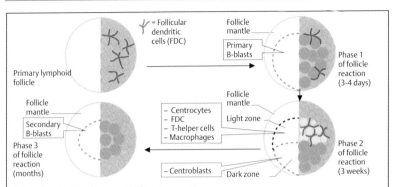

A. B-cell activation: the germinal center reaction

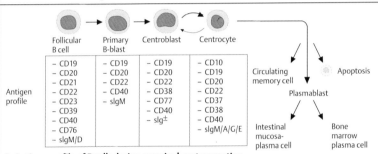

B. Antigen profile of B cells during germinal center reaction

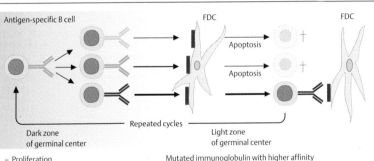

- Proliferation
- Point mutation in
  V-region of H/L-chains

Mutated immunoglobulin with higher affinity
binds antigen-presenting FDC and survives

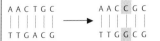

= Amino acid switch = 10-fold increase in affinity

C. Selection of high-affinity antibodies through hypermutation in the germinal center

Fundamental Principles

25

A. Immunoglobulin Structure

B-cell antigen receptors are immunoglobulins expressed on the surface of mature B cells. The receptors are produced by terminally differentiated B cells (plasma cells) and secreted as antibodies into the blood. Immunoglobulins are glycoproteins composed of two identical heavy (H) chains and two identical light (L) chains. Their molecular weights are in the range 50 000–70 000 Da and 25 000 Da, respectively. There are two types of light chains, denoted kappa (κ) and lambda (λ).

Cysteine residues form bridges between the individual chains of an immunoglobulin molecule. An enzyme (papain) separates two identical antigen-binding fragments (Fab fragments) from a non-antigen-binding fragment known as the Fc (crystallizable) fragment. Fc fragments possess binding sites for complement factor C1q (see p. 58).

Light chains consist of two large regions of approximately equal size. The constant region (C_L) varies little from one immunoglobulin to another. The amino acid sequence of the variable region (V_L), on the other hand, exhibits an enormous degree of variability. Both the constant and the variable domains consist of about 110 amino acids (AA). Heavy chains consist of one variable (V_H) domain with around 110 AA and three constant (C_H) domains, except in the case of IgM and IgE, which have four constant domains. The different domains of a given immunoglobulin molecule have a similar globular structure characterized by the presence of multiple β-pleated sheets and disulfide bonds.

B. Immunoglobulin "Superfamily"

Globular domains of similar structure are characteristic of an entire series of molecules of the immune system referred to as an immunoglobulin superfamily. The superfamily comprises immunoglobulins as well as T-cell receptors (TCR), class I and class II major histocompatibility complex (MHC) molecules, a large number of MHC-recognition antigens present on natural killer cells, molecules involved in cell-to-cell interactions (e.g., CD4, CD8, CD19, and CD22 antigens), adhesion molecules (e.g., CD56), and polymeric immunoglobulin receptors (poly-IgR). Poly-IgR is responsible for the passage of IgA and IgM through epithelial cells. The superfamily also includes many other antigens whose function has not yet been characterized.

C. Determination of Antigen Specificity by Hypervariable Regions

The variable domains of heavy and light chains contain regions with extremely variable amino acid sequences. Hence the name "hypervariable regions."

Hypervariable regions consist of 6–8 amino acids around positions 30, 50, and 93 of light chains and around positions 32, 55, and 98 of heavy chains. They determine the specificity of antigen binding and are referred to as *complementarity-determining regions* (CDR); see section **A**. The substitution of a single amino acid in this region is crucial for the binding of a particular antigen.

The effector function of a given immunoglobulin is determined by the constant region. In other words, the constant region determines the degree of complement binding, interaction with specific receptors (Fc receptors) of various cells, and transplacental transfer.

Immunoglobulins are proteins and their amino acid sequence can be immunogenic for different individuals and different species, so they can act as an antigen. In fact, they can even act as a "self-antigen"—they have *isotypic*, *allotypic*, and *idiotypic* determinants. *Isotypic determinants* are responsible for the differences between the different immunoglobulin classes and subclasses and between heavy and light chains. *Allotypic determinants* are variations in the constant regions of immunoglobulins of the same isotype, owing to allelic variations in the genes found among different individuals. *Idiotypic determinants* are the individual determinants of any given antibody molecule in accordance with the variability of the immunoglobulin's CDR region.

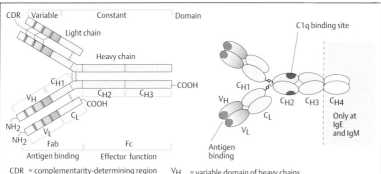

CDR = complementarity-determining region
Fab = antigen-binding fragment
Fc = crystallizable fragment

V_H = variable domain of heavy chains
V_L = variable domain of light chains
$C_{H/L}$ = constant domain of heavy / light chains

A. Immunoglobulin structure

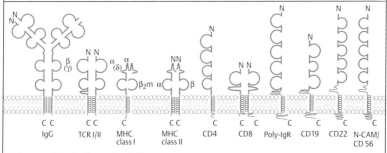

B. Immunglobulin-"superfamily"

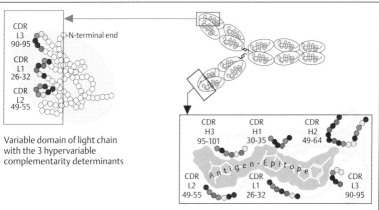

Variable domain of light chain
with the 3 hypervariable
complementarity determinants

C. Hypervariable regions determine the antigen specificity

A. Protein Electrophoresis

In an applied electric field, serum proteins separate into fractions consisting of albumin, α_1-, α_2-, β-, and γ-globulins. IgG immunoglobulins migrate into the γ-globulin fraction, while other immunglobulins, particularly IgM and IgD, have a lower electrophoretic mobility and are therefore found mainly in the β-globulin fraction, but even in the α_2-fraction.

B. Different Types of Immunoglobulins

Circulating antibodies are produced and secreted by plasma cells in the bone marrow, in mucosa-associated lymphoid tissue and in lymph nodes. IgA immunoglobulins predominate in the saliva, secretions from the bronchial and urinary tracts, tear fluid, colostrum, and breast milk, where they provide protection against bacteria.

Immunoglobulins are expressed on the surface of mature B cells when they serve as surface antigen receptors. Some endogenous immunoglobulins are bound to other cells (e.g., granulocytes, mast cells, monocytes/macrophages, and epithelial cells), usually via Fc receptors.

C. Immunoglobulin Structure and Features

IgG immunoglobulins comprise the largest portion of serum immunoglobulins. They are divided into four subclasses (IgG1, IgG2, IgG3, and IgG4) which are distinguished by differences in their γ chains, as is denoted by the numerical suffixes γ1 to γ4. The heavy chains have one variable domain and three constant domains. The molecular weight of IgG amounts to a total of ca. 150 000 Da. The light chains (ca. 212 amino acids) contribute around 23 000 Da, and the heavy chains (ca. 450 amino acids) around 50 000–70 000 Da in the various subclasses. IgG3 is heavier than all other IgG subclasses because it contains a long series of disulfide bonds in the so-called *hinge region*. It is especially good at binding complement. All IgG antibodies occur as monomers.

Serum IgA immunoglobulins usually also occur as monomers but can also be present as dimers (about 15 %); they rarely occur as polymers. IgA dimers are held together by a J chain. There are two IgA subclasses (IgA1 and IgA2) that are distinguished by differences in the disulfide bonds in their hinge region. IgA molecules are very high in carbohydrates and do not bind complement.

IgM usually occurs in pentameric form (molecular weigh ca. 900 000 Da). It infrequently occurs as other polymeric complexes, and rarely occurs in monomeric form. The IgMs represent the classical surface immunoglobulins on the cell membrane of mature B cells. IgM molecules have four constant domains. IgM pentamers (like the IgA dimers) are fastened together by J chains. IgM has a high affinity for complement binding.

IgD, like IgM, is one of the most common membrane immunoglobulins in human B cells. Its function in serum is unknown.

Only very small amounts of free IgE are detectable in serum. It usually binds to basophilic granulocytes and mast cells and, in individuals with allergies, to epithelial cells in the mucosal lining of the bronchial and gastrointestinal tracts. IgE plays an important role in the defense against parasites and in immediate hypersensitivity reactions (see p. 66).

D. Transport of IgG through the Intestinal Epithelium

Newborns are not fully immunocompetent (immunoglobulin production begins at 6 months). While at birth antibodies from the mother are still present in the blood (IgG crosses the placenta), breasst milk is a good source of antibodies for the first months of life. IgG molecules from the breast milk are absorbed by specialized epithelial cells in the intestine of the infant and passed on to the blood via a pH gradient.

E. Secretion of IgA

Secretory IgA molecules occur as dimers with an additional secretory component (ca. 70 000 Da). This involves a certain portion of the membrane receptor that binds IgA on the extraluminal side of the epithelial cell. The receptor undergoes cleavage, and the portion that was bound to IgA is released along with the immunoglobulin.

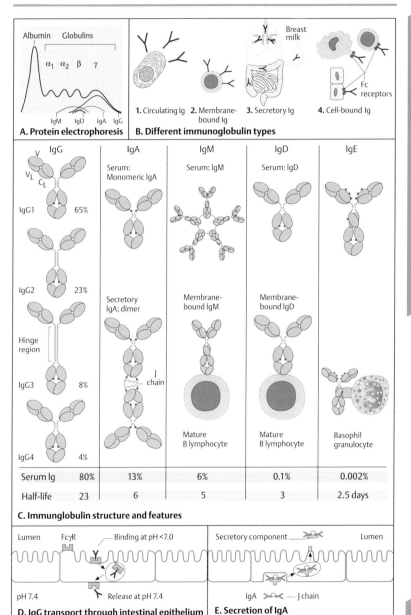

A. Protein electrophoresis

Albumin | Globulins

α_1 α_2 β γ

IgM IgD IgA IgG

B. Different immunoglobulin types

Breast milk

1. Circulating Ig
2. Membrane-bound Ig
3. Secretory Ig
4. Cell-bound Ig

Fc receptors

C. Immunglobulin structure and features

IgG

V
V_L C_L

IgG1 — 65%
IgG2 — 23%

Hinge region

IgG3 — 8%
IgG4 — 4%

IgA

Serum: Monomeric IgA

Secretory IgA; dimer

J chain

IgM

Serum: IgM

Membrane-bound IgM

Mature B lymphocyte

IgD

Serum: IgD

Membrane-bound IgD

Mature B lymphocyte

IgE

Basophil granulocyte

	IgG	IgA	IgM	IgD	IgE
Serum Ig	80%	13%	6%	0.1%	0.002%
Half-life	23	6	5	3	2.5 days

D. IgG transport through intestinal epithelium

Lumen | FcγR — Binding at pH <7.0

pH 7.4 — Release at pH 7.4

E. Secretion of IgA

Secretory component — Lumen

IgA — J chain

Fundamental Principles

29

An individual can produce at least 10^{11} different antibodies. This great diversity is attributable mainly to the large number of genes that encode the variable regions on immunoglobulins.

A. Organization and Rearrangement of H Genes of Immunoglobulins

The genes that code for immunoglobulin heavy (H) chains are located on chromosome 14. In the germline configuration of immature cells, these genes are located in four regions (variable, diversity, joining, constant). Around 50 functionally active V genes code for amino acids (AA) 1 to 95 in the variable region, 10–30 D genes code for AA 96 to 101 in the diversity region, and 6 J genes code for AA 102 to 110 in the joining region. In addition, the constant region of the heavy chain is determined by 9 C genes: μ for IgM, $\gamma 1$ for IgG1, and $\gamma 2$ for IgG2, etc. Each V gene is headed by a leader (L) sequence. During the process of maturation, a D gene becomes linked with a J gene (D-J rearrangement) via deletion of the DNA portion between them. An mRNA molecule is transcribed from the DJ sequence and the gene for the constant region of the IgM molecule (C_μ), so a precursor DJ-C_μ protein is synthesized (see p. 32). During the course of further maturation, the V gene sequences are rearranged in such a way that a V gene (together with the corresponding L segment) is brought next to the rearranged DJ gene (V-DJ rearrangement). VDJ-C_μ mRNA is now transcribed from this, and a VDJ-C_μ protein is synthesized. Cleavage of the L sequence ultimately yields the μ heavy chain of the immunoglobulin. The total of ca. 50 V genes, 10–30 D genes, and 6 J genes yields a recombination potential of around 3×10^3 to 9×10^3 for the amino acid sequences of the variable region of heavy chains. This process is referred to as *somatic recombination*.

B. Organization of κ Light Chain Genes

The genes for κ light chains are located on chromosome 2. Around 35–40 functionally active V genes (together with the corresponding L genes) code for amino acids 1 to 95 of the variable region of κ light chains; 5 J genes code for amino acids 96 to 110. V genes are brought next to J genes during the process of DNA rearrangement. A precursor mRNA is transcribed from a VJ sequence, together with the sequence from the constant region of the κ light chain (C_κ). The L sequence then splits off from the protein.

A total of 35–40 V genes and 5 J genes can code for approximately 175–200 different κ light chain specificities.

C. Organization of λ Light Chain Genes

The organization of λ light chain genes on chromosome 22 is not fully understood. There are a number of genes for the constant region, and the J sequences lie directly in front of the C genes. There are presumably just as many genes for the λ chain as for the κ chain.

Because every heavy chain is linked with a κ or λ chain, there are, theoretically, 5.2×10^5 ($175\times3\times10^3$) to 1.8×10^6 ($200\times9\times10^3$) different κ-bearing antibody recombinations. The projected number of different λ-bearing immunoglobulins is probably similar. The actual number of possible antibody molecules is, however, much higher. This is attributable to several reasons, such as: (1) mutations at the DNA level during ontogenesis; (2) errors in the course of deletion and recombination of V, D, and J genes, during the course of which nucleotides are inserted from DNA sequences that are not normally transcribed; (3) the synthesis of new immunoglobulins with enhanced affinity due to the switching of amino acids via point mutation during germinal center reactions (see p. 24).

D. Immunoglobulin Class-Switching

Immunoglobulins of different classes are synthesized during an immune response. The maturing B cells first produce IgM immunoglobulins. Over the course of time, the rearranged VDJ sequences are positioned directly adjacent to other C genes. Every C gene is preceded by a so-called switching (S) sequence that controls the rearrangement process by recombining with other S sequences due to the high level of homology. The C_μ sequences located between the VDJ sequences and the new C genes are deleted in the process.

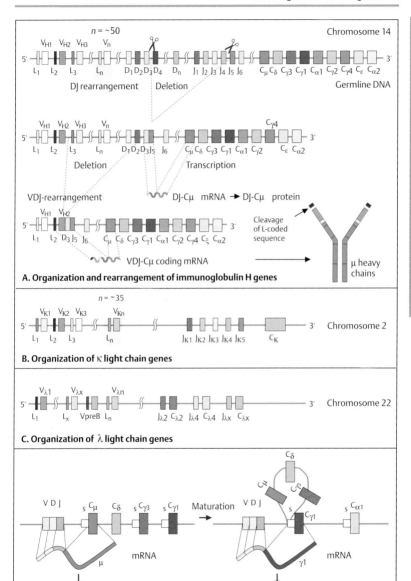

A. Organization and rearrangement of immunoglobulin H genes

B. Organization of κ light chain genes

C. Organization of λ light chain genes

D. Immunoglobulin class-switching

A. B-Cell Differentiation Scheme

Various stages of B-cell differentiation can be defined with the help of antibodies directed against surface antigens. The antigens CD19 and CD22 are the earliest specific B-cell markers. CD22 is initially expressed only in cytoplasm but, as the maturation process continues, it is also expressed on the cell surface. Progenitor B cells also express stem cell-associated antigens, such as CD34 and CD117 (c-kit/stem cell growth factor receptor) and CD10. Since CD10 was first detected in the cells of leukemia patients, it is referred to as common acute lymphoblastic leukemia-associated (CALLA) antigen. Mature circulating cells are CD10-negative, but CD10 is expressed on germinal center cells. The expression of CD20 starts approximately at the level of pre-B-II cells.

CD23 (low affinity Fc-IgE receptor) and CD21 are markers of mature B cells. CD21 is also a receptor for the Epstein–Barr virus and for the C3d fragment of complement.

B. Immunoglobulin Modulation during B-Cell Differentiation

Immunoglobulins are expressed on the surface of mature B cells and are secreted in large amounts by plasma cells. The amino acid sequences for the different parts of the complete immunoglobulin are determined in the precursor cells during the course of B-cell ontogeny.

In progenitor B cells (pro-B cells), still unmodified DNA is found at heavy and light chain loci in the so-called germline configuration. In addition to genes for the lambda light chain, two other genes (VpreB and $\lambda 5$) that code for the corresponding light chain-like proteins (surrogate light chains) are also located on chromosome 22. The surrogate light chains are first expressed on the cell membrane together with a 130 kDa glycoprotein complex. They presumably bind to cellular or soluble ligands and transport the signals for further B-cell development to the cell interior.

More differentiated B cells (pre-B-I cells) have rearranged D_H and J_H genes at the H locus of chromosome 14. A DJ-C_μ protein is coded during the process of DJ-C_μ mRNA transcription (see p. 30). The protein transmits a negative feedback signal to stop the further synthesis of DJ-C_μ proteins. VpreB/$\lambda 5$ chains can associate both with p130 glycoproteins as well as with DJ-C_μ proteins on the cell membrane.

Pre-B-II cells have already rearranged V_H-D_H-J_H and synthesize a VDJ-C_μ protein corresponding to a complete μ chain. This chain (H_μ) is expressed on the cell membrane together with the VpreB/$\lambda 5$ surrogate chain, which functions as the signal to start rearranging the light chain. Immature B cells are defined by the simultaneous expression of the μ heavy chains in association with VpreB/$\lambda 5$ surrogate chains (H_μ/VpreB) and with normal kappa or lambda light chains (complete IgM/κ [H_μ/L_μ] or IgM/λ [H_μ/L_μ] immunoglobulins). If rearrangement at a light chain locus is successful and a light chain is synthesized, further rearrangement at the L loci will be suppressed. If a cell has undergone productive rearrangement at the κ locus, for example, rearrangement at the λ locus will be suppressed and vice versa. Rearrangement at the λ locus is still possible, however, if rearrangement at the κ locus was aborted. This mechanism ensures the production of only one type of light chain by the B cell (*light chain restriction*).

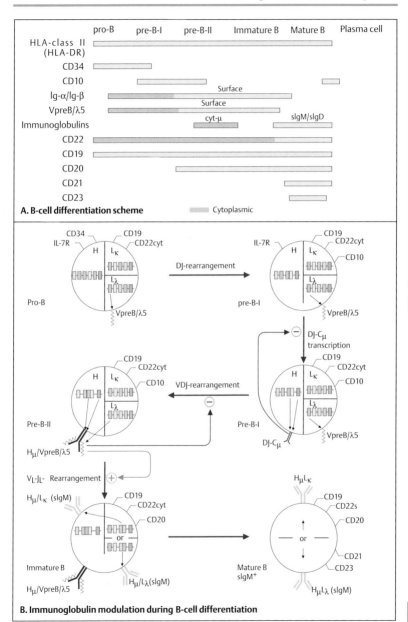

A. B-cell differentiation scheme

B. Immunoglobulin modulation during B-cell differentiation

The binding of an antigen to surface immuno-globulins triggers a cascade of biochemical signals within a B cell. Since immunoglobulins have only a very short intra-cytoplasmic tail, they are dependent on accessory molecules, similar to the CD3 complex of the T-cell receptor. Ig-α (CD79a) and Ig-β (CD79b) chains assume this function. These chains are structurally similar to TCR γ, δ, and ε chains and they form, together with the immunoglobulins, the B-cell receptor (BCR) complex.

CD10 is referred to as *common acute lymphoblastic leukemia-associated* (CALLA) *antigen* because it was first found on lymphoblasts of patients with the common variant of acute lymphatic leukemia (common ALL). CD10 is an extracellular zinc-binding metalloproteinase that can catalyze the cleavage of various peptides, such as substance P, endothelin, oxytocin, bradykinin, and angiotensins I and II. It is expressed on stromal cells, on immature T and B cells in the bone marrow, and on germinal center cells in secondary lymphoid organs.

CD19 is expressed on the membrane of all B lymphocytes and is thus a marker of the entire B cell series. CD19 unites with CD21, CD81, and Leu-13 to form a co-receptor that modulates the signals transduced by the BCR complex. This activity is especially important in immature B cells.

CD20, a "pan-B-cell marker" expressed on all B cells except progenitor B cells, is structurally similar to an ion channel. Its transmembrane segment crosses the cell membrane four times and seems to be associated with the cytoskeleton.

CD21 is a low-affinity receptor for the complement cleavage products iC3b and C3d. It also serves as the Epstein–Barr virus receptor. Together with CD19, CD81, and Leu-13, CD21 is functionally associated with the B-cell receptor.

CD22, like CD3 on T cells, exhibits bimodal expression. CD22 is expressed on the cell membrane only in mature B cells, but is present within the cytoplasm of all B cells. It functions as an adhesion molecule that interacts with *sialylglycoconjugates*. Ligation of CD22 leads to the downregulation of signal transmission by BCR complexes, mediating an inhibitory effect.

CD23 is the B-cell-associated receptor for the Fc fragment of IgE. The binding of CD23 to IgE or to immune complexes containing IgE induces feedback inhibition of IgE synthesis. An autocrine/paracrine B-cell growth factor occurs as a cleavage product of CD23.

CD40 is mainly expressed by B cells, but also by dendritic cells (DC), follicular dendritic cells (FDC), hematopoietic progenitor cells, epithelial cells, and carcinoma cells. CD40 is a member of the TNF receptor family. A TNF-related glycoprotein that is mainly expressed on activated CD4$^+$ T cells (CD40 ligand, CD154) provides an important survival signal for B cells. The germinal centers cannot develop completely if CD40/CD40 ligand interaction is defective. If this is the case, IgM is the only immunoglobulin the B cells can produce because of a blocked immunoglobulin class-switching (hyper-IgM syndrome).

CD72, like CD23, is a member of the *asialoglycoprotein* receptor family. Like CD19, it is a broad B-cell marker, but its function is not yet understood. Earlier evidence that CD72 functions as a ligand for CD5 has not yet been confirmed.

CD80 and **CD86** are not B-cell lineage-specific. They are expressed on other antigen-presenting cells, such as monocytes and dendritic cells. The interaction of CD80/CD86 with their ligands on T cells (CD28 and CTLA-4) is crucial for the complete activation or deactivation of T cells (see p. 36).

Molecule	Molecular weight(kDa)	Gene locus (chromosome)	Cell expression	Function
sIg	150–900	14 (H-chains) 2 (κ-chain) 22 (λ-chain)	Mature B cells	Antigen binding part of B-cell antigen receptor (BCR)
Ig-α(CD79a) Ig-β(CD79b)	34 39	19q132 17q23	Pre-B cells Mature B cells	sIg-associated molecules signal transducing part of BCR
CD10 (CALLA)	100	3q21-q27	Pre-B cells B cells of germinal center Granulocytes	Neutral endopeptidase
CD19	95	16p11.2	All B cells incl. progenitor B cells	With CD21-, CD81- Leu-13 co-receptor for BCR
CD20	35–37	11q-q13	Pre-B cells Mature B cells	Ion channel subunit
CD21	140	1q32	Mature B-cells Follicular dendritic cells (FDC)	C3d/EBV-receptor (CR2) BCR-association, signal transduction
CD22	135	19q13.1	All B cells (cytoplasm) Mature B cells (surface)	B-cell adhesion molecule (B-B and B-T interaction) modulation of BCR
CD23	45	19p13.3	Mature B cells FDC Act. monocytes eosinophils	Low-affinity Fcε receptor (FcεRII) cleavage product = B-cell growth factor
CD40	48	20q12-q13.2	Pre-B cells Mature B cells Dendritic cells (DC)	Interaction with CD40 ligand (T cell) Anti-apoptosis signal
CD72	43–39	9p	All cells of B-cell lineage Macrophages	Adhesion molecule
CD80/86	60	3q21	B cells, act. monocytes Dendritic cells (DC)	T-APC interaction (ligands for CD28/CTLA-4)

A. Important B-cell antigens

Fundamental Principles

A. Molecules Involved in Interactions between T Cells and APCs

Several adhesion and accessory molecules promote the interaction of T cells with antigen-presenting cells (APCs), such as B cells, dendritic cells (DCs), and monocytes.

Leukocyte function-associated antigen-1 (LFA-1), a ubiquitous antigen, binds to intercellular adhesion molecule-1 (ICAM-1). CD2 binds to LFA-3, a glycoprotein, which is mainly expressed on endothelial cells, epithelial cells, and connective tissue. The CD40/CD40-ligand interaction transmits a survival signal to germinal center B cells and induces DCs to mature and produce large quantities of IL-12. The adhesion of B cells to T cells is further stabilized by interactions of the CD106 antigen, or **v**ascular **c**ell **a**dhesion **m**olecule-1 (VCAM-1), which is also expressed on endothelial cells, with the CD49d antigen, also called **v**ery **l**ate **a**ntigen-4 (VLA-4) on activated T cells. The interaction of the T-cell molecule CD28 with CD80/CD86 on APCs has a stimulatory effect, whereas the interaction of CD152, or **c**ytotoxic **T**-lymphocytes **a**ntigen-4 (CTLA-4), with the same antigens has an inhibitory effect.

B. Several Signals Are Needed for T-Cell Activation

Antigen recognition by the T-cell receptor (TCR) provides a first activating signal for a T cell, but it is not sufficient to induce full activation. In the absence of a second signal, the T cell becomes tolerant or anergic. The second signal is provided by the interaction of the CD28 antigen, which is constitutionally expressed on resting T cells, with the co-stimulatory molecules B7.1 (CD80) or B7.2 (CD86) on APCs. On activation by both signals, the antigen CTLA-4 (CD152) is upregulated in T cells within 24-48 hours. CTLA-4 is a higher-affinity receptor for CD80/CD86; it competes with CD28 and inhibits cell cycle progression. This negative signal is probably emitted by CTLA-4 to end T-cell activation in order to prevent an exaggerated immune response. A further inhibitory receptor is known as programmed death gene-1 (PD-1), which can interact with two B7 family members: PD-L1 or B7-HI and PD-L2 or B7-DC.

Terminally differentiated DCs can produce large quantities of IL-12 on CD40/CD40-ligand interaction, inducing the release of interferon-γ (IFN-γ) and the differentiation of CD4+ cells into T$_H$1 cells. IL-12 is also a direct and potent stimulus of cytotoxic T lymphocytes (CTLs) and natural killer cell (NK) function. IFN-γ stimulates antimicrobial and proinflammatory activity of macrophages and enhances the activation of CTLs.

C. ICOS in T-Cell Activation

Unlike CD28, the CD28 homologous inducible T-cell co-stimulator (ICOS) is not constitutively expressed on resting T cells but only after activation via TCR/CD3 complex. Engagement of ICOS, like CD28, can mediate potent co-stimulation of T cells and promote proliferation. Recent studies indicate that stimulation via ICOS can induce both T$_H$1 and T$_H$2 differentiation. ICOS interacts with the ICOS ligand ICOSL, which is also known as B7h, B7RP-1, and B7-H2. ICOSL is expressed constitutively on B cells, DCs, macrophages, and endothelial cells, and it is upregulated by TNF-α or inflammatory stimuli.

D. Superantigen Stimulation

Superantigens are mainly bacterial products (e.g., staphylococcal enterotoxins) or viral proteins that induce nonselective T-cell activation. The response of T cells to superantigens is not clonal; a large number of different T cells are activated. While a highly specific interaction of the processed peptide embedded in the MHC complex with the α and β chain of the TCR is mandatory during antigen specific T-cell activation, superantigens do not require intracellular processing. They bind as whole proteins to the outer side of the V$_\beta$ region of several TCRs. Around 100 times more T cells react with superantigens than with normal antigens. Some superantigens induce activation of up to 10% of peripheral blood T cells. On superantigen activation, CD4+ T cells release a high amount of cytokines, which can mediate toxic effects in the host.

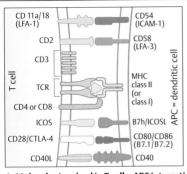

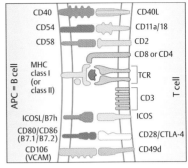

A. Molecules involved in T cell – APC interaction

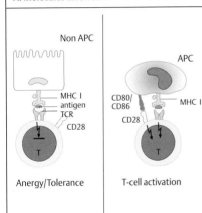

1. Signal 1 only

2. Co-stimulation via CD28

B. Several signals needed for T-cell activation

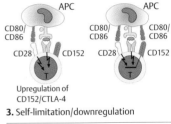

3. Self-limitation/downregulation

4. Effector cell induction

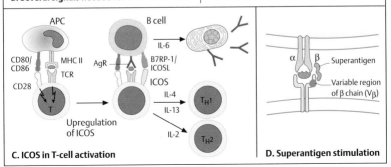

C. ICOS in T-cell activation

D. Superantigen stimulation

Natural killer (NK) cells make up around 10% of the lymphocytes in the blood. They lack the re-arrangement of genes coding for antigen receptors found in T and B lymphocytes. NK cells do not attack cells that express normal levels of MHC class I molecules, but they kill cells with foreign MHCs, as well as cells with decreased or absent MHC I expression. This is an event that is frequently seen in viral infections and cancer. NK cells can be identified in peripheral blood as large lymphocytes with azurophilic (red) granules (large granular lymphocytes, LGLs).

A. Development of NK Cells

Common NK-cell/T-cell progenitors expressing CD7, CD2, and sometimes CD5 are found in the bone marrow, in the fetal liver, and in the thymus. IL-15, which is produced abundantly by bone marrow stromal cells, is crucial for NK-cell differentiation; IL-2 and IL-18 promote the further maturation of NK cells.

The low-affinity receptor for the Fc portion of IgG (CD16) and the CD56 adhesion molecule are typical NK cell markers.

B. Target Recognition by NK Cells

Most activating and inhibitory NK cell receptors are coded for by genes on chromosome 19. Activating receptors, such as NKp46, NKp30, and NKp44 (natural cytotoxicity receptors, NCRs), allow NK cells to "dock" onto target cells. They belong to the immunoglobulin (Ig) super-family and have short intracytoplasmic tails. Therefore, they need to associate with transducing polypeptides, such as the ζ chain, FcεRIγ, and DAP12, in order to trigger NK cell activity. Their ligands are still unknown. A fourth triggering receptor is NKG2D, a C-type lectin homodimer, which associates with the transducing molecule DAP10. The NKG2D receptor interacts with MHC class I-related proteins called MICA and MICB, which are expressed weakly in normal cells but are upregulated in stressed cells and in tumor cells. These proteins are similar to classical MHC I molecules but do not bind peptides and do not associate with β_2-microglobulin.

Many receptors are involved in the recognition of classical MHC molecules. In contrast to antigen-specific T cells, these receptors usually recognize a whole set of different HLA class I alleles but not the peptide/MHC complex. They can be grouped in two large families:

killer cell immunoglobulin-like receptors (KIRs) and immunoglobulin-like transcripts (ILTs, also known as leukocyte immunoglobulin-like receptors, LIRs). While KIRs are expressed only on NK cells and on a subgroup of T cells, ILTs/LIRs are also expressed on monocytes, dendritic cells, and B cells. These receptors can mediate activation or inhibition, depending mainly on the structure of their intracytoplasmic tails. In most cases, a long cytoplasmic tail indicates the presence of an immunoreceptor tyrosine-rich inhibitory motif (ITIM). ITIM triggers a specific phosphatase, which, in turn, blocks the intracellular transduction of signals from activating receptors. Receptors with a short cytoplasmic tail lack ITIM and associate with transducing polypeptides, such as the adapter molecules DAP12 or FcRγ, which contain immunoreceptor tyrosine-based activating motif (ITAM), in order to transduce activating signals. More than a dozen different receptors have been defined for both the KIR and LIR families. A third class of NK cell receptors belongs to the C-type lectin-like receptor family (such as the already mentioned activating NKG2D receptor). Although most NK receptors exist in both activating and inhibitory isoforms, it appears that inhibitory signals by ITIM-bearing receptors largely prevail over the activating signals. Some inhibitory molecules with their corresponding ligands are shown in **C**.

D. Cytolytic Mechanisms of NK Cells

Nonsecretory lysis is involved when the target cells have apoptosis receptors, such as the CD95 antigen (also called Fas or APO-1) (**D.1**), which triggers a type of "cell suicide," referred to as programmed cell death or apoptosis (see p. 74).

The most common mechanism of lysis by NK cells is the release of lytic granules (**D.2**). The granules contain perforin, a protein that creates pores in the membrane of the host cell, and granzymes, a group of different proteinases. In the presence of perforin, granzyme B reaches the cell nucleus, where it activates caspases (important apoptosis-promoting proteins), inducing cell death. NK cells can destroy antibody-coated cells. Binding of the antibody to the Fc receptor on a NK cell (CD16) activates the cytolytic program of antibody-dependent cell-mediated cytotoxicity (ADCC) by inducing the release of proteolytic enzymes (**D.3**).

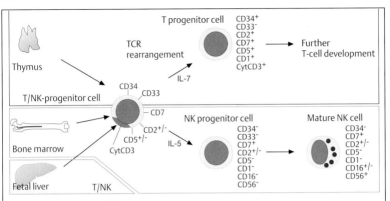

T progenitor cell
CD34+
CD33-
CD2+
CD7+
CD5+
CD1+
CytCD3+

Thymus

TCR rearrangement

IL-7 → Further T-cell development

T/NK-progenitor cell

CD34 CD33
CD7
CD2+/-
CD5+/-
CytCD3

Bone marrow

IL-5

NK progenitor cell
CD34-
CD33-
CD7+
CD2+/-
CD5-
CD1-
CD16-
CD56-

Mature NK cell
CD34-
CD7+
CD2+/-
CD5-
CD1-
CD16+/-
CD56+

Fetal liver

T/NK

A. Development of NK cells

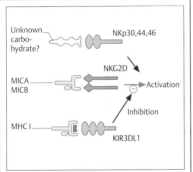

Unknown carbo-hydrate? — NKp30,44,46

MICA MICB — NKG2D → Activation

MHC I — KIR3DL1 → Inhibition

B. Target recognition by NK cells

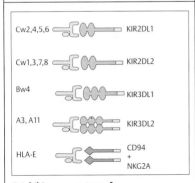

Cw2,4,5,6 — KIR2DL1

Cw1,3,7,8 — KIR2DL2

Bw4 — KIR3DL1

A3, A11 — KIR3DL2

HLA-E — CD94 + NKG2A

C. Inhibitory receptors of NK cells

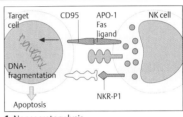

Target cell — CD95 APO-1 Fas ligand — NK cell

DNA-fragmentation

NKR-P1

Apoptosis

1. Nonsecretory lysis

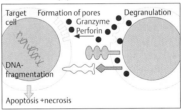

Target cell — Formation of pores — Degranulation
Granzyme
Perforin

DNA-fragmentation

Apoptosis +necrosis

2. Secretory lysis

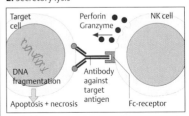

Target cell — Perforin Granzyme — NK cell

DNA fragmentation

Antibody against target antigen

Fc-receptor

Apoptosis + necrosis

3. ADCC (antibody-dependent cellular cytotoxicity)

D. Cytolytic mechanisms of NK cells

A. The Phagocyte System

Granulocytes, monocytes, and dendritic cells (DCs) have phagocytic capabilities (from the Greek word *phagein* = to eat). They all derive from blood progenitor cells: the cytokine granulocyte colony-stimulating factor (G-CSF) promotes the differentiation into granulocytes, while granulocyte-macrophage colony-stimulating factor (GM-CSF), IL-4, and tumor necrosis factor-α (TNF-α) promote differentiation into monocytes and DCs. The normal fate of circulating monocytes (their half-life in the blood is only a few hours) is to differentiate into tissue phagocytes. The macrophages remain in the tissue for the rest of their lifetime (up to years). Monocytes are larger than lymphocytes. They have a nucleus that is horseshoe-shaped or bizarrely shaped, and they have a broad rim of cytoplasm with granules containing enzymes (peroxidase and hydrolases). DCs are large, mobile cells with long cytoplasmic processes (some >10 μm). DCs are seldom found in the blood; their precursors migrate into the skin to form the Langerhans cells of the epidermis and dermal DCs, or into the lymph nodes, where they give origin to interdigitating dendritic cells (IDC) in the T-cell areas and to germinal center dendritic cells (GCDC). A different lineage of DCs, called lymphoid DC or type-2 DC, differentiates from progenitor cells in the presence of IL-3 and the cytokine Flt3L. They locate in the paracortical region of the lymph nodes. It has been suggested that they constitute the thymic DC population.

B. Mechanisms of Endocytosis

Uptake of small fluid particles (pinocytosis, from the Greek word *pinein* = to drink) begins with the formation of membrane indentations, which is driven by a protein complex called *clathrin*. Clathrin-coated vesicles, or "coated pits," fuse with lysosomes, where the antigens are digested. In macropinocytosis, the cell can absorb large drops up to 0.5 μm in size. Water is expelled through channels, called aquaporins. Polymerization of the cytoskeleton protein actin is needed for the formation of larger phagocytic vesicles. Langerhans cells of the skin utilize Birbeck granules (small vesicles with a typical narrow neck) for phagocytosis. Some bacteria (e.g., *Legionella pneumophila*) are internalized by coiling phagocytosis, whereby a cytoplasmic protrusion, called pseudopodium, spirals around the bacterium to form a "coiling phagosome." The membranes of the pseudopodium then fuse, releasing the pathogen within the cytoplasm.

C. Fc-Mediated Phagocytosis.

Several receptors can bind the Fc portion of immunoglobulins (see p. 43). Receptors for IgG, IgA, and IgE are called FcγR, FcαR, and FcϵR respectively. These receptors signal through immunoreceptor tyrosine-based activation motifs (ITAMs), which are intracytoplasmic domains consisting of two tyrosine (Y) residues separated by 9-12 amino acids. On ligation, the tyrosines in these ITAM domains become phosphorylated, leading to the recruitment of the tyrosine kinase Syk, which then triggers different intracellular signal cascades, leading to transcriptional activation, cytoskeletal rearrangement, and release of inflammatory mediators. FcγRII-A has itself an ITAM motif in its intracellular portion, while FcγRI and FcγRIII lack ITAMs in their cytoplasmic tails. They interact respectively with γ- and ζ-transducing proteins, which contain the ITAMs needed for signal transduction.

D. Mannose Receptor

Macrophages and DCs can recognize the sugars mannose and fucose, which are present on different pathogens, through the mannose receptor (MR), a molecule with a long extracellular portion consisting of multiple (at least 8) lectin-like domains. MR ligation leads to the release of cytokines, such as IL-1β, IL-6, GM-CSF, TNF-α, and IL-12.

E. Complement Receptor-Mediated Phagocytosis

Serum complement proteins coat (opsonize) altered red blood cells or bacteria. The complement receptors CR1, CR3, and CR4 are present on monocytes and macrophages. CR1 binds to the complement fractions C3b, C4b, and C3bi. CR3 and CR4 (see p. 43) bind specifically to C3bi. Complement-coated particles, such as senescent red blood cells, sink directly into the cell, almost without pseudopodia formation. In this process, the proteins vinculin, paxillin, and F-actin are involved. There is no release of proinflammatory cytokines.

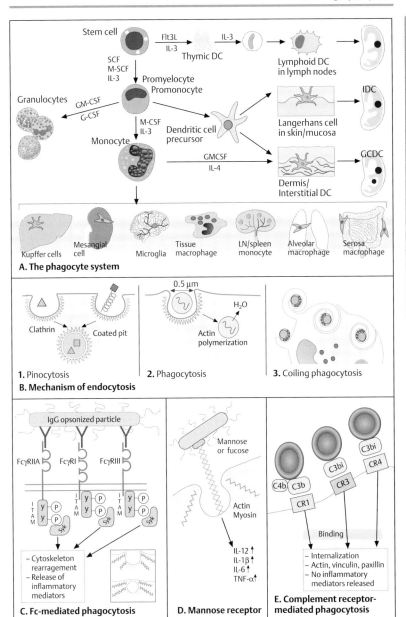

Stem cell

Flt3L
IL-3

Thymic DC

IL-3

Lymphoid DC
in lymph nodes

SCF
M-SCF
IL-3

Promyelocyte
Promonocyte

Granulocytes

GM-CSF
G-CSF

M-CSF
IL-3

Dendritic cell
precursor

IDC

Langerhans cell
in skin/mucosa

Monocyte

GMCSF
IL-4

Dermis/
Interstitial DC

GCDC

Kupffer cells   Mesangial
cell   Microglia   Tissue
macrophage   LN/spleen
monocyte   Alveolar
macrophage   Serosa
macrophage

A. The phagocyte system

Clathrin   Coated pit

1. Pinocytosis

0.5 μm

H_2O

Actin
polymerization

2. Phagocytosis

3. Coiling phagocytosis

B. Mechanism of endocytosis

IgG opsonized particle

FcγRIIA   FcγRI   FcγRIII

ITAM   ITAM   ITAM

Syk   Syk   Syk

– Cytoskeleton
rearragement
– Release of
inflammatory
mediators

C. Fc-mediated phagocytosis

Mannose
or fucose

Actin
Myosin

IL-12 ↑
IL-1β ↑
IL-6 ↑
TNF-α ↑

D. Mannose receptor

C4b   C3b   C3bi   C3bi   CR4

CR1   CR3

Binding

– Internalization
– Actin, vinculin, paxillin
– No inflammatory
mediators released

**E. Complement receptor-
mediated phagocytosis**

Fundamental Principles

41

A. Function of Monocytes and Macrophages.

Monocytes and macrophages are important accessory cells for the generation of highly specific adaptive immune responses but also crucial mediators of the innate immune response. They can also be activated in response to cytokines (e.g., interferon-γ; IFN-γ) released by T cells. **Activation** of monocytes and macrophages leads to the secretion of different cytokines, such as IL-1, TNF-α, and IL-6, which are responsible for systemic (generalized) effects. Both killing of phagocytosed bacteria and release of cytokines are mediated by nitric oxide (NO), a cellular metabolite product with a broad range of effects. IL-1, TNF-α, and IL-6 cause the liver to release "acute-phase proteins," such as C-reactive protein and mannan-binding lectin, which opsonize pathogens and facilitate their elimination. IL-1, TNF-α, and IL-6 also act on the hypothalamus region of the brain, inducing fever and mobilization of neutrophils from the bone marrow to the blood (leukocytosis). IL-1 and TNF-α increase vascular permeability, facilitating migration of cells into tissue. **Chemotaxis** is mediated by IL-8, which synergizes with the increased vascular permeability in recruiting granulocytes and causing **tissue inflammation**. Granulocytes and macrophages cooperate in the **phagocytosis** of pathogens and removal of damaged tissue (**scavenger function**) by means of proteolytic digestion, followed by tissue repair, which is facilitated by new vessel formation (angiogenesis). TNF-α and IFN-γ synergize in inducing synthesis of the reactive nitrogen metabolite NO, which is responsible for some of the **effector functions** of monocytes and macrophages, e.g., killing of intracellular bacteria and tumor cells. Other reactive oxygen intermediates (NO radicals, $NO^{\cdot}$, NO^{+}), as well as proteases, participate in these processes. Monocytes are important in **antigen presentation** to T cells (see p. 36). By releasing the cytokines IL-10 and IL-12, they act as crucial regulators of T-cell responses in the **modulation** of T_H1 vs. T_H2 responses.

B. Monocytes and Dendritic Cell Antigens

Monocytes have three important adhesion receptors: leukocyte function-associated antigen-1 (**LFA-1**) and complement receptors 3 and 4 (**CR3** and **CR4**). These antigens are members of the *integrin* family, a large family of molecules consisting of two polypeptide subunits (α and β chains) that are noncova-

lently bound. LFA-1, CR3, and CR4 have identical 95 kDa β chains that are recognized by anti-**CD18** antibodies. The three α chains are larger molecules of 180 kDa (**CD11a**), 170 kDa (**CD11b**), and 150 kDa (**CD11c**).

A genetically related absence of the β chain leads to a leukocyte adhesion defect, which is reflected by an extremely high susceptibility to infections.

CD14 and **CD68** are expressed on monocytes in the peripheral blood (CD14) and on tissue macrophages (CD68). CD14 is a receptor for the complex of lipopolysaccharide (LPS) and LPS-binding protein. Bacterial LPS is a powerful mitogen, which leads to an increased release of inflammatory mediators and to increased microbicidal activity. CD68 is a lysosomal/endosomal glycoprotein.

Monocytes express receptors for the Fc portion of IgG immunoglobulins. There are three types of receptors characterized by high (FcγRI = **CD64**), medium (FcγRII = **CD32**), and low affinity (FcγRIII = **CD16**). CD64 is predominantly expressed in monocytes, CD32 in granulocytes, and CD16 in natural killer (NK) cells. Granulocytes also express an isoform of the CD16 molecule, which is anchored in the membrane by glycosylated phosphatidylinositol (GPI). IgG1 and IgG3 bind very strongly to Fc receptors, whereas IgG2 and IgG4 create weak bonds. Murine antibodies can also bind to human Fc receptors; IgG2a and IgG3 bind very well, but IgG1 does not.

The **CD40**, **CD80**, and **CD86** antigens are co-stimulatory molecules for antigen presentation (see p. 36). They are expressed on B cells, monocytes, and dendritic cells (DCs).

The **CD83** antigen is useful for the characterization of the maturation stage of DCs as it is positive only on mature DCs. It is also present on some germinal center B cells and on activated T cells. It seems to play a role in cell adhesion.

The **CD206** antigen, or **mannose receptor**, is a C-type lectin (lectins bind to carbohydrates) that is expressed on macrophages and DCs. It binds with high affinity to mannose-sugar residues, which are present on many pathogens (bacteria, viruses). A similar structure called **CD205** is found on DCs and serves as an antigen uptake receptor.

The **CD1a** antigen is a MHC class I-like molecule, which is used for the presentation of lipid antigens, typically expressed on immature DCs and Langerhans cells.

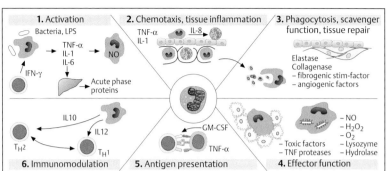

1. Activation | **2.** Chemotaxis, tissue inflammation | **3.** Phagocytosis, scavenger function, tissue repair

Bacteria, LPS — TNF-α / IL-1 / IL-6 → NO

IFN-γ

Acute phase proteins

TNF-α, IL-1 → IL-8

Elastase
Collagenase
– fibrogenic stim-factor
– angiogenic factors

IL10 / IL12

T_H2 | T_H1

GM-CSF

TNF-α

– NO
– H₂O₂
– O₂
– Lysozyme
– Hydrolase

– Toxic factors
– TNF proteases

6. Immunomodulation | **5.** Antigen presentation | **4.** Effector function

A. Function of monocytes/macrophages

Molecule	Molecular-weight (kDa)	Gene locus (chromosome)	Cell expression	Function
CD11a / CD18 LFA-1	CD11a: 180 CD18: 95	16p11-13.1 21q22.3	Monocytes, MΦ, lymphocytes (T-B), granulocytes	Cell–cell and cell–matrix adhesion, ligand for ICAM-1, ICAM-2
CD11b / CD18 CR3	CD11b: 170 CD18: 95	16p11-13.1 21q22.3	Myeloid cells, NK cells	Cell–cell and cell–matrix adhesion, ligand for iC3b, C4b, ICAM-1
CD11c / CD18 CR4	CD11c: 150 CD18: 95	16p11-13.1 21q22.3	Macrophages, myeloid cells	Cell–cell adhesion, ligand for iC3b, C4b, ICAM-1, LPS, fibrinogen
CD14	55	5q31	Monocytes, MΦ, granulocytes, (B cells)	Receptor for LPS and LPS/LPB complex
or CD16 (FcRIII)	50–80	1q23	Monocytes, MΦ, NK cells, granulocytes (GPI)	Low-affinity Fc-IgG receptor
CD32 (FcRII)	40	1q23-24	Phagocytes, B cells, platelets	Intermediate-affinity Fc-IgG receptor
CD64 (FcRI)	72	1q21	Monocytes, MΦ	High affinity Fc-IgG receptor
CD40	48	20q12-q13.2	Pre-B cells, mature B cells dendritic cells (DC)	Interaction with CD40 ligand (T cell), anti-apoptosis signal
CD80/86	60	3q21	B cells, act. macrophages, dendritic cells (DC)	T-APC interaction (ligands for CD28/CTLA-4)
CD83	45	6p23	Mature dendritic cells, some B cells and T cells	Adhesion receptor
Mannose receptors	180	10p13	Phagocytes, lymphoid endothelium	Pattern recognition receptor
CD1a	43–49	1q22-23	Thymocytes, DC	Antigen presentation (glycolipids)
CD68	110	17p13	Monocytes, MΦ, granulocytes, basophils, LGL lymphocytes	Lysosomal and endosomal glycoprotein

B: Monocytes and DC antigens

Dendritic cells (DCs) make up less than 0.5% of all mononuclear cells in the blood but are present in all organs. DCs have long cytoplasmic processes and only a few intracytoplasmic organelles but a large number of mitochondria. They have a high level of mobility. Only DCs can prime naive T cells.

A. Different Dendritic Cell Populations

DCs belong to the myeloid lineage. They differentiate from hematopoietic progenitor cells in response to TNF-α, IL-4, and GM-CSF. In the skin, DCs are found in the epidermis (Langerhans cells, LCs) and in the dermis. LCs have characteristic inclusions (*Birbeck granules*), probably endosomes, which play a role in antigen uptake. After capturing antigens in the skin, LCs begin maturation in response to inflammatory cytokines, such as TNF-α, and migrate to the T-cell region of lymph nodes, where they activate antigen-specific T cells. Mature monocytes can differentiate into interstitial DCs in various organs; a crucial step in this process is the interaction with adhesion molecules and chemokines of endothelial cells during transendothelial migration. Monocyte-derived DCs and interstitial DCs migrate preferentially to the germinal centers of lymph nodes, where they can activate both T and B cells. Mature DCs are rarely found in peripheral blood, but a small percentage (0.1–0.5%) of blood mononuclear cells has morphological and immunological features of immature DCs, i.e., smaller cytoplasmic protrusions, low levels of MHC molecules, and low levels of co-stimulatory molecules and the DC-associated antigen CD83. These cells, called **pre-DC-1**, express myeloid antigens, such as CD13, CD11c, and CD1c, as well as BDCA-3. Once isolated in vitro, they differentiate into typical DCs in response to IL-4, GM-CSF, and TNF-α. They secrete large amounts of IL-12 (type-1 DC or DC-1).

Some rare mononuclear cells of the blood respond to IL-3 and Flt3L, giving origin to a cell population that lacks the myeloid CD13 and CD33 antigens, while expressing some T-cell-associated antigens, such as CD2, CD5, and CD7, and the newly defined antigens BDCA-2 and BDCA-4, as well as Toll-like receptor 9 (TLR9). These cells migrate to the paracortical region of lymph nodes in close association with high endothelial venules. Given their positivity for T-cell-associated antigens and their morphology, these cells were described in the past as "plasmacytoid T cells," later also as "plasmacytoid monocytes." They are now called **pre-DC-2**: in response to CD40 ligation and IL-3, they acquire typical dendritic morphology and secrete high levels of IFN-α and IL-10 (type-2 DC or DC-2, or **i**nterferon **p**roducing **c**ells, **IPC**).

B. Life Cycle of a Dendritic Cell

Antigens absorbed through the skin are processed by Langerhans cells, which then migrate into the efferent lymph tract as *veiled cells*, transporting the antigen to the regional lymph nodes. Here, they prime and activate CD4+ T cells. Activated T cells acquire high levels of the CD40 ligand antigen (CD154), which in turn binds to CD40 on DCs. Further co-stimulation is provided by CD28, which interacts with CD80/86. Activated T cells head for the antigen entry site. They secrete cytokines, such as IL-2 and IFN-γ, which promote T-cell proliferation and further cell recruitment, finally leading to the accumulation of T cells, macrophages, and other inflammatory cells. This reaction (delayed-type hypersensitivity) can be detected about 48 hours after inoculation of the antigen. It is manifested by the formation of reddish papules (see pp. 66 and 91).

C. Recruitment of Dendritic Cell Precursors and Dendritic Cell Migration

The epithelia of tonsils and gut secrete the chemokine MIP-3α, which is the ligand for the chemokine receptor CCR6 present on immature DCs (and also on T cells that migrate into gut epithelia). MIP-3α is induced during inflammatory processes and mediates chemoattraction for immature DCs and Langerhans cells. On maturation, DCs lose CCR6 expression, so they escape from the local gradient of MIP-3α and acquire the chemokine receptor CCR7. This makes them responsive to the chemokines MIP-3β and SLC (**s**econdary **l**ymphoid **t**issue **c**hemokine), which are released and bound by lymphatic vessels, endothelial cells, and stromal cells of the lymph nodes. T cells are also driven to the lymph nodes by this chemokine gradient. In the T-cell area of lymph nodes, DCs can interact with antigen-specific T cells. Lymph node-resident DCs themselves produce SLC and MIP-3β, leading to further T-cell recruitment (**C2**) and DC attraction, which results in an amplification of the immune response.

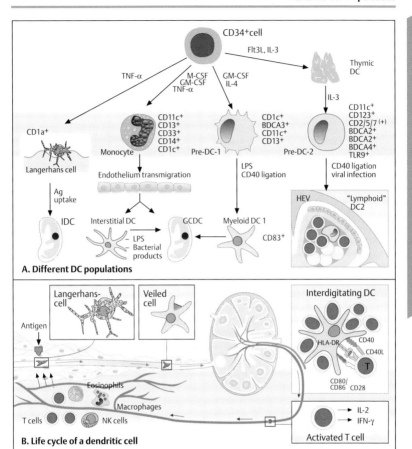

A. Different DC populations

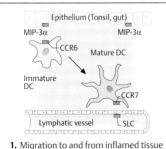

B. Life cycle of a dendritic cell

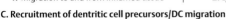

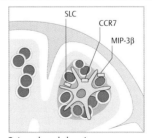

1. Migration to and from inflamed tissue   2. Lymph node homing

C. Recruitment of dendritic cell precursors/DC migration

A. Dendritic Cell Maturation: Changes in Phenotype and Function

The phenotype of dendritic cells (DCs) changes according to their maturation stage. Immature DCs express high levels of the myeloid antigens CD13 and CD33; of the chemokine receptors CCR1, CCR5, and CCR6; and of Fc receptors. They have only low levels of the co-stimulatory molecules CD40, CD80, and CD86 and do not express the antigen CD83 and the lysosome-associated membrane protein (**LAMP**). Some immature DCs, in particular the Langerhans cells of the skin, express abundantly the CD1a antigen. The levels of MHC I and MHC II molecules are low because the molecules are recycled from the cell surface into lysosomes at a high rate. Presented peptides are therefore available for T-cell recognition only for a short time. Immature DCs have high phagocytic and antigen uptake activity but, owing to their low levels of co-stimulatory molecules, they have poor antigen-presenting capability. Inflammatory stimuli (e.g., TNF-α, IL-1, IL-6, LPS, bacteria, and viruses) induce maturation of DCs. The turnover of MHC II molecules drops tenfold to a hundredfold. Consequently, peptides derived from captured antigens are available for T-cell recognition for several hours. Since the expression of co-stimulatory molecules is highly upregulated, mature DCs efficiently stimulate T cells. Upregulation of adhesion molecules, such as DC-SIGN, a C-type lectin that interacts with ICAM-3 on naive T cells, further contributes to T-cell stimulation. Final maturation is induced by CD40 ligation, which induces DCs to produce large amounts of IL-12.

B. Polarization of TH Response by Dendritic Cells: Lineage Duality vs. Plasticity

DCs are important regulators of the immune response. They can divert the immune response toward a T_H1-type or a T_H2-type response. In the presence of high levels of IL-12, T cells are driven toward T_H1, with secretion of IFN-γ, IL-2, and a predominantly inflammatory T-cell response. In contrast, a low concentration of IL-12 facilitates the differentiation of T_H2 cells, which secrete IL-4 and IL-10 and promote differentiation of B cells into plasma cells secreting IgM, IgG2, and IgG4. It is still unclear whether the ability to secrete high levels of IL-12 is a "constitutive" characteristic of type-1 myeloid-derived DCs (DC-1) in contrast to the typical lymphoid-type DCs or DC-2, which differentiate in response to Flt3 ligand and IL-3 (upper part of panel **B**). It is also possible that both types of DCs can produce different levels of IL-12, depending on the stimulus: bacterial products such as LPS and unmethylated CpG oligonucleotides, CD40 ligation, and the presence of a high DC/T-cell ratio induce DCs to secrete high amounts of IL-12. Conversely, in the presence of IL-10, TGF-β, prostaglandin PGE_2, and a low DC/T-cells ratio, DCs secrete only low levels of IL-12—the immune response is driven toward a T_H2 type (lower part of panel **B**).

Typically, DC-1 express the antigen BDCA-3, mannose receptors, CD1, as well as the Toll-like receptors (TLR) 2 and 4. DC-2, or "lymphoid DC," express the antigens CD123 (IL-3 receptor α-chain), BDCA-2, and BDCA-4, as well as TLR7 and TLR9. Type-2 DCs have a low phagocytic capacity, and they secrete type-I interferons (IFN-α and IFN-β) and are also called "interferon-producing cells" (IPC). Final maturation of DC-2 is induced by viral antigens in the presence of IL-3, while LPS and bacterial antigens are important stimuli for the maturation of type-1 DCs. CD40 ligation is important for both cell types.

C. Feedback Regulation of DC-1 and DC-2

Differentiation of T cells into T_H2 cells induces the secretion of IL-4. This cytokine is important for the generation of DC-1, while it inhibits the differentiation of type-2 DCs from precursor cells. In this way, a certain balance of T_H1/T_H2 responses is maintained despite the type of initial stimulus.

D. Tolerogenic Potential of Immature Dendritic Cells

Antigen uptake by immature DCs in the skin, mucosa, and even in tumors may induce antigen-specific tolerance rather than T-cell activation if further maturation stimuli (e.g., TNF, LPS) are missing. In these conditions, co-stimulatory molecules are not upregulated; IL-10 is produced instead of IL-12. Antigens presented under these conditions are likely to be tolerated. This mechanism could provide an important mechanism for avoiding autoimmunity but also an escape mechanism by which tumor-associated antigens induce tolerance rather than immunity.

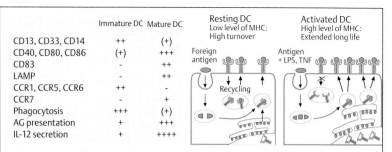

	Immature DC	Mature DC
CD13, CD33, CD14	++	(+)
CD40, CD80, CD86	(+)	+++
CD83	-	++
LAMP	-	++
CCR1, CCR5, CCR6	++	-
CCR7	-	+
Phagocytosis	+++	(+)
AG presentation	+	+++
IL-12 secretion	+	++++

A. DC maturation: changes in phenotype and function

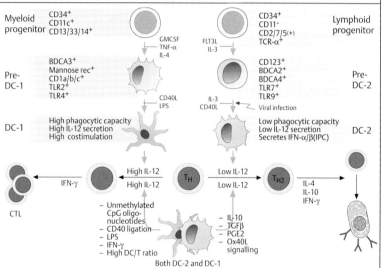

B. Polarization of TH responses by DCs: lineage duality vs. plasticity

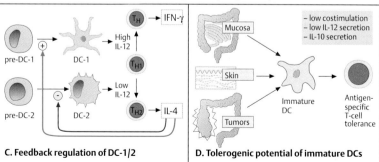

C. Feedback regulation of DC-1/2

D. Tolerogenic potential of immature DCs

Fundamental Principles

47

A. Genomic Organization of the HLA Complex

Transplant studies in experimental animals revealed that transplants that are not genetically identical are rejected. This was attributed to the antigens of the major histocompatibility complex (MHC). The corresponding structures were discovered in humans in the 1950s. Human MHC antigens are called *human leukocyte antigens* (HLA) because antibodies against human leukocytes were easier to detect in the human system after transplantation. The antigens have now been detected in virtually all nucleated cells. The HLA system is characterized by an extremely high level of polymorphism, i.e., it codes for genetic features that occur in more than one phenotypic form and that are passed on according to Mendel's laws. This polymorphism of the MHC system results in highly comprehensive antigen presentation. The genes for the human MHC are encoded on the short arm of chromosome 6.

HLA antigens are divided into two groups, *class I* and *class II*. As with other specificities, the classes denote the historical order of their discovery, and not their actual configuration on the chromosome. Class I antigens form complexes of antigens located at three other adjacent gene loci (HLA-A, HLA-B, HLA-C). These antigens were first defined serologically. *HLA-D antigens*, on the other hand, were discovered in cellular studies of mixed leukocyte cultures. HLA-D forms complexes comprising HLA-DR (D-related), HLA-DQ, and HLA-DP antigens.

Unlike the class I antigens, whose heavy chains are associated with the same light chain (β_2-microglobulin, which is not encoded on chromosome 6), different gene loci code for the α chain (DRA, DQA, DPA) and β chain (DRB, DQB, DPB) of the class II antigens. The number and structure of these loci vary from one individual to the next, depending on the HLA haplotype. Combining the different β chains of the DR antigens, for example, yields the various groups shown in (**4**). Other structurally related genes are in the vicinity of the DP, DQ, and DR genes (**3**). These are, in many cases, untranslated pseudogenes without any known function.

The configuration of the actual gene structure is divided into a number of exons that form the various domains. The genes that code for complement factors C2, C4, and Bf are located between the MHC class I and II genes (**2**). The expression products of these genes were originally called *class III antigens* (**1**). These genes also demonstrate extensive polymorphism which is made even more complex by gene duplication and/or length variation in C4 genes. Other important genes are scattered throughout the HLA complex, e.g., genes for TNF-α, TNF-β, the related lymphotoxin LTB, and enzymes CYP21a and CYP21b. The illustration does not show the genes for transport proteins TAP1 and TAP2, which are located between DP and DQ. The products of their expression are important for transport of antigenic peptides to the HLA molecule.

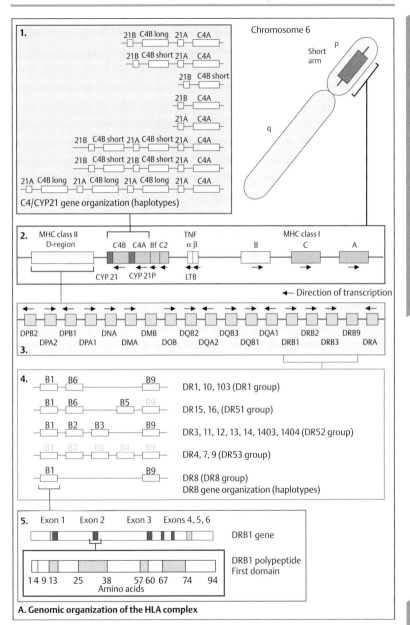

1. Chromosome 6

21B C4B long 21A C4A
21B C4B short 21A C4A
21B C4B short
21B C4A
21A C4A
21B C4B short 21A C4B short 21A C4A
21B C4B short 21B C4B short 21A C4A
21A C4B long 21A C4B long 21A C4B long 21A C4A

C4/CYP21 gene organization (haplotypes)

Short arm p

q

2. MHC class II D-region | C4B C4A Bf C2 | TNF α β | B C A — MHC class I

CYP 21 CYP 21P LTB

← Direction of transcription

3. DPB2 DPA2 DPB1 DPA1 DNA DMA DMB DOB DQB2 DQA2 DQB3 DQB1 DQA1 DRB2 DRB3 DRB1 DRB9 DRA

4.
B1 B6 B9 — DR1, 10, 103 (DR1 group)
B1 B6 B5 B9 — DR15, 16, (DR51 group)
B1 B2 B3 B9 — DR3, 11, 12, 13, 14, 1403, 1404 (DR52 group)
B1 B7 B8 B4 B9 — DR4, 7, 9 (DR53 group)
B1 B9 — DR8 (DR8 group)
DRB gene organization (haplotypes)

5. Exon 1 Exon 2 Exon 3 Exons 4, 5, 6

DRB1 gene

DRB1 polypeptide First domain

1 4 9 13 25 38 57 60 67 74 94
Amino acids

A. Genomic organization of the HLA complex

A. HLA Molecule (Schematic Representation)

Each HLA class I molecule consists of a 44 kDa heavy chain and a 12 kDa light chain known as β_2-microglobulin. The α chain is a transmembrane protein consisting of three domains (α_1, α_2, and α_3, with 90 amino acids each), plus a transmembrane fragment (25 AA) and an intracellular fragment (30 AA). The α chains form noncovalent bonds with the extracellular β_2-microglobulin.

Each class II HLA molecule consists of two chains, namely, a 33–35 kDa α chain and a 26–28 kDa β chain. Both chains have two extracellular domains weighing 90–100 kDa each (designated α_1, α_2 and β_1, β_2) which unite with a transmembrane fragment containing 20–25 amino acids and with an intracellular fragment consisting of 8–15 amino acids. The α_2 and β_2 domains are preserved, whereas the α_1 and β_1 domains are highly polymorphic. The latter domains consist of a "base plate" made of beta-pleated sheets, to the side of which alpha helices bind. This, altogether, yields a basketlike structure for antigen accommodation (see also **B**).

B. Structure of HLA Class I Molecules

The spatial structure of HLA antigens can be demonstrated by means of x-ray structural analysis, as is schematically shown for a class I molecule. Each of the α_1 and α_2 domains consists of four antiparallel beta-pleated sheets, the C-terminal ends of which bind to alpha helices. This induces the development of an antigen-combining structure that corresponds to a peptide-combining groove (see figure). The T-cell receptor now recognizes its matching HLA antigen (MHC receptor) as well as the peptide contained in its groove (*trimolecular complex*). The bond between the antigen-bearing cell and the T cell is stabilized by "helper molecules," such as CD8 in the case of cytotoxic T cells.

C. HLA Class I Alleles

The HLA antigens were traditionally named in the order of their discovery as A, B, and C (class I) antigens and D antigens and assigned numbers within the individual groups. As a result, the designations became too varied and confusing. After the exact structure of the genes was identified by molecular biological methods, a uniform international nomenclature for them was introduced. The new designation for HLA class I molecules consists of a code for the gene region and an identification number, separated by an asterisk. All currently known and traditionally defined alleles are listed in the table.

HLA DR, DQ, and DP Alleles in the HLA System (tables on pp. 52, 53)

These tables contain analogous classifications of the class II antigens. The nomenclature is still rather complicated owing to the polymorphic nature of the α and β chains. The subregion HLA-DR, for example, contains a gene for the α chain (DRA1) and for several β chains (DRB1, DRB2, DRB3, DRB4, DRB5, DRB6, and DRB9), which do not all occur simultaneously (see **3** on p. 45). The subregion HLA-DP contains the coding genes DPA1 and DPB1, and the subregion HLA-DQ contains the coding genes DQA1 and DQB1. The designation for the gene or subregion is followed by an asterisk, then the identification number of the allele, immediately followed by the number of the subtype. HLA-DRB1*0101 therefore means: DRB1 locus (coded for β chain 1), allele 01, subtype 01. The table on p. 52 lists the traditional nomenclature (e.g., DR4) followed by the cellular type designation and other codes for oligonucleotide typing.

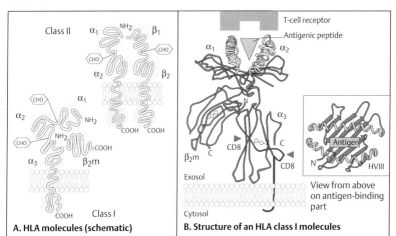

A. HLA molecules (schematic)

B. Structure of an HLA class I molecules

HLA-A alleles		HLA-B alleles		HLA-C alleles	
New nomen-clature	Old nomen-clature	New nomen-clature	Old nomen-clature	New nomen-clature	Old nomen-clature
A*0101	A1	B*0701	B7, B7.1	Cw*0101	Cw1
A*0201	A2, A2.1	B*0702	B7, B7.2	Cw*0201	Cw2, Cw2.1
A*0202	A2, A2.2F	B*0801	B8	Cw*02021	Cw2, Cw2.2
A*0203	A2, A2.3	B*1301	B13, B13.1	Cw*02022	Cw2, Cw2.2
A*0204	A2	B*1302	B13, B13.2	Cw*0301	Cw3
A*0205	A2, A2.2Y	B*1401	B14	Cw*0501	Cw5
A*0206	A2, A2.4a	B*1402	Bw65 (14)	Cw*0601	Cw6
A*0207	A2, A2.4b	B*1501	Bw62 (15)	Cw*0701	Cw7
A*0208	A2, A2.4c	B*1801	B18	Cw*0702	Cw7, JY328
A*0209	A2, A2-ZB	B*2701	B27, 27f	Cw*1101	Cw11
A*0210	A2, A2-LEE	B*2702	B27, 27e, 27K, B27.2	Cw*1201	Cx52
A*0301	A3, A3.1	B*2703	B27, 27d, 27J	Cw*1202	Cb-2
A*0302	A3, A3.2	B*2704	B27, 27b, 27C, B27.3	Cw*1301	CwBL18
A*1101	A11, A11E	B*2705	B27, 27a, 27W, B27.1	Cw*1401	Cb-1
A*1102	A11, A11K	B*2706	B27, 27D, B27.4		
A*2401	A24 (9)	B*3501	B35		
A*2501	A25 (10)	B*3502	B35		
A*2601	A26 (10)	B*3701	B37		
A*2901	A29 (w19)	B*3801	B38 (16), B16.1		
A*3001	A30 (w19), A30.3	B*3901	B39 (16), B16.2		
A*3101	A31 (w19)	B*4001	Bw60 (40)		
A*3201	A32 (w19)	B*4002	B40, B40*		
A*3301	Aw333 (w19), Aw33.1	B*4101	Bw41		
A*6801	Aw68 (28), Aw68.1	B*4201	Bw42		
A*6802	Aw68 (28), Aw68.2	B*4401	B44 (12), B44.1		
A*6901	Aw69 (28)	B*4402	B44 (12), B44.2		
		B*4601	Bw46		
		B*4701	Bw47		
		B*4901	B49 (21)		
		B*5101	B51 (5)		
		B*5201	Bw52 (5)		
		B*5301	Bw53		
		B*5701	Bw57 (17)		
		B*5801	Bw58 (17)		
		B*7801	B'SNA'		

C. HLA class I alleles

Fundamental Principles

New nomenclature	Old nomenclature	New nomenclature	Old nomenclature
DRB1-alleles		**DRB1-alleles**	
DRB1*0101	DR1, Dw1	DRB1*1304	DRw6, DRw13
DRB1*0102	DR1, Dw20	DRB1*1305	DRw6, DRw13
DRB1*0103	DR' BR', Dw' BON'	DRB1*1401	DRw6, DRw14, Dw9, Drw6b
DRB1*1501	DR2, DRw15, Dw2	DRB1*1402	DRw6, DRw14, Dw16
DRB1*1502	DR2, DRw15, Dw12	DRB1*1403	DRw6, DRw14
DRB1*1601	DR2, DRw16, Dw21	DRB1*1404	DRw6, DRw6b.2
DRB1*1602	DR2, DRw16, Dw22	DRB1*1405	DRw6, DRw14
DRB1*0301	DR3, DRw17, Dw3	DRB1*0701	DR7, Dw17
DRB1*0302	DR3, DRw18,	DRB1*0702	DR7, Dw'DB1'
DRB1*0401	DR4, Dw4	DRB1*0801	DRw8, Dw8.1
DRB1*0402	DR4, Dw10	DRB1*08021	DRw8, Dw8.2
DRB1*0403	DR4, Dw13, 13.1	DRB1*08022	DRw8, Dw8.2
DRB1*0404	DR4, Dw14, 14.1	DRB1*08031	DRw8, Dw8.3
DRB1*0405	DR4, Dw15	DRB1*08032	DRw8, Dw8.3
DRB1*0406	DR4, Dw'KT2'	DRB1*0804	DRw8
DRB1*0407	DR4, Dw13, 13.2	DRB1*09011	DR9, Dw23
DRB1*0408	DR4, Dw14, Dw14.2	DRB1*09012	DR9, Dw23
DRB1*0409	DR4	DRB1*1001	DRw10
DRB1*0410	DR4		
DRB1*0411	DR4		
DRB1*1101	DR5, DRw11, Dw5, DRw11.1	**Other DRB alleles**	
DRB1*1102	DR5, DRw11, DRw11.2	DRB3*0101	DRw52a, DW24
DRB1*1103	DR5, DRw11, DRw11.3	DRB3*0201	DRw52b, Dw25
DRB1*1104	DR5, DRw11	DRB3*0202	DRw52b, Dw25
DRB1*1201	DR5, DRw12, Dw'DB6'	DRB3*0301	DRw52c, Dw26
DRB1*1202	DR5, DRw12, DRw12b	DRB4*0101	DRw53
DRB1*1301	DRw6, DRw13, Dw18, DRw6a	DRB5*0101	DR2, DRw15, Dw2
DRB1*1302	DRw6, DRw13, Dw19, DRw6c	DRB5*0102	DR2, DRw15, Dw12
DRB1*1303	DRw6, DRw13, Dw'HAG'	DRB5*0201	DR2, DRw16, Dw21
DRB1*1304	DRw6, DRw13	DRB5*0202	DR2, DRw16, Dw22

A. HLA-DR, HLA-DQ, and HLA-DP alleles in the HLA system (class II alleles)

New nomenclature	Old nomenclature	New nomenclature	Old nomenclature
DQA1 alleles		**DPA1 alleles**	
DQA1*0101	DQA 1.1, 1.9	DPA1*0101	LB14/LB24, DPA1
DQA1*0102	DQA 1.2, 1.19, 1.AZH	DPA1*0102	pSBa-318
DQA1*0103	DQA 1.3, 1.18, DRw8-Dqw1	DPA1*0103	DPw4a1
DQA1*0201	DQA 2, 3.7	DPA1*0201	DPA2, pDAa13B
DQA1*03011	DQA 3, 3.1, 3.2		
DQA1*03012	DQA 3, 3.1, 3.2, DR9-DQw3	**DPB1 alleles**	
DQA1*0302	DQA 3, 3.1, 3.2, DR9-DQw3	DPB1*0101	DPw1, DPB1, DPw1a
DQA1*0401	DQA 4.2, 3.8	DPB1*0201	DPw2, DPB2.1
DQA1*0501	DQA 4.1, 2	DPB1*02011	DPw2, DPB2.1
DQA1*05011	DQA 4.1, 2	DPB1*02012	DPw2, DPB2.1
DQA1*05012	DQA 4.1, 2	DPB1*0202	DPw2, DPB2.2
DQA1*05013	DQA 4.1, 2	DPB1*0301	DPw3, DPB3
DQA1*0601	DQA 4.3	DPB1*0401	DPw4, DPB4.1, DPw4a
		DPB1*0402	DPw4, DPB4.2, DPw4b
DQB1 alleles		DPB1*0501	DPw5, DPB5
DQB1*0501	DQw5 (w1), DQB 1.1, DRw10-DQw1.1	DPB1*0601	DPw6, DPB6
DQB1*0502	DQw5 (w1), DQB 1.2, 1.21	DPB1*0801	DPB8
DQB1*05031	DQw5 (w1), DQB 1.3, 1.9, 13.1	DPB1*0901	DPB9
DQB1*05032	DQw5 (w1), DQB 1.3, 1.9, 13.2	DPB1*1001	DPB10
DQB1*0504	DQB 1.9	DPB1*1101	DPB11
DQB1*0601	DQw6 (w1), DQB 1.4, 1.12	DPB1*1301	DPB13
DQB1*0602	DQw6 (w1), DQB 1.5, 1.2	DPB1*1401	DPB14
DQB1*0603	DQw6 (w1), DQB 1.6, 1.18	DPB1*1501	DPB15
DQB1*0604	DQw6 (w1), DQB 1.7, 1.19	DPB1*1601	DPB16
DQB1*0605	DQw6 (w1), DQB 1.8, 1.19b	DPB1*1701	DPB17
DQB1*0201	DQw2, DQB 2	DPB1*1801	DPB18
DQB1*0301	DQw7 (w3), DQB 3.1	DPB1*1901	DPB19
DQB1*0302	DQw8 (w3), DQB 3.2		
DQB1*03031	DQw9 (w3), DQB 3.3		
DQB1*03032	DQw9 (w3), DQB 3.3		
DQB1*1401	DQw4, DQB 4.1, Wa		
DQB1*0402	DQw4, DQB 4.2, Wa		

	DW4	DRB1*0401
	DW10	DRB1*0402
	DW13	DRB1*0403
	DW14	DRB1*0407
DR4	DW15	DRB1*0404
	DW"KT2"	DRB1*0408
		DRB1*0405
		DRB1*0406

B. HLA-DR, DQ, and DP alleles in the HLA system (continued)

Fundamental Principles

A. MHC Class II-Dependent Antigen Processing

Exogenous antigens, including foreign molecules or microorganisms, must be internalized, digested into peptide fragments, and bound to the peptide-binding groove of MHC molecules before antigen-specific CD4+ T cells recognize them. Through receptor-mediated endocytosis or phagocytosis (see p. 40), exogenous antigens are conveyed into endosomal vesicles. These develop from parts of the internalized cell membrane and have a neutral pH, so acidic proteases are inactive. Within hours, the pH of the endosome decreases, and internalized proteins are digested by cystein proteases called cathepsins. The endosomes then fuse with vesicles containing MHC class II molecules. Recently synthesized transmembrane proteins, such as MHC molecules, are translocated from the cytosol to the endoplasmic reticulum (ER), where they are folded and assembled correctly. They first occur as dimers of α and β chains. A third chain, the gamma or "invariant" chain (**Ii**-chain), binds noncovalently to an MHC II α-β heterodimer blocking its binding site. This prevents the binding of endogenously synthesized peptides, which are abundant in the ER (see also p. 56). The part of the invariant chain that blocks the groove of the α-β heterodimer is called **cl**ass-II associated **i**nvariant chain **p**eptide (**CLIP**). The protein **calnexin** retains the complex within the ER until assembly is correct, then dissociates and allows the complex of MHC II/Ii to leave the ER via small coatomer-coated vesicles. These fuse with the Golgi apparatus on dissociation of the coatomer-coated protein. The invariant chain targets the MHC complexes to transport vesicles of the "trans-Golgi network," which traffic to endosomal vesicles. The invariant chain is cleaved, leaving only the small CLIP fragment bound to the binding site of the MHC II heterodimer. The compartment where fusion of the transport vesicles with the endosomes occurs is called **M**HC class **II** compartment (**MIIC**). An MHC class II-like molecule, called HLA-DM, induces release of the CLIP peptide from the binding groove of the MHC and stabilizes the empty MHC II heterodimer until an appropriate exogenous peptide is bound. Finally, HLA-DM dissociates and the peptide/MHC II complex is transported to the cell membrane. Peptides that were unable to bind to MHC molecules are degraded in lysosomes.

B. Anchor Amino Acids in MHC II Peptides.

The peptide-binding groove of MHC class II molecules is open at both ends, so the size of peptides that can bind ranges typically from 12 to 24 amino acid residues. Both chains of the MHC II molecule interact with the side chains of the peptide and determine binding affinity. Each class II allele has different side chain contacts, allowing only peptides with certain amino acids to bind into particular key positions (anchor positions). The anchor position closest to the NH_2 terminus (position 1) accepts only aromatic or large aliphatic amino acids—this is essential for high-affinity peptide binding. Other important, although less critical anchors, are the amino acids at peptide position 4, 6, and 9. On the other hand, side chains of certain amino acids can interfere with peptide binding (inhibitory amino acids). Anchor positions are the most important contact sites of the peptide with the MHC II molecule, so it is not surprising that the same key positions are critical for binding inhibition. Amino acids that favor or inhibit peptide binding to HLA-DRB1*0401 are shown in **C**. The CLIP peptide of the invariant chain can bind promiscuously to different MHC II alleles: it has methionine at position 1 and side chains that are accepted by all DR alleles in positions 2-9. Computer programs can now predict binding motifs for a particular HLA-DR allele from the protein sequence.

D. T-Cell Activation via MHC II

The peptide/MHC class II complex can activate CD4+ T cells and induce the proliferation and secretion of various cytokines. Tumor necrosis factor-α (TNF-α) released by the antigen presenting cell plays an important role in this process. It leads to the formation of oxygen radicals that are able to kill intracellular microorganisms. Furthermore, activated CD4+ T cells can stimulate antibody formation in B cells. Both mechanisms are directed at the elimination of extracellular pathogens.

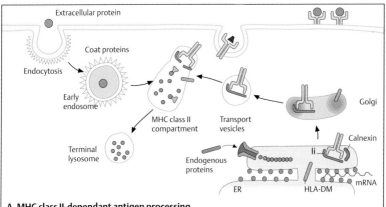

A. MHC class II-dependant antigen processing

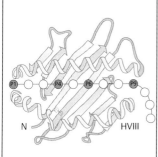

B. Anchor AA in MHC II peptides

	Anchor AA	Inhibitory AA
P1	Phe, Ile, Leu, Met, Val, Trp, Tyr	
P4	Asp, Met, Gln, Ser	Gly, Lys, Pro, Arg, Trp, Tyr
P6	Ser, Thr, Val	Gln, Phe, Gly, His, Lys, Leu, Met, Tyr
P9	Ser	Asp, Gln, Leu, Asn, Pro

C. Allele-specific motifs in DRB1*0401-binding peptides

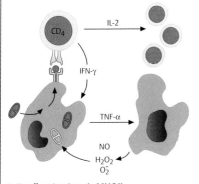

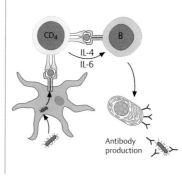

D. T-cell activation via MHC II

A. Processing and Presentation of Endogenous Antigens

MHC class I-presented peptides derive from proteins that are present in the cytoplasm. This allows the immune system to recognize cells that have been infected by viruses or by intracellular bacteria. Theoretically, this also allows recognition of mutated proteins of cancer cells.

In order to preserve cell viability, damaged, denatured, unassembled, or misfolded proteins must be eliminated. Normal proteins also need to be constantly degraded and replaced (with half-lives ranging from a few minutes to several days or weeks). Proteins are tagged for destruction by the protein ubiquitin. Multiubiquitinated proteins are recognized by the proteasome, a large protease complex with a molecular weight of 2000 kDa. It is barrel-shaped and made of a core unit of 20S (650 kDa) as well as of two additional outer rings of 19S (each 700 kDa in size). The four rings of the 20S proteasome consist of two inner β units and two α units, all of them consisting of seven different subunits, which surround a central chamber where proteolysis occurs.

The majority of peptides processed by the proteasome are quickly degraded into single amino acids by cytosolic or nuclear enzymes. Only a few peptides (mostly with a size of 8–10 amino acids) are transported into the endoplasmic reticulum (ER) by a heterodimer/protein complex called **t**ransporter associated with **a**ntigen **p**rocessing (**TAP**). In the ER, peptides bind to the peptide-binding groove of MHC class I proteins if the side chains of their amino acids fit properly with the amino acids of the binding groove of the MHC I α chain. Initially, the α chain is bound by "chaperon" proteins, such as calnexin, calreticulin, Erp57, which regulate peptide binding. Taparin bridges the α chain to TAP. Two or three pockets in each MHC molecule accept only particular amino acids (e.g., aliphatic amino acids, basic amino acids). These are called anchor residues. They differ for different MHC I alleles, since each allele has a different sequence of the α chain. In most cases, the amino acids in position 2 and 9 are crucial for binding. Anchor residues of peptides that bind with high affinity to three frequent HLA alleles are shown in **B**. Peptides with a different amino acid in these positions may bind, but with a lower affinity.

The restrictions dictated by the anchor residues are responsible for the fact that out of a whole protein only a small number of peptides bind with high affinity to a particular HLA-allele (**C**). However, since each individual may have up to six different HLA alleles (maternal and paternal alleles of HLA-A, -B, and -C), a broad spectrum of peptides can still be presented. Computer programs available through the Internet can predict binding epitopes of a given protein for the most common HLA haplotypes.

Lymphoid tissue and cells exposed to IFN-γ have a slightly different proteasome complex as some of the β subunits are substituted by subunits with different substrate preferences, such as LMP2, LMP7, and MECL1 (immunoproteasome, **D**). The proteolytic activity of the immunoproteasome appears to be enhanced compared with the constitutive proteasome, which is in accordance with the higher antigen-processing requirements of antigen-presenting cells and of virus-infected cells exposed to IFN-γ. Proteins processed by the immunoproteasome can generate a whole different set of peptides.

T-cell recognition can be prevented by "immune escape" mechanisms (**E**): defects—e.g., mutations, in the sequence of TAP proteins—can prevent the transport of peptides into the ER so that empty MHC I molecules are generated that are unstable and dissociate quickly from the cell membrane. Viral proteins, such as the Herpes Virus proteins US2 and US11, can induce active export of MHC molecules from the ER, preventing loading of viral peptides in the MHC molecules. Indeed, low levels of MHC I are frequently found in viral infections.

Since many endogenous "self" peptides are presented to T cells by MHC I molecules, two major mechanisms exist to prevent autoreactivity. In the thymus, presentation of self-antigens by thymic epithelia or dendritic cells can lead to clonal deletion of antigen-specific T cells (central tolerance by thymic deletion, **F** and p. 12). In the periphery, recognition of self-antigens by antigen-specific T cells that may have survived thymic selection leads to abortive activation or apoptosis because of a lack of co-stimulatory molecules (peripheral tolerance, **G**).

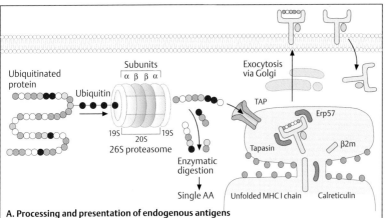

A. Processing and presentation of endogenous antigens

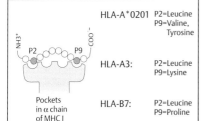

HLA-A*0201 P2=Leucine
P9=Valine,
Tyrosine

HLA-A3: P2=Leucine
P9=Lysine

HLA-B7: P2=Leucine
P9=Proline

Pockets in α chain of MHC I

B. Binding motifs

MAPP**QVLAFGLLL**AAATATFAAAQEECVLENY
KLAVNCFVNNNRQCQCTSVGAQNTVICSKL
AAKCLVMKAEMNGSKLGRRAKPEGALQNND
GLYDPDCDESGLFKAKQCNGTSTCWCVNTA
GVRRTDKDTEITCSERVRTYWIIIELKHKAREK
PYDSKSLRLTALQKEITT**RYGLDPKFITSILYENN
VITI**DLVQNSQQKTQNDVDIADVAYYVEKDV
KGESLFSHKKMDLTVNGEQLDLDPGQTLIYY
VDEKAPEFSMQ**GLKAGVIAV**IVVVVIA**VVAGI
VVL**VISRKKRMAKIEKAEIKEMGEMHRELNA

C. HLA-A2-binding epitopes of a 314 AA protein

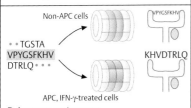

Non-APC cells

•• TGSTA
VPYGSFKHV
DTRLQ •••

VPYGSFKHV

KHVDTRLQ

APC, IFN-γ-treated cells

D. Immunoproteasome

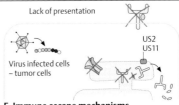

Lack of presentation

Virus infected cells – tumor cells

US2
US11

E. Immune escape mechanisms

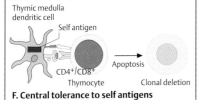

Thymic medulla dendritic cell

Self antigen

CD4+/CD8+
Thymocyte

Apoptosis

Clonal deletion

F. Central tolerance to self antigens

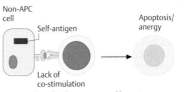

Non-APC cell

Self-antigen

Lack of co-stimulation

Apoptosis/ anergy

G. Peripheral tolerance to self-antigens

Fundamental Principles

57

A. Complement Activation

The "complementary" activity of serum is required for the lysis of cells or bacteria by antibodies. A number of proteases referred to as *complement components* are responsible for this serum activity. Historically, these proteins are designated with the letter "C" followed by a number. The majority of complement proteins are *zymogens*, i.e., inactive proenzymes that become activated after proteolysis. The cleavage products are labeled with an additional lower-case letter.

The C3 protein, which is present in plasma at concentrations of 1 g/l, plays a central role. There are two complement activation pathways (classical and alternative). Both lead to the formation of a proteolytic complex referred to as *C5 convertase.*

The *classical complement pathway* is antibody-dependent. Clustered immunoglobulins such as those in immune complexes have a high affinity for the C1q portion of mannan-binding C1 protein. C1q binding induces a conformational change in C1. This leads to the activation of C1r and C1s, which catalyzes the proteolysis of serum protein C4, yielding a C4a and a C4b fragment. C4b, the largest fragment, binds to complement protein C2, which is then broken down by C1s into C2a and C2b fragments. The C2a fragment remains bound to C4b, thus producing the C3 convertase C4b2a. C4b2a catalyzes the proteolysis of C3 into C3a and the highly reactive C3b fragment. The C5 convertase C4b2a3b is synthesized as the final product of classical complement pathway activation.

Small quantities of C3 are continuously hydrolyzed to C3a and C3b in plasma. The *alternative complement pathway* can be activated when C3b binds to the surface of a microorganism. Due to interaction with C3b, plasma factors B and D catalyze the cleavage of factor B into Ba and Bb fractions. Together with C3b, factor Bb forms the C3bBb complex, another C3 convertase. Binding with properdin (factor P) stabilizes the C3bBb complex. The stabilized complex catalyzes the continued and complete proteolysis of C3 (amplification). C3bBb binds other C3b fragments, ultimately producing C3bBb3b, the C5 convertase of the alternative complement pathway.

B. Lytic Terminal Sequence

Two proteolytic C5 convertases are the terminal products of the classical and alternative complement activation pathways. In each pathway, C3b serves as the binding site for the C5 serum protein, which is split into C5a and C5b fragments by proteolysis. C5b is capable of binding complement proteins C6 and C7. C5b67 is a hydrophobic trimolecular complex that becomes well anchored in the lipid double layer of the cell membrane. Complement proteins C8 and C9 can bind to C5b67, yielding a C5b6789 or C5b-C9 complex. C9 forms polymeric complexes containing up to 14 monomeric C9 molecules. The overall complex is known as the *membrane attack complex (MAC)*, which creates pores in the cell membrane. Endogenous cells have a surface protein-mediated protective mechanism that protects them from MAC-induced lysis. CD59, for example, is bound to the cell membrane by glycosylphosphatidylinositol (GPI) anchoring. Since GPI-bound molecules remain "soluble" in the lipidic cell membrane, they have a high level of "lateral mobility." CD59 molecules inhibit the insertion and polymerization of CD9. Dysfunction of GPI-anchored proteins can lead to increased susceptibility of erythrocytes to lysis by autologous complement in diseases such as paroxysmal nocturnal hemoglobinuria (PNH).

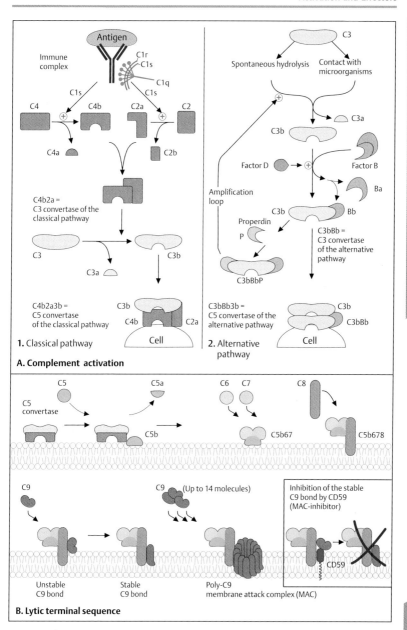

A. Complement activation

1. Classical pathway

2. Alternative pathway

Immune complex

Antigen

C1r
C1s
C1q

C1s — C4 → C4b
C4a

C1s — C2a — C2 → C2b

C4b2a =
C3 convertase of the
classical pathway

C3 → C3b
C3a

C4b2a3b =
C5 convertase
of the classical pathway

C3b
C4b — C2a
Cell

C3

Spontaneous hydrolysis — Contact with microorganisms

C3a

C3b

Factor D → Factor B

Ba

Amplification loop

C3b — Bb

Properdin P

C3bBb =
C3 convertase
of the alternative
pathway

C3bBbP

C3bBb3b =
C5 convertase of the
alternative pathway

C3b
C3bBb
Cell

B. Lytic terminal sequence

C5

C5 convertase → C5b

C5a

C6 C7 → C5b67

C8 → C5b678

C9 → Unstable C9 bond

Stable C9 bond

C9 (Up to 14 molecules) → Poly-C9 membrane attack complex (MAC)

Inhibition of the stable C9 bond by CD59 (MAC-inhibitor)

CD59

Fundamental Principles

59

A. Protection of Autologous Cells by Regulation of Complement Activity

The serum contains a number of regulatory proteins that prevent complement from attacking normal cells. One of these proteins is a protease (C1) inhibitor that inactivates C1r and C1s. Congenital C1 inhibitor deficiency leads to chronic and spontaneous complement activation, which manifests as severe and recurrent episodes of edema (angioneurotic edema).

There are also a number of complement-controlling proteins, such as *decay-accelerating factor* (DAF) and *complement receptor type I* (CR1). DAF inhibits the binding of C2 to C4b (**1**) and promotes the dissociation of existing C4b2a complexes (**2**). Complement receptor CR1 has effects similar to those of DAF; it also promotes the cleavage of C4b by enzyme factor I (FI; **3**). Factor I catalyzes the cleavage of C3b at multiple sites. This first yields the intermediate iC3b, then ultimately the fragments C3c and C3dg. The C3dg fragment remains cell membrane-bound. FI also needs the help of CR1 to fulfill this function.

B. Biological Effects of Complement Factors: Inflammatory Effects

Cleavage of C3 and C5 yields two small fragments (C3a and C5a) that induce the degranulation of basophils and mast cells. These cleavage products are known as *anaphylatoxins*. C5a is very potent (almost 100 times stronger than C3a). C4a, on the other hand, has much weaker anaphylatoxin activity (approximately one-tenth that of C3a). Anaphylatoxin activity is mediated by receptors that induce smooth-muscle contractions, increased vessel permeability, and the degranulation of basophils and mast cells. This activity also induces chemotaxis and activation of granulocytes, resulting in the release of proteolytic enzymes and the production of free radicals.

C. Biological Effects of Complement: Immunological Effects

The terminal sequence of complement leads to direct lysis of bacteria by means of pore formation (**1**). The process of coating microorganisms with complement intermediates (*opsonization*) leads to increased phagocytosis of the microorganisms. This activity also prevents the accumulation of a dangerous excess of antibody-rich immune complexes.

There are four types of complement receptors:

- **CR1** or CD35, which is mainly expressed by erythrocytes, neutrophils, monocytes and macrophages; it binds to C3b, C4b, and iC3b, and promotes phagocytosis. The CR1 receptors on the erythrocytes play an important role in the elimination of immunocomplexes from the circulation (**2**). The immune complexes are transported to the liver and the spleen, where macrophages bearing both CR1 and Fc receptors can remove them from the surface of the erythrocytes.
- **CR2**, which is expressed as CD21, primarily on B lymphocytes, but also on some T cells and epithelial cells. It binds to C3d, iC3b, and C3dg. CR2 in B cells is part of the B-cell co-receptor complex. It also serves as receptor for Epstein–Barr viruses.
- **CR3** or CD18/CD11b. This, like **CR4** (CD18/CD11c), is a member of the integrin family. Both of these complement receptors are expressed on cells of the myeloid lineage, including monocytes, macrophages, dendritic cells, granulocytes, and both bind to iC3b.

Immune complexes bearing cleavage products of complement are efficiently removed from the circulation, mainly by phagocytosis induced by complement receptor-bearing cells. Complement receptors and complement proteins on the cell membrane also promote cell–cell interaction (**3**). Interaction between follicular dendritic cells and B cells via complement receptors and Fc receptors plays an important role in the generation of memory B cells (**4**).

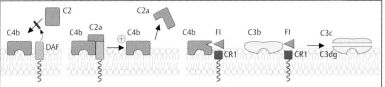

1. Blockage of binding
2. Dissociation of C2a and C4b, enhanced by DAF or CR 1
3. Cleavage of C4b and C3b by CR1/FI

A. Regulation of complement effects: protection of autologous cells

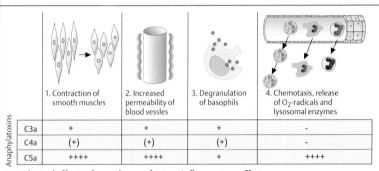

	1. Contraction of smooth muscles	2. Increased permeability of blood vessels	3. Degranulation of basophils	4. Chemotaxis, release of O_2-radicals and lysosomal enzymes
C3a	+	+	+	−
C4a	(+)	(+)	(+)	−
C5a	++++	++++	+	++++

Anaphylatoxins

B. Biological effects of complement factors: inflammatory effects

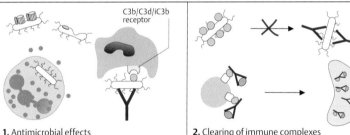

1. Antimicrobial effects

2. Clearing of immune complexes

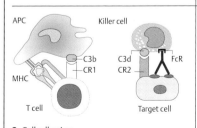

3. Cell adhesion

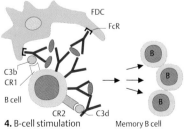

4. B-cell stimulation

C. Biological effects of complement: immunological effects

Fundamental Principles

A. Pathogen-Associated Molecular Patterns and Pattern Recognition Receptors

The evolutionarily ancient system of innate immunity recognizes molecular structures, called **p**athogen-**a**ssociated **m**olecular **p**atterns (PAMPs), which are highly conserved among microorganisms but not expressed by host tissues. They are recognized by specific **p**attern **r**ecognition **r**eceptors (**PRR**), which are expressed mostly on phagocytes.

A typical PAMP is bacterial DNA, which shows a high frequency of unmethylated pairs of cytosine and guanosine dinucleotides (CpG). These oligonucleotides are recognized by Toll-like receptor 9 (TLR9). There are at least ten members of the Toll family of receptors. It is now evident that TLR4 is the receptor for lipopolysaccharide (LPS), the major compound of cell walls of Gram-negative bacteria. LPS-binding protein (LBP) plays a role as an opsonin (i.e., tagging the molecule for better clearance), and CD14 is an opsonic receptor for complexes of LPS and LBP. If the dose of LPS exceeds physiological levels, LPS can also be taken up by endocytosis via scavenger receptors. In contrast to Gram-negative bacteria, Gram-positive bacteria typically expose peptidoglycans at the cell surface, which are recognized by TLR2. Other ligands for TLR2 are lipoproteins, lipopeptides, peptidoglycans, and lipoarabinomannan. The latter is a glycolipid that is present in mycobacteria and can be presented via CD1 molecules to T cells. The yeast cell wall constituents zymosan and mannan also bind to mannose receptors that mediate phagocytosis. This process is facilitated by mannose-binding protein or lectin, which work as opsonins.

B. Pattern Recognition Receptors

Pattern recognition receptors can be divided into three groups: secreted, endocytic, and signaling receptors.

Secreted pattern recognition molecules are opsonins that bind to microbial cell walls to tag them for degradation by the complement system or by phagocytes (**B1**). The best-known receptor of this class is mannose-binding lectin, which is secreted by the liver as an "acute-phase" protein. It recognizes carbohydrates on bacteria, yeast, and some parasites and viruses. Mannose-binding lectin contains two mannan-binding lectin-associated proteases (MASP 1 and 2) that are related to C1r and C1s of the classic complement pathway. Their activation cleaves C3, the third component of complement, which initiates the cascade of complement activation (see p. 58).

Endocytic pattern recognition receptors are expressed on the surface of phagocytes and mediate the uptake and transport to lysosomes (**B2**). After lysosomal degradation and antigen processing, the microbial peptides can be presented to T cells via MHC class II molecules (adaptive immunity). The mannose receptor and scavenger receptors belong to the class of endocytic pattern recognition receptors. The mannose receptor recognizes frequent motifs of mannose typically expressed in microbes; the scavenger receptor binds to bacteria walls, thereby clearing them from circulation.

The last group, the signaling pattern recognition receptors, encompasses the members of the Toll-like family (**B3**). The best-studied pathway is the one mediated by TLR4 after recognition of LPS. MD-2 is a molecule that binds to the extracellular domain of TLR4 and is required for TLR4 signaling. TLR4 has a cytoplasmic domain similar to that of the IL-1 receptor. Indeed, common signaling steps include binding of the adapter molecule MyD88, activation of the IL-1 receptor-associated kinase (IRAK) and of the adapter molecule TNF receptor-associated factor 6 (TRAF6), the involvement of mitogen-activated protein kinases (MAPK), and the final release of the transcription factor NFκB from its inhibitory protein IκB to induce transcription of immune response genes.

C. Dendritic Cells as a Link between Innate and Adaptive Immunity

Dendritic cells (DCs) express both signaling PRRs, such as TLRs, and endocytic PRRs, such as scavenger receptors. TLRs sense LPS as part of the cell wall of Gram-negative bacteria and mediate signaling that results in the secretion of proinflammatory cytokines and chemokines. The innate immune response is activated within hours. Through scavenger receptors, bacteria are phagocytosed and destroyed. In addition, TLRs induce DC maturation and upregulation of co-stimulatory molecules, such as CD80/CD86, which promote the presentation of microbial peptides. After 3-5 days, stimulation by DCs results in sufficient numbers of clonally expanded antigen-specific T-effector and T-helper cells, the components of adaptive immunity.

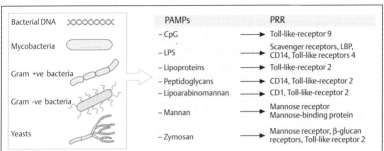

A. Pathogen-Associated Molecular Patterns and Pattern Recognition Receptors

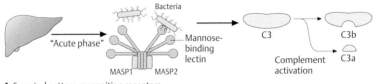

1. Secreted pattern recognition receptors

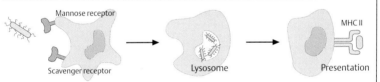

2. Endocytic pattern recognition receptors

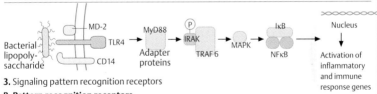

3. Signaling pattern recognition receptors

B. Pattern recognition receptors

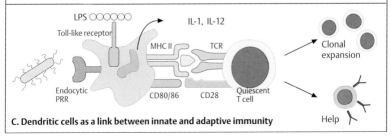

C. Dendritic cells as a link between innate and adaptive immunity

Fundamental Principles

A. Leukocyte Adhesion and Extravasation

Lymphocytes leave the circulation by passing through the endothelium. In the postcapillary venules of lymph nodes and Peyer's patches, a specialized endothelium made up by unusually high endothelial cells, called **h**igh-**e**ndothelial **v**enules (**HEV**), allows migration of resting leukocytes. Migration is enhanced in inflamed tissues. As a first step, the circulating leukocytes engage adhesion molecules in order to slow down. This step is called "tethering" and is mediated by selectins. L-selectin is expressed on leukocytes, whereas endothelial cells express E-selectin as well as P-selectin (which are also found on platelets). All selectins bind sialomucin-like glycoproteins of the sialyl-Lewis^x type, such as **P**-**s**electin **gl**ycoprotein **l**igand-1 (**PSGL-1**), an essential ligand for P-selectin but also for E-selectin and L-selectin. In addition, L-selectin binds to addressins, such as **p**eripheral **n**ode **ad**dressin (**PNAd**), a specific feature of peripheral lymph nodes, and **m**ucosal **ad**dressin **c**ell **a**dhesion **m**olecule-1 (**MAd-CAM-1**), typical for Peyer's patches. The adhesion bonds dissociate and build up over and over, resulting in a slow rolling motion. Tethering and rolling of leukocytes is further supported by α integrins, such as $α_4β_1$ (also referred to as VLA-4) and $α_4β_7$. However, selectin-mediated bonds are not sufficient to permanently arrest the cells. Endothelial cells secrete chemokines that bind to specific chemokine **r**eceptors, which have seven **t**ransmembrane **d**omains (**7TMR**) expressed on rolling leukocytes. After the rapid activation of $β_2$ integrins, e.g., $α_Lβ_2$ (LFA-1, CD11a/CD18) or $α_Mβ_2$ (Mac-1, CD11b/CD18), as well as $α_4$ integrins, the integrins bind several adhesion molecules that belong to the immunoglobulin superfamily, such as ICAM-1 (CD54), ICAM-2 (CD102), VCAM-1 (CD106), and MAdCAM-1. This provides a tighter bond of the leukocytes, which finally arrest and migrate through the endothelium.

B. T-Cell Migration

To find antigens, T lymphocytes periodically migrate to the secondary lymphoid organs. When T lymphocytes roll along the endothelium after initiation of selectin-mediated adhesion, they encounter the **s**econdary **l**ymphoid tissue **c**hemokine (**SLC**) on HEVs. SLC is produced by HEVs but also by stromal cells in the T-cell zone of secondary lymphoid organs.

T cells express the chemokine receptor CCR7, a receptor for SLC and for the **E**pstein–Barr virus-induced receptor **l**igand **c**hemokine (**ELC**), which is also referred to as **m**acrophage **i**nflammatory **p**rotein-3β (**MIP-3β**). T-cell migration is driven by SLC produced by stromal cells and ELC made by dendritic cells and macrophages in the lymph node T zone. Memory T cells have a low expression of CCR7 compared with naive T cells, which may contribute to their reduced trafficking through lymph nodes. Yet, if restimulated by antigen, they quickly react to SLC and ELC again. T_H2 cells also have a weak expression of CCR7, so they do not migrate to the T-cell zone but are rather found at the edge of B-cell areas, where they can provide help to B cells.

C. B-Cell Migration

B cells may encounter antigens in blood, lymph nodes, or the spleen. They can also recognize antigens on the surface of antigen-presenting cells or **f**ollicular **d**endritic **c**ells (**FDC**) within follicles. B lymphocytes are attracted into lymph nodes by **B l**ymphocyte **c**hemoattractant (BLC) produced by FDCs and stromal cells. The corresponding receptor for BLC on B lymphocytes is the chemokine receptor CXCR5.

D. Dendritic Cell Migration into Inflamed Tissue

At sites of inflammation, microbial antigens are captured by the Langerhans cells (LC) of the epidermis. Microbial components, such as **l**ipo**p**oly**s**accharide (LPS), initiate maturation of LC, which then migrate to the dermal lymphatic vessels. LPS induces secretion of inflammatory cytokines, such as TNF-α, and chemokines, such as MIP-1α, MCP-1, IL-8, and RANTES, by dermal dendritic cells (DCs) and macrophages. Immature DCs that express the corresponding chemokine receptors CCR1, CCR2, CCR5, CCR6, and CXCR1 are attracted. During maturation, these receptors are downregulated so that DCs can leave the site of infection. At the same time, maturing DCs upregulate the chemokine receptors CCR7 and CXCR4. Mature DCs that express CCR7 are attracted by endothelial cells of dermal lymphatic vessels that express the CCR7 ligand SLC and are then driven to the subcapsular sinuses of regional lymph nodes. Here, they are guided by a gradient of both ELC and SLC to the T-cell areas.

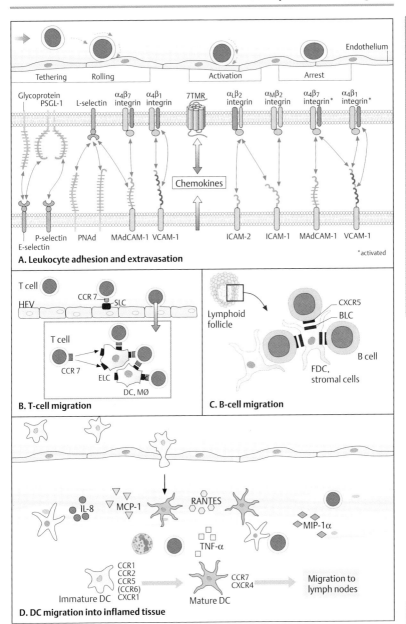

A. Leukocyte adhesion and extravasation

Tethering | Rolling | Activation | Arrest

Endothelium

Glycoprotein PSGL-1 | L-selectin | $\alpha_4\beta_7$ integrin | $\alpha_4\beta_1$ integrin | 7TMR | $\alpha_L\beta_2$ integrin | $\alpha_M\beta_2$ integrin | $\alpha_4\beta_7$ integrin* | $\alpha_4\beta_1$ integrin*

Chemokines

E-selectin | P-selectin | PNAd | MAdCAM-1 | VCAM-1 | ICAM-2 | ICAM-1 | MAdCAM-1 | VCAM-1

*activated

B. T-cell migration

T cell
HEV
CCR 7 — SLC
T cell
CCR 7
ELC
DC, MØ

C. B-cell migration

Lymphoid follicle
CXCR5
BLC
B cell
FDC, stromal cells

D. DC migration into inflamed tissue

IL-8
MCP-1
RANTES
MIP-1α
TNF-α
Immature DC
CCR1 CCR2 CCR5 (CCR6) CXCR1
Mature DC
CCR7 CXCR4
Migration to lymph nodes

Overreactions to foreign antigens can lead to tissue damage. Such responses are known as *hypersensitivity reactions*, which are divided into four types. Type I–III reactions are mediated by antibodies, whereas type IV reactions are mediated by T cells.

A. Types of Hypersensitivity Reactions

Type I: immediate reaction. Some antigens (allergens), such as insect venom, foods, pollen, and dust mite, can induce the formation of IgE antibodies in individuals with a corresponding predisposition (atopics; see also p. 204). The IgE antibodies bind via Fc receptors to mast cells (sensitization). If the individual is reexposed to the allergen, cross-linkage of the membrane-bound IgE occurs. This results in the immediate release of mediators (e.g., histamine, kininogen), which induce vasodilation, smooth-muscle contraction, mucus secretion, edema, and/or skin blisters. Most allergens are small proteins that can easily diffuse through the skin or mucosa. They are frequently proteases and are active at very low doses. IL-4 favors differentiation of T_H2 cells. The exact mechanism that leads B cells to produce IgE is not known.

Type II: antibody-mediated cytotoxic reaction. The immunization of individuals to erythrocyte antigens during pregnancy is a typical example of a type II reaction (see also p. 116). Children who inherit the RhD erythrocyte antigen from their father can induce immunization against the RhD+ antigen in their RhD- mother. Sensitization usually occurs at birth when fetal blood cells come into contact with the maternal immune system. In any subsequent pregnancies, maternal anti-RhD antibodies of the IgG type can pass into the placenta and cause severe hemolysis of fetal RhD+ erythrocytes.

Other examples: Drugs (e.g., penicillin) can passively bind to erythrocytes. Antibodies directed against penicillin then lead to lysis of the erythrocytes (see also p. 124). The formation of antibodies directed against the basement membrane (BM) of the glomerulus can develop during the course of kidney inflammation (see also p. 226). Lung damage accompanied by pulmonary hemorrhage and renal inflammation (glomerulonephritis) may occur due to cross-reaction of these antibodies with the basement membrane of the lung (Goodpasture's syndrome).

Type III: immune complex-mediated reaction. Antibody–antigen complexes (immune complexes) can form during an immune response. Immune complexes can settle in vessel walls, the basement membrane of the lungs and/or kidneys, and in the joints (synovia). They can induce inflammatory processes in these structures by binding complement factors C3a and C5a (anaphylatoxins).

A particular type III reaction is the Arthus reaction: when an antigen has penetrated the skin of an individual who has preformed IgG antibodies, the immune complexes can bind to Fc receptors of most cells inducing degranulation—inflammatory cells are recruited and complement is activated, leading to the release of C5a and local inflammation, platelet accumulation, and eventually to blood vessel occlusion with necrosis.

Type IV: delayed-type hypersensitivity reaction. Haptens are molecules of very small molecular weight (often < 1 kDa). They are too small to function as antigens, but they can penetrate the epidermis and bind to certain proteins in the skin (carrier proteins). Hapten–carrier complexes are bound by antigen-presenting cells of the skin (Langerhans cells), which then migrate to regional lymph nodes (see also p. 45). T-cell stimulation then occurs at the lymph node. The so-called *sensitization phase* lasts ca. 10–14 days. If the individual is reexposed to the hapten, antigen-specific T cells migrate to the skin, where they accumulate and proliferate. They also cause edema formation and local inflammation with the help of cytokines. Compounds containing nickel or chrome and chemicals such as those found in rubber are typical triggers of type IV hypersensitivity reactions (see also p. 202).

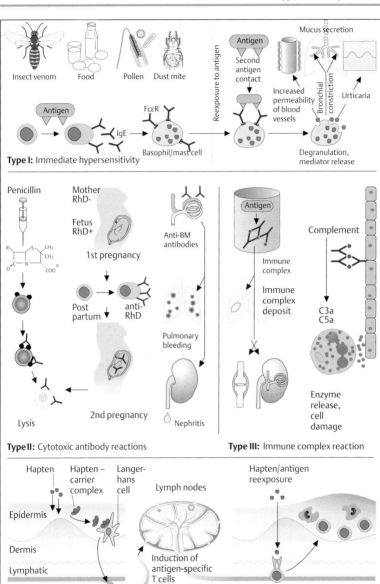

Type I: Immediate hypersensitivity

Type II: Cytotoxic antibody reactions

Type III: Immune complex reaction

Type IV: Delayed type hypersensitivity (DTH)

A. Types of hypersensitivity reactions

A. Induction of T-Cell Tolerance by Antigen-presenting Dendritic Cells

The following experimental model demonstrates the induction of tolerance by central mechanisms. Splenic tissue sections were removed from a strain A adult mouse, and preparations containing dendritic cells were made. The cells were incubated with the *mature* T cells of a strain B mouse. As expected, this induced the activation and reaction of the strain B cells. This was not the case when *foreign* strain A cell preparations were incubated with *immature* strain B thymus cells. Hence, a specific nonreaction (*tolerance*) occurred. Tolerance apparently developed due to the prenatal contact with the foreign dendritic cells. Thus, the prenatal phase and immediate postnatal period are of critical importance in the induction of tolerance, i.e., for the prevention of later autoimmunity (see also pp. 12 and 56).

B. Peripheral Mechanisms for Induction of Tolerance

The prenatal and immediate postnatal selection mechanisms start to function when a potential autoantigen passes into the thymus before birth. Autoreactive T cells with no antigens present in the thymus escape from negative selection. They can, however, be "bridled" by peripheral tolerance mechanisms, e.g., regulator cells (see also p. 72). No immune reaction is possible before this mechanism has failed.

Apart from the active mechanisms of suppression, it is also important that potentially autoreactive T cells are unable to recognize their antigens if they are "hidden" (in the extravascular or intravascular space) or were not suitably presented by professional antigen-presenting cells (ignorance model, see also p. 70). The fact that most organ cells do not bear accessory T-cell-activating molecules is also important. Therefore, no immune response can develop, even when the cell is bound via the TCR.

On the other hand, contact with self-antigens can lead to the depletion of reactive cells, to TCR modulation and, ultimately, to anergy.

C. Transgenic Mice

Important hypotheses concerning the reasons for the *induction and preservation of tolerance* were derived from studies in transgenic mice and rats. In these studies, one or more foreign genes were introduced into the germline of the animals by microinjecting DNA that codes for these genes in the pro-nuclei of fertilized eggs. The eggs were then implanted in sham-pregnant mice. The offspring that developed from these embryo were "transgenic." In other words, the foreign gene was permanently integrated into their germline genes and transmitted to progeny. This experimental system has one decisive advantage over the previous experimental models. The gene product with the tolerance-inducing feature of interest is present in the developing organism right from birth. It does not need to be artificially implanted at a later time.

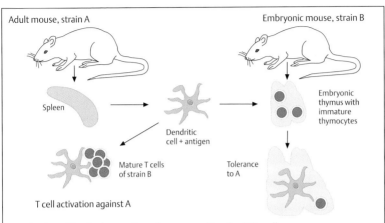

Adult mouse, strain A

Embryonic mouse, strain B

Spleen

Dendritic cell + antigen

Embryonic thymus with immature thymocytes

Mature T cells of strain B

Tolerance to A

T cell activation against A

A. Induction of T-cell tolerance by antigen-presenting dendritic cells

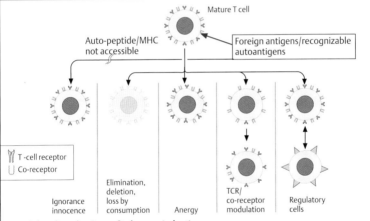

Mature T cell

Auto-peptide/MHC not accessible

Foreign antigens/recognizable autoantigens

T-cell receptor

Co-receptor

Ignorance innocence

Elimination, deletion, loss by consumption

Anergy

TCR/ co-receptor modulation

Regulatory cells

B. Peripheral mechanisms of tolerance induction

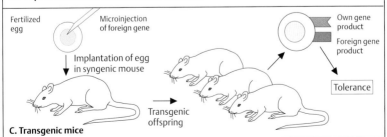

Fertilized egg

Microinjection of foreign gene

Own gene product

Foreign gene product

Implantation of egg in syngenic mouse

Transgenic offspring

Tolerance

C. Transgenic mice

A. Induction of Autoimmune Response by Virally Induced T-Cell Activation

Autoreactive T cells cannot be activated by target cells in the absence of a co-stimulatory signal (see also p. 68). T-cell activation and destruction of the target cells can only occur after the antigen has been presented to the T cells by "professional" antigen-presenting cells (APCs), e.g., in infection.

The previously described experiment produced double-transgenic mice with T cells that all bore the same T-cell receptor directed against a lymphocytic choriomeningitis virus (LCMV) protein. The gene for the viral protein was additionally linked to the insulin promoter and introduced into animals of the same strain. Hence, all islet cells expressed this protein via their MHC molecules. In theory, the islet cells should have been killed quickly since they all bore a molecule recognized by cytotoxic T cells. In practice, however, prenatal tolerance did not develop because the transgenic gene product apparently had not entered the thymus. No T-cell reaction occurred, and the animals did not develop diabetes mellitus. Direct infection of the animals with the LCM virus, on the other hand, led to T-cell activation and destruction of islet cells. Only then did the cytotoxic T cells receive a (co-stimulatory) signal via antigen-presenting cells and activated T-helper cells.

B. Induction of Antibody Formation with T-Cell Help after Autoantibody-mediated Antigen Presentation

Autoreactive B cells cannot be activated to form antibodies without the help of T cells. With the help of their cell-based immunoglobulin, however, they are able to recognize, bind, process, and present molecules containing endogenous antigen (*autoantigen*) and foreign antigen components. Once such an antigen has been processed, the B cells present the foreign component of the antigen to T cells via their MHC molecule. The T cells then transmit signals for B-cell help. In this case, the B cells are those that recognize an autoantigen and, thus, secrete the corresponding autoantibodies.

C. Induction of Autoimmunity via Molecular Mimicry

According to the *molecular mimicry hypothesis*, a certain antigen, such as a viral or bacterial antigen, has a great degree of similarity with endogenous structures. Because of mistaken identity, the body then attacks foreign as well as endogenous molecules when infected with the antigen.

D. Induction of an Autoimmune Reaction after Viral Infection due to Aberrant MHC Class II Antigens

In many autoimmune diseases, HLA class II antigens are found on target cells that do not exhibit the corresponding cell systems in healthy individuals. IFN-γ-related induction could be a possible mechanism in such "aberrant" class II antigen expression. A virus infects a certain cell group, and its surface molecules are identified as foreign by specific T lymphocytes. During the defense process, the T lymphocytes secrete IFN-γ, which leads to the induction of class II antigens in previously uninvolved cells. This "aberrant" expression of class II antigens might prompt autoreactive T cells, in association with class II antigens that are not normally expressed, to identify autoantigens on the cell surface as foreign and, ultimately, to destroy endogenous cells.

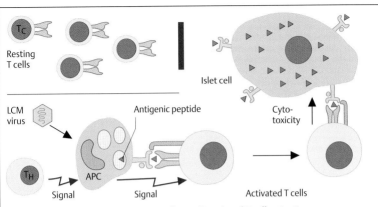

A. Induction of an autoimmune response by virally induced T-cell activation

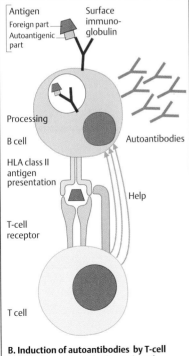

B. Induction of autoantibodies by T-cell help after autoantibody-mediated antigen presentation

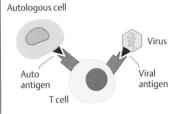

C. Induction of an autoimmune reaction by molecular mimicry

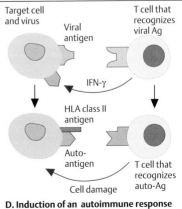

D. Induction of an autoimmune response after viral infection by aberrant MHC class II antigens

Fundamental Principles

71

A. Induction of Autoimmunity through the Loss of Regulatory Mechanisms

Peripheral regulatory mechanisms still exist after early deactivation of autoreactive T-cell clones in the thymus has occurred (see p. 11). Both CD8+ and CD4+ T cells can have a regulatory function. Autoimmunity can develop after the loss of such regulator cells.

In addition to these cellular mechanisms, there are also humoral mechanisms for preserving tolerance. Anti-idiotypic antibodies directed against determinants of the hypervariable region of other antibodies form an *anti-idiotypic network* (according to N. Jerne) that contributes to tolerance. Disturbances in the network caused by the loss of anti-idiotypic antibodies or the predominance of pathogenic autoantibodies lead to the loss of tolerance. External supplementation, e.g., by administering normal immunoglobulins, can restore the balance of the network.

B. Organ-Specific and Non-Organ-Specific Autoimmune Diseases

Autoimmune diseases may be directed against very specific organ determinants or against various tissue structures (systemic autoimmune disease).

C. Sequestered Antigens

The concept of sequestered antigens was derived from the observation that after eye injuries, for example, the healthy eye suddenly develops symptoms of *sympathetic ophthalmia*. Thus, certain regions of the body are not accessible to the immune system or are "sequestered." This not only affects proteins in the lens of the eye, but also the cartilage and testicular tissue. Once this isolation is broken, e.g., due to injury or severe inflammation, the immune system has access to the tissue it then identifies as "foreign."

D. Relationship between Diseases and the HLA System

Two conditions must exist in order for autoimmune diseases to develop: a genetic component and environmental factors (*realization factors*). Environmental factors can lead to the manifestation of an autoimmune disease when there is a genetic basis (predisposition) for the disease. Because certain HLA constellations are associated with the transmission of a high susceptibility to certain diseases, the *HLA system* (see pp. 44–51) is an important determinant of the genetic component. Certain HLA antigens are often associated with specific determinants of some autoimmune diseases (the old nomenclature is used in the table for simplicity). Spondylarthritis, for example, is so closely associated with the HLA-B27 antigen that diagnosis of the disease is greatly helped by the detection of this important determinant. Some of the most important associations are listed below.

- *Class I association*: seronegative spondylarthritis and HLA-B27;
- *Class II association*: rheumatoid arthritis (chronic polyarthritis) and HLAs DR4 and DR1; type I diabetes mellitus and HLAs DR3 and DR4; narcolepsy and HLA-DR2.

Narcolepsy and HLA-DR2 are so frequently associated that the *relative risk* cannot be calculated mathematically: relative risk = (number of patients with HLA antigen×number of controls without HLA antigen)÷(number of patients without HLA antigen×number of controls with HLA antigen).

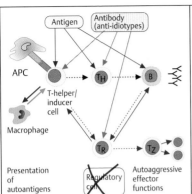

A. Induction of autoimmunity by loss of regulatory mechanisms

APC

T-helper/inducer cell

Macrophage

T$_H$

B

T$_R$

T$_Z$

Antigen

Antibody (anti-idiotypes)

Presentation of autoantigens

Regulatory cell

Autoaggressive effector functions

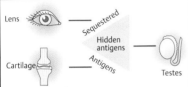

C. Sequestered antigens

Lens

Cartilage

Hidden antigens

Sequestered

Antigens

Testes

B. Organ-specific and non-organ-specific autoimmune diseases

Organ-specific diseases	Non-organ-specific diseases
Brain MS	**Brain** SLE
Cartilage Polychondritis	**Nose** Wegener's granulomatosis
Thyroid gland Hashimoto's thyroiditis, primary myxedema, thyrotoxicosis (Graves' disease)	**Lung** Scleroderma, MCTD, Wegeners' granulomatosis
Stomach Pernicious anemia	**Muscle/skin** Dermato-myositis
Liver PBC, autoimmune hepatitis	**Kidney** SLE, Wegeners' granulomatosis
Pancreas Juvenile diabetes	
Intestine Crohn's disease, ulcerative colitis	**Joints** Rheumatoid arthritis
Bone marrow Autoimmune hemolytic anemia, ITP	**Skin** Scleroderma, SLE
Skin Pemphigus	

Disease	Allele*	Frequency (%)		Relative risk
		Patients	Controls	
Behçet's disease	B5	41	10	6,3
Ankylosing spondylitis	B27	90	9	87,4
Reiter's syndrome	B27	79	9	37,0
Acute anterior uveitis	B27	52	9	10,4
Subacute thyroiditis	B35	70	15	13,7
Psoriasis vulgaris	Cw6	87	33	13,3
Dermatitis herpetiformis	DR3	85	26	15,4
Celiac sprue	DR3	79	26	10,8
Graves' disease	DR3	56	26	3,7
Diabetes mellitus type I	DR3 and/or DR4	91	57	7,9
Myasthenia gravis	DR3	50	26	2,5
Systemic lupus erythematosus	DR3	70	26	5,8
Idiopathic membr. nephropathy	DR3	75	26	12,0
Narcolepsy	DR2	100	25	N.D.
Multiple sclerosis	DR2	59	25	4,1
Rheumatoid arthritis	DR4	50	19	4,2
Hashimoto's thyroiditis	DR5	19	6	3,2
Pernicious anemia	DR5	25	6	5,4
Juvenile chronic arthritis	DRw8	23	8	3,6

D. Associations between diseases and the HLA system (*old nomenclature)

Fundamental Principles

Cells must constantly die to ensure the normal development of an organism and to maintain the balance between the generation and loss of cells (*homeostasis*). This activity is regulated by *programmed cell death*, a type of "cell suicide," the morphological correlative of which is apoptosis. Apoptosis plays an important role for the correct function of the immune system.

A. Differences between Necrosis and Apoptosis

Cell necrosis occurs as the result of severe injuries due, for example, to burns, oxygen deficiency (e.g., heart attack), and trauma. In necrosis, the cell membrane loses its integrity. As a result, the cell starts to swell, and the cell contents, together with a number of toxic substances, are released into the surrounding tissue, thus inducing an inflammatory reaction.

Apoptosis, on the other hand, is a very subtle process. The first signs of apoptosis are chromatin condensation and shrinkage of the cell. The cell membrane then develops small bulges in a process known as *zeiosis* (*blebbing*). The cell then begins to expel its contents into vesicles, some of which contain parts of the fragmented and condensed (pyknotic) cell nucleus. The vesicles are ingested and degraded by macrophages. Since the cytoplasmic enzymes and toxic metabolites are always surrounded by membranes, no inflammatory reaction occurs.

B. Regulation of Apoptosis

Apoptosis is a genetically regulated process that requires energy and protein synthesis. Apoptotic cell fragmentation can be induced by a number of signals, including physiological stimuli, such as antigen receptor binding. This takes place, for example, when the stimulus occurs without the accessory signals (see p. 36).

Surface molecules, such as CD95 (APO-1 or Fas antigen), are important mediators of apoptosis. CD95 is a member of the tumor necrosis factor (TNF)/nerve growth factor (NGF) family of receptor proteins. When activated by APO-1/Fas ligands, CD95 triggers an apoptotic signal in a number of cells. Apoptosis can be triggered by the loss of cell–cell contact (*anoikis*) or the withdrawal of growth factors by glucocorticoids, hyperthermia, and granzyme (see p. 38). A common intracellular mediator may be oxidative stress, which causes nuclease activation. This leads to the cleavage of DNA into fragments. In DNA electrophoresis, this fragmentation process yields a ladder-like pattern that has been identified as a typical feature of apoptosis (**C**).

Apoptosis is accompanied by the activation of a number of genes. One of the most important is *interleukin-1β converting enzyme* (ICE). The c-*myc*, *p53*, and *nur77* genes are also upregulated in the initial phase of an apoptotic process. The *bcl-2* gene, on the other hand, codes for a protein that prevents apoptosis. High titers of the protein can be found in the follicular cortex of cells that have successfully rearranged their immunoglobulin genes, while the protein cannot be detected in the germinal center, where the rate of apoptosis is very high. Products of the *bax* and *bad* genes are bcl-2 protein antagonists, and activation of these products is associated with apoptosis. The *bax* gene forms complexes with bcl-2 protein, thereby inactivating it. bcl-X protein, which occurs in two forms: an anti-apoptotic long-splice variant (bcl-X_L) and a pro-apoptotic, short-splice variant (bcl-X_S), is related to bcl-2. Downregulation of *bax* and other apoptosis-promoting genes may play a role in the development of neoplasms.

C. Caspase Activation by Mitochondria

Apoptosis-inducing agents, such as ceramide, oxidants, *bax*, calcium, and activated caspases can release the protein cytochrome *c* from mitochondria. Caspases are **c**ysteine **a**spartate proteases that cleave cellular proteins, resulting in cell death. After being released into the cytosol, cytochrome *c* binds to its adapter molecule Apaf-1, which activates pro-caspase 9. This complex is called apoptosome. Caspase 9 in turn activates downstream caspases 3 and 7, resulting in DNA fragmentation and apoptosis. Caspases can be inhibited by IAPs (inhibitors of apoptosis proteins).

D. Phagocytosis of Apoptotic Cells

During apoptosis, phosphatidylserine (PS) is exposed at the cell surface. Scavenger receptors A and endotoxin receptor CD14 can bind to PS. The vitronectin receptor cooperates with the thrombospondin (TSP) receptor CD36 to bind TSP. Triggering of these receptors induces actin rearrangement, leading to internalization of apoptotic cells. The release of proinflammatory cytokines or chemokines is downregulated.

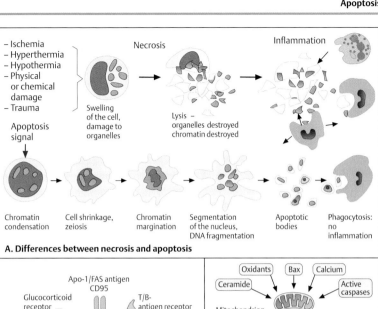

Necrosis

- Ischemia
- Hyperthermia
- Hypothermia
- Physical or chemical damage
- Trauma

Inflammation

Swelling of the cell, damage to organelles

Lysis – organelles destroyed chromatin destroyed

Apoptosis signal

Chromatin condensation

Cell shrinkage, zeiosis

Chromatin margination

Segmentation of the nucleus, DNA fragmentation

Apoptotic bodies

Phagocytosis: no inflammation

A. Differences between necrosis and apoptosis

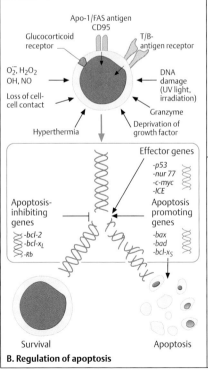

Apo-1/FAS antigen CD95

Glucocorticoid receptor

T/B-antigen receptor

O_2^-, H_2O_2 OH, NO

DNA damage (UV light, irradiation)

Loss of cell-cell contact

Granzyme

Hyperthermia

Deprivation of growth factor

Effector genes

-p53
-nur 77
-c-myc
-ICE

Apoptosis-inhibiting genes

-bcl-2
-bcl-x_L
-Rb

Apoptosis promoting genes

-bax
-bad
-bcl-x_S

Survival

Apoptosis

B. Regulation of apoptosis

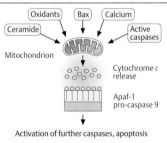

Oxidants   Bax   Calcium

Ceramide

Active caspases

Mitochondrion

Cytochrome c release

Apaf-1 pro-caspase 9

Activation of further caspases, apoptosis

C. Caspase activation by mitochondria

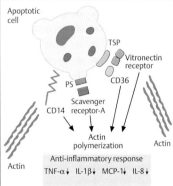

Apoptotic cell

TSP

Vitronectin receptor

PS

CD36

CD14

Scavenger receptor-A

Actin polymerization

Actin

Actin

Anti-inflammatory response
TNF-α↓ IL-1β↓ MCP-1↓ IL-8↓

D. Phagocytosis of apoptotic cells

A. Heidelberger Precipitation Curve

Precipitation techniques are used to measure antigen or antibody concentrations. The tests can be performed in solid phase (radial immunodiffusion, immunoelectrophoresis) or liquid phase systems (turbidimetry, nephelometry).

The *Heidelberger precipitation curve* can be described as follows. Soluble immune complexes form in the antibody excess zone (low Ag/Ab ratio) of the curve. The amount of complexes formed is proportional to the antigen concentration. The region of equivalence is reached as increasing concentrations of the antigen are added. A visualizable precipitate made of insoluble immune complexes forms at equivalence. Mainly soluble immune complexes are present in the subsequent region of antigen excess. The concentration of the complexes increases as the antigen concentration rises. This simulates an antigen concentration that is too low. The test sample must therefore be diluted in order to keep the antigen concentration in the ascending part of the curve to ensure that the results are proportional to the antigen concentration.

B. Precipitation and Agglutination

Precipitation reactions. Immune complexes form due to interaction between an antibody and molecular antigens. In immune precipitation, the antigen is diluted by diffusion in a sample with a known antibody concentration until the point of precipitation occurs, i.e., until the antigen/antibody ratio reaches the equivalence zone.

Agglutination reactions. Immune complexes form due to interaction between an antibody and particulate antigens. A distinction is made between direct agglutination (e.g., hemagglutination test for determination of blood type and Widal's bacterial agglutination test) and indirect agglutination tests (e.g., latex agglutination test and Boyden's passive hemagglutination test).

C. Precipitation Reactions in Fluid Phase

Turbidimetry. An antigen sample is placed in a cuvette and allowed to react with an excess of an antiserum containing the corresponding antibody. Soluble immune complexes form. The change in turbidity in the cuvette is measured by photometry. To determine the end point, the increase in absorption within a certain time is used as the measure of antigen concentration.

Nephelometry. This technique is also based on the reaction principle of immune complex formation due to antigen–antibody interaction. The cuvette is irradiated with laser light, which scatters from the immune complexes. Lenses are used to focus the scattered light onto a photometer. Using the measured signals, the unknown antigen concentration can then be determined from a standard curve.

D. Simple Radial Immunodiffusion (Mancini Method)

In this test, an agar plate is homogeneously coated with a gel containing the appropriate antibody. The antigen sample is placed in wells of the plate. The antibody diffuses radially into the gel and is thereby diluted. Immune complexes form precipitates in the region of equivalence. In the Mancini method, the antigen concentration is said to be proportional to the square of the diameter (d^2) of the ring of precipitation. The unknown antigen concentration is determined from a standard curve obtained with known concentrations of the antigen.

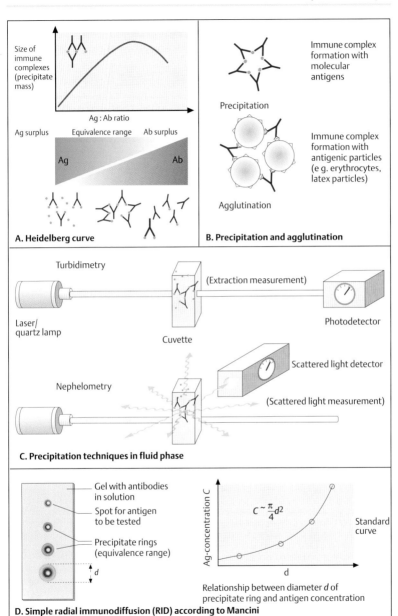

A. Heidelberg curve

Size of immune complexes (precipitate mass)

Ag : Ab ratio

Ag surplus   Equivalence range   Ab surplus

Ag   Ab

B. Precipitation and agglutination

Immune complex formation with molecular antigens

Precipitation

Immune complex formation with antigenic particles (e g. erythrocytes, latex particles)

Agglutination

Turbidimetry

(Extraction measurement)

Laser/ quartz lamp

Photodetector

Cuvette

Scattered light detector

Nephelometry

(Scattered light measurement)

C. Precipitation techniques in fluid phase

Gel with antibodies in solution

Spot for antigen to be tested

Precipitate rings (equivalence range)

Ag-concentration C

$C \sim \frac{\pi}{4} d^2$

Standard curve

Relationship between diameter *d* of precipitate ring and antigen concentration

D. Simple radial immunodiffusion (RID) according to Mancini

Laboratory Applications

A. Radial Double Immunodiffusion (Ouchterlony Method)

In this test, both antigen and antibody diffuse radially toward each other in aqueous agarose gel. Visible bands of precipitation form at the sites where the antigen and antibody meet. This method is a very effective way to test the identity of unknown antigens based on the symmetry of precipitation patterns. Identity of two antisera (with respect to the unknown antigen) occurs when the two bands of precipitation fuse to form a single line. The bands cross when there is nonidentity, and a so-called spur forms in partial identity.

B. Electroimmunodiffusion (Countercurrent Electrophoresis)

When a sample is adjusted to a given pH (e.g., pH 8.2 for the test antigen: extractable nuclear antigens, ENA), the antigen and antibody migrate in opposite directions through the gel due to differences in their electric charges. Immune complexes form during the transmigration process if the corresponding antibody is present in the patient's serum. The immune complexes form lines of precipitation that can be visualized by staining.

C. Immunoelectrophoresis

Immunoelectrophoresis is a combination of protein electrophoresis and immunoprecipitation. The test and reference samples are first separated by electrophoresis. The antiserum diffuses perpendicularly to the direction of separation. Due to the formation of precipitating immune complexes, sharply defined lines of precipitation form in the range of equivalence. Proteins can be identified based on the intensity, shape, and position of the precipitation lines.

Immunoelectrophoresis is used in patients with suspected monoclonal and polyclonal gammopathies. Polyclonal immunoglobulins are uniformly distributed throughout the gamma-globulin fraction after electrophoretic separation. Monoclonal immunoglobulins form a local gradient in the gamma-globulin fraction (M gradient), leading to the formation of a distinctive indentation pattern.

D. Rocket Electrophoresis (Electrophoresis in Antibody-containing Gel)

In this technique, antigens migrate through a gel containing an antibody toward an anode. This leads to the formation of long, rocket-shaped precipitates (rockets) that can be visualized by staining. This method permits quantitation of the antigen concentration by comparing the test specimen to a simultaneously measured standard.

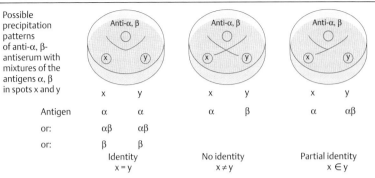

Possible precipitation patterns of anti-α, β-antiserum with mixtures of the antigens α, β in spots x and y

	x	y
Antigen	α	α
or:	αβ	αβ
or:	β	β
	Identity	
	x = y	

x	y
α	β
No identity	
x ≠ y	

x	y
α	αβ
Partial identity	
x ∈ y	

A. Radial double diffusion (Ouchterlony)

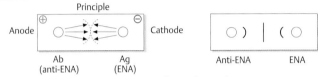

Principle

Anode ⊕ ... ⊖ Cathode

Ab (anti-ENA) Ag (ENA)

Anti-ENA ENA

B. Transmigration electrophoresis (countercurrent electrophoresis)

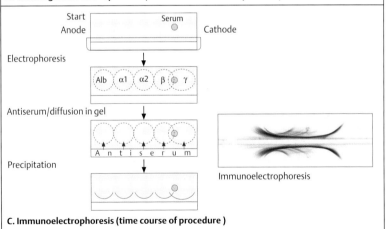

Start

Anode Serum Cathode

Electrophoresis

Alb α1 α2 β γ

Antiserum/diffusion in gel

A n t i s e r u m

Precipitation

Immunoelectrophoresis

C. Immunoelectrophoresis (time course of procedure)

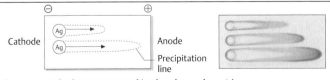

Cathode ⊖ Ag Ag ⊕ Anode

Precipitation line

D. Electrophoresis in antibody-containing gel (rocket electrophoresis)

A. Agglutination Techniques

1 **Hemagglutination**: detection of agglutinating antibodies in a serum sample. *Complete antibodies* are immunoglobulins of the IgM class. They bind to the antigen determinants of red blood cells as pentamers and induce agglutination of the antigens. They are called complete (natural) antibodies because they can induce agglutination due to their pentameric structure. Antibodies against blood group antigens are a type of complete antibodies.

Incomplete antibodies also exist (IgG antibodies). These antibodies bind to the antigen determinant of RBCs but cannot induce agglutination. Hemagglutination occurs when the distance between red blood cells is reduced by adding a supplement (albumin) or a solution with a low ionic charge, thus allowing the IgG antibody (incomplete antibody) to bridge the gap between the cells. The formation of antibodies against Rh+ red blood cells in Rh-negative patients, e.g., after an Rh-incompatible blood transfusion, is a good example.

2 **Latex agglutination**: In this method, a latex particle is allowed to react with the unknown antibody. In the illustrated example (rheumatoid factor screening), IgG binds to the latex particle. Agglutination of the latex particle occurs if rheumatoid factor (IgM anti-IgG) is present in the serum sample (positive reaction).

Bacterial agglutination (not illustrated). *Antibody detection* (*Widal method*): Bacterial suspensions incubated in serial dilutions of the patient's serum serve as the antigen. Agglutination occurs if the antibody corresponding to the antigen is present in the patient's serum. *Antigen detection* (Gruber method): Bacterial cultures are incubated with class-specific and type-specific antibodies. This method is used for bacterial type determination.

B. Complement-binding Reaction (CBR)

This method involves the binding and activation of complement by antigen–antibody complexes for determination of antibodies in serum or cerebrospinal fluid. Antigen and complement corresponding to the target antibody are added to the serum sample (complement-free due to inactivation). Complement will be bound and consumed if the antibody is present in the serum sample. Test red blood cells coated with test antibodies (immune complexes) are used as the indicator system. When the test is positive, no complement-mediated hemolysis of the indicator system occurs since the complement was consumed. If the test is negative, complement is still available to induce lysis of the test RBCs of the indicator system.

One of the drawbacks of this method is false-positive results due to, for example, to self-inhibition of serum due to rheumatoid factors, immune complexes, etc. This is reflected as a positive reaction of the control sample (patient serum alone without the addition of antigen).

Other materials may also contaminate the antigen and form immune complexes with the target antibody in the patient's serum, thus inducing complement binding. This is also reflected as a positive reaction of the control antigen.

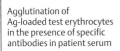

Agglutination of Ag-loaded test erythrocytes in the presence of specific antibodies in patient serum

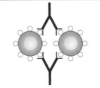

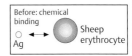

Before: chemical binding

Ag ⟷ Sheep erythrocyte

1. Hemagglutination

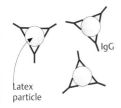

Latex particle

IgG

RF (IgM anti-IgG)

IgM-RF in patient serum

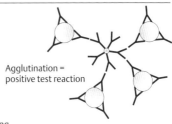

Agglutination = positive test reaction

2. Latex agglutination in rheumatoid factor screening

A. Agglutination techniques

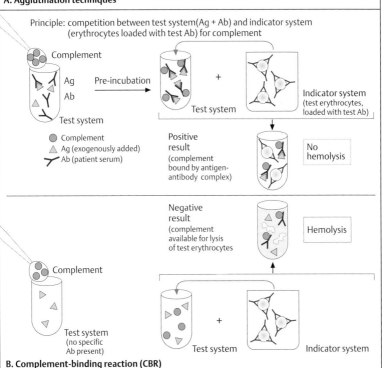

Principle: competition between test system (Ag + Ab) and indicator system (erythrocytes loaded with test Ab) for complement

Complement

Ag
Ab

Pre-incubation

Test system

Test system

+

Indicator system (test erythrocytes, loaded with test Ab)

● Complement
△ Ag (exogenously added)
⅄ Ab (patient serum)

Positive result (complement bound by antigen-antibody complex)

No hemolysis

Negative result (complement available for lysis of test erythrocytes)

Hemolysis

Complement

Test system (no specific Ab present)

Test system

+

Indicator system

B. Complement-binding reaction (CBR)

Laboratory Applications

A. Enzyme-Linked Immunosorbent Assay (ELISA)

The enzyme immunoassay is a method of quantitative analysis in which one of the reagents is labeled with an enzyme. This may be either the antigen or the antibody.

In the illustrated example, a well of the carrier medium (usually a microtiter plate) is coated with the antigen corresponding to the target antibody. If this antibody is present in the test sample (e.g., serum), it will bind to the antigen. An enzyme-conjugated secondary antibody (e.g., sheep anti-human IgG, Fab fragment) binds to the target antibody in the subsequent reaction step. In the presence of the enzyme, the substrate is transformed in a color staining reaction. The antibody concentration in the test sample can be determined by comparing the color reaction product with that of standards of known concentration.

Sandwich ELISA is a method of antigen determination. The antibody for the target antigen is bound to the solid phase of a microtiter well. The amount of bound antigen in the sample is determined by adding an enzyme-conjugated secondary antibody. The secondary antibody forms a sandwich complex and binds to the antigen.

B. C1q Solid-Phase ELISA

In this method, C1q is covalently bound to chemically activated polystyrene microtiter strips. Circulating immune complexes in the sample (e.g., serum) bind to C1q. An enzyme-labeled antibody against human IgG is used to detect the immune complexes. A color staining reaction occurs after addition of a corresponding substrate. The intensity of the reaction is proportional to the concentration of circulating immune complexes in the sample.

C. Radioimmunoassay (Classical Method)

The classical radioimmunoassay (RIA) is based on the principle of competitive binding. In the illustrated example, the antigen corresponding to the target antibody is immobilized in the solid phase of the microtiter well. The unlabeled antibodies in the serum sample and the radioactively labeled antibodies now compete for antigen binding sites. Antibody still free in solution is subsequently removed by washing. The higher the number of unlabeled antibodies in the serum, the lower the number of labeled antibodies able to bind to the antigen. Hence, the measured radioactivity will be low when the serum antibody titer is high and vice versa.

D. Immunoblotting (Western Blot)

In Western blotting, proteins are separated according to molecular weight by means of sodium dodecyl sulfate (SDS)–polyacrylamide gel electrophoresis (SDS-PAGE). All proteins obtain a negative charge due to the presence of SDS (SDS binding). The addition of 2-mercaptoethanol diminishes internal disulfide bonds. Since they lose their characteristic charge and form during electrophoretic separation, the proteins are separated according to their molecular weight.

The proteins are then "blotted," that is, transferred from the gel to an immobilizing nitrocellulose (NC) membrane, where they can be recognized by specific antibodies in the membrane. Antibodies against *Borrelia burgdorferi* are used in the example. One of the main advantages of Western blotting is its ability to identify a specific antibody after protein separation.

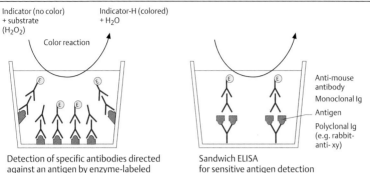

Detection of specific antibodies directed against an antigen by enzyme-labeled secondary antibodies (conjugate)

Sandwich ELISA for sensitive antigen detection (e.g. cytokines)

Anti-mouse antibody
Monoclonal Ig
Antigen
Polyclonal Ig (e.g. rabbit-anti- xy)

 Antibody   Antigen   Secondary antibody, enzyme linked

A. Enzyme-linked immunosorbent assay (ELISA)

C1q
Ig
Anti-human Ig with subsequent color reaction

B. C1q solid-phase ELISA

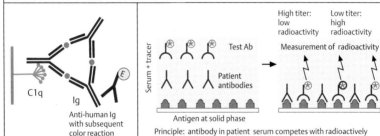

High titer: low radioactivity   Low titer: high radioactivity

Measurement of radioactivity

Test Ab
Patient antibodies
Antigen at solid phase

Principle: antibody in patient serum competes with radioactively labeled test antibody

C. Radioimmunoassay (classical method)

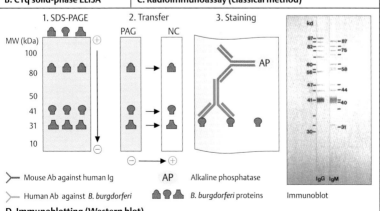

1. SDS-PAGE   2. Transfer   3. Staining

MW (kDa)
100
80
50
41
31
10

PAG   NC

AP

kd
97 — — 87
82 — — 75
60 — — 58
56 —
47 — — 44
41 — — 40
— 31
30 —

IgG IgM

Immunoblot

>— Mouse Ab against human Ig

>— Human Ab against *B. burgdorferi*

AP   Alkaline phosphatase

B. burgdorferi proteins

D. Immunoblotting (Western blot)

Laboratory Applications

83

A. Fluorescence emission

Certain materials have the property of absorbing energy when exposed to light of a given wavelength. The light that is emitted has a lower energy and therefore a different color than the incident light. The emitted light is called fluorescence. Fluorescein isothiocyanate (FITC) is the most commonly used fluorescent dye. FITC is stimulated by high-energy blue light at wavelengths of 450–500 nm and emits yellow-green fluorescence at a lower wavelength (500–550 nm).

The exciter filter on a fluorescence microscope restricts the passage of light to a defined wavelength (e.g., 470 nm). The filtered light is projected onto the fluorescent sample. Fluorescent light emitted at wavelengths of 520–550 nm is then passed though a dichroic mirror and a bandpass barrier filter, thereby making it visible under the microscope.

B. Immunofluorescence

In *direct immunofluorescence*, the antibodies are already conjugated with a fluorescent dye. In *indirect fluorescence*, on the other hand, a fluorochrome-labeled secondary antibody is added in a second step after the antigen-specific primary antibody has been bound. Direct immunofluorescence can be used to study two or more antigens at a time. Indirect immunofluorescence improves the visualization of weakly expressed antigens because several molecules of the labeled antibody can bind to the primary antibody. The sample can be fixed to make the cell membrane permeable enough for identification of intracytoplasmic antigens. This is also an effective way to stain cells in suspension, tissue sections, or cytospins. (**B.2**)

C. Flow Cytometry

In flow cytometry (**C.1**), cell suspensions are loaded in a vibrating flow chamber with a nozzle that expels them in droplets, each containing a single cell. The droplets pass a laser beam and scatter light as the beam strikes them. This scattering is measured by a photomultiplier tube (PMT) detector. *Forward-angle light scatter* (FSC) correlates with cell size. *Orthogonal light scatter* or side scatter, defined as 90° light scatter (90°LS) with respect to the beam axis, correlates with cellular granularity and with the plasma/nucleus ratio of the cells.

This method permits differentiation between large cells with a high plasma/nucleus ratio and a granular cytoplasm (granulocytes) and small cells with a large nucleus (lymphocytes). Monocytes have intermediate properties (**C.2**).

D. Flow Cytometry Histograms

The sorted cell populations can also be analyzed for other parameters, such as fluorescence. The immunofluorescence of lymphocytes and monocytes in the sample can be separately analyzed. The intensity of cell fluorescence roughly correlates with the antigen density on the cell surface and can be quantified using a photomultiplier tube (PMT) detector (**D.1**).

A number of antibodies directed against different antigens and conjugated to different fluorescent dyes can be analyzed simultaneously. Some of the most common dyes used in flow cytometry are fluorescein isothiocyanate (FITC) and phycoerythrin (PE). Both dyes are excited by laser light at a wavelength of 488 nm, but their fluorescence emissions peaks vary. FITC peaks in the green emission range, whereas PE peaks in the red emission range. Assuming there are two target antigens of interest, fluorescent dyes can be used to differentiate and identify antigen-positive cell populations that express both of the target antigens (emit both red and green fluorescence) or only one of the target antigens (either red or green), and identify antigen-negative cell populations that do not express either of the antigens (no fluorescence), as shown in the right panel. The example shows double staining for CD3 and CD4. Four populations can be detected: CD4$^+$ T cells (helper T lymphocytes), CD4$^-$ T cells (most will be CD8-positive lymphocytes), CD4$^+$ CD3$^-$ cells (most will be monocytes), and double negative cells, including B lymphocytes, NK cells, and some monocytes.

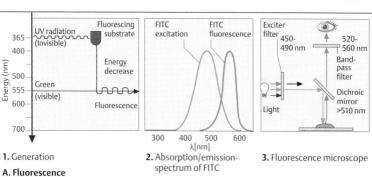

1. Generation

A. Fluorescence

2. Absorption/emission-spectrum of FITC

3. Fluorescence microscope

1. Direct immunofluorescence

2. Double fluorescence

3. Indirect immunofluorescence

B. Immunfluorescence

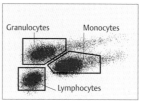

4. Intracytoplasmic fluorescence

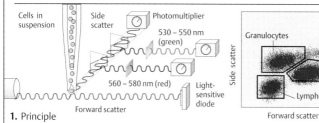

1. Principle

C. Flow cytometry

2. Separation of cell fractions

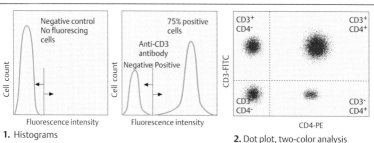

1. Histograms

D. Flow cytometry: Histograms

2. Dot plot, two-color analysis

A. Immunohistological Staining

Tissue samples for histological analysis are routinely fixed in formalin. Since formalin fixation may alter the antigen determinants of many cellular structures, specimens must be shock frozen to yield cryostat sections more suitable for immunohistochemical staining. Cryopreserved sections are incubated with antibodies against the target antigen for 20–30 minutes at +4 °C. Mouse monoclonal antibodies are most commonly used. The specimens are then washed, and a secondary antibody against mouse immunoglobulin is added. The secondary antibodies are often biotinylated, that is, conjugated to biotin, a vitamin with an extremely high affinity for the protein streptavidin. A complex made of streptavidin and the enzyme peroxidase is used for staining. The enzyme therefore comes into close proximity to the target antigen. The addition of a chromogenic substrate, such as diaminobenzidine (DAB) or aminoethylcarbazole (AEC), leads to a color staining reaction that accurately reflects the distribution of the target antigen in the tissue sample.

The *APAAP method* is another common immunohistochemical staining technique. The primary antibody (usually a murine antibody) binds to the target antigen. An anti-mouse Ig antibody ("bridging" antibody) is then added, followed by a complex consisting of alkaline phosphatase (AP) and a monoclonal mouse antibody directed against alkaline phosphatase. The latter antibody is referred to as an anti-AP (AAP) antibody. The AP–AAP complex binds to the target antigen via bridging antibodies. The subsequent enzymatic reaction with a chromogenic substrate leads to antigen-dependent precipitation of dye in the sample. The sensitivity of APAAP staining can be enhanced by repeating the bridging reaction. Examples of this immunohistochemical staining technique are shown in illustrations (**4**) and (**5**). In (**4**), a single tumor cell can be visualized among negative bone marrow cells using an antibody against epithelial cells. In (**5**), CD22 antibodies produce an excellent stain of B lymphocytes in the follicle mantle, thus making it possible to visualize the structure of the germinal center.

B. Fluorescence In-situ Hybridization

Fluorescence in-situ hybridization (FISH) is used to identify molecular structures on the DNA or RNA level. The DNA double helix is rup-tured by treating the test specimens with heat, chemicals, or solutions with an alkaline pH. DNA probes directed against specific DNA sequences are used. DNA probes are complementary DNA sequences labeled with a marker molecule. The DNA probes hybridize with DNA in the sample, and the marker molecule on the probe renders hybridization visible.

Specific RNA probes are also available. These probes permit the identification of RNA for specific cell products, such as cytokines, at the single-cell level. The most common marker substances are fluorescein and biotin, but other immune complexes (e.g., digoxigenin–anti-digoxigenin antibodies) are also used.

C. Example: FISH Staining in 8:21 Translocation

In the interphase, the ETO gene on chromosome 8 and the AML-1 gene on chromosome 21 of normal cells can be visualized using DNA probes labeled with FITC or PE respectively.

Translocation of a small segment of chromosome 21 to chromosome 8 and vice versa occurs in some cases of acute myeloid leukemia (see p. 128). A segment of the FITC-labeled AML-1 gene is brought next to the PE-labeled ETO gene. The fusion of the two genes can be visualized due to the juxtaposition of the red and green fluorescence.

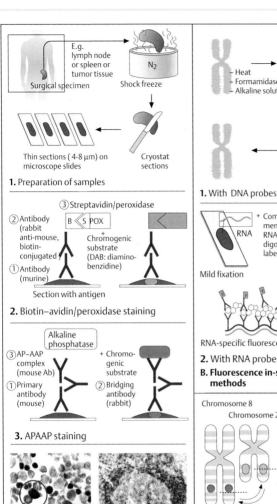

1. Preparation of samples

③ Streptavidin/peroxidase

② Antibody (rabbit anti-mouse, biotin-conjugated)

+ Chromogenic substrate (DAB: diamino-benzidine)

① Antibody (murine)

Section with antigen

2. Biotin–avidin/peroxidase staining

Alkaline phosphatase

③ AP–AAP complex (mouse Ab)

① Primary antibody (mouse)

+ Chromogenic substrate

② Bridging antibody (rabbit)

3. APAAP staining

4. Detection of tumor cells in the bone marrow

5. Staining of the follicle mantle with CD22 Abs

A. Immunohistological staining

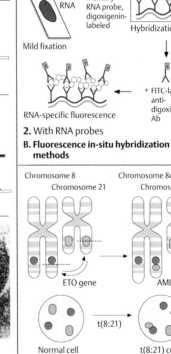

- Heat
- Formamidase
- Alkaline solutions

Rupture of H-bonds: single-strand DNA

Hybridization

Fluorochrome-labeled complementary DNA-probe

1. With DNA probes

Mild fixation

+ Complementary RNA probe, digoxigenin-labeled

Hybridization

+ FITC-labeled anti-digoxigenin Ab

RNA-specific fluorescence

2. With RNA probes

B. Fluorescence in-situ hybridization methods

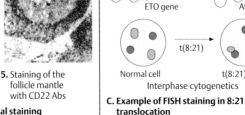

Chromosome 8
Chromosome 21

Chromosome 8q-
Chromosome 21q+

ETO gene

AML 1 gene

Normal cell

t(8:21)

t(8:21) cell

Interphase cytogenetics

C. Example of FISH staining in 8:21 translocation

A. Isolation of Mononuclear Cells from Peripheral Blood

Mononuclear cells in the peripheral blood can be separated from other cells by density gradient centrifugation. A Ficoll-Hypaque solution (density of 1.077 g/L) is placed in a test tube, and diluted heparinized blood is layered on top. The tube is then centrifuged. Low-density cells (lymphocytes and monocytes) now float on top of the solution, and all other blood components form a pellet at the bottom of the tube. The mononuclear cells at the Ficoll–plasma interface can be removed with a pipette. After incubation of the cell material in culture flasks, the monocytes adhere to the plastic walls of the bottle. This makes it possible to capture lymphocytes selectively.

B. Separation of T and B Lymphocytes (Rosette Formation)

T lymphocytes express adhesion molecules, such as the CD2 molecule. CD2 interacts with LFA-3 (CD58) on the surface of sheep red blood cells (SRBC). After treatment with an enzyme, such as neuraminidase or 2-aminoethyli-sothiouronium bromide (AET), the adhesion molecule on the RBC surface more readily interacts with T lymphocytes. Several SRBC can bind to a single T cell, thereby forming "rosettes." Rosette-forming cells can be isolated by density gradient centrifugation on Ficoll. A fraction of approximately 95% pure T lymphocytes can be isolated after hypotonic lysis of the red blood cells.

Cells that do not form rosettes float on top of the Ficoll layer and can also be isolated. These cells primarily consist of B cells and other non-T cells.

C. Antibody-Mediated Separation of Cell Fractions

Culture flasks or plastic dishes can be coated with antibodies at an alkaline pH (*panning*). When a cell mixture is incubated on top of the antibody-coated surface, the cells that express the target antigen will adhere to the plastic walls of the bottle or dish. Antigen-negative cells can easily be removed by decanting.

The antigen-positive cells can be removed by mechanical means or by enzymatic digestion.

By coating antibodies onto small beads that contain iron (available in different sizes), it is possible to capture either antigen-positive or antigen-negative cell fractions. This method is called *immunomagnetic separation*. A magnet that attracts the iron-loaded cells is used to separate antigen-bearing cells. This is a very effective method for removing unwanted cells from a solution. As little as a single contaminating tumor cell can be separated from 1000 normal cells by immunomagnetic separation. In other words, a 3–4 log depletion of unwanted cells can be achieved.

D. Cell Separation by Flow Cytometry

Normal flow cytometry was described on page 84. A *fluorescence-activated cell sorter* (FACS) is a specialized flow meter in which the fine cell-containing droplets are electrically charged under computer guidance. Droplets with fluorescent cells are positively charged, and those with nonfluorescent cells (e.g., antigen-negative cells) are negatively charged. The stream of cells is guided through electric deflection plates, where the antigen-positive and antigen-negative cells are separated, then guided into separate collection tubes. The purity of cells separated by FACS is up to 99%.

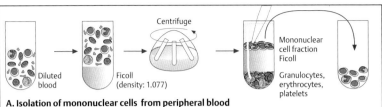

A. Isolation of mononuclear cells from peripheral blood

Diluted blood → Ficoll (density: 1.077) → Centrifuge → Mononuclear cell fraction Ficoll; Granulocytes, erythrocytes, platelets

Sheep erythrocytes

Mononuclear cells — Binding of sheep erythrocytes to T cells: rosette formation — Centrifuge — Ficoll — Non-T fraction (B lymphocytes, monocytes); T lymphocytes, sheep erythrocytes

B. Separation of T and B lymphocytes: Rosette formation

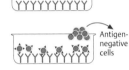

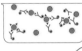

Plastic surface coated with antibodies

Antigen-bearing cells adhere — Antigen-negative cells

1. Panning method

Antibody labeled with iron beads

Antigen-bearing cells attracted by magnet — Magnet — Antigen-negative cells

2. Immunomagnetic separation

C. Antibody-mediated separation of cell fractions

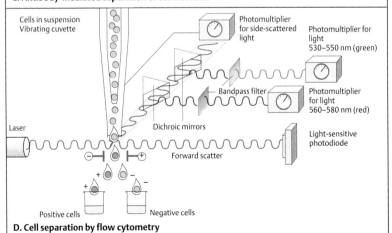

Cells in suspension Vibrating cuvette

Photomultiplier for side-scattered light

Photomultiplier for light 530–550 nm (green)

Bandpass filter

Photomultiplier for light 560–580 nm (red)

Dichroic mirrors

Laser

Forward scatter

Light-sensitive photodiode

Positive cells — Negative cells

D. Cell separation by flow cytometry

A. Activation Tests

T cells are activated and induced to proliferate on contact with specific antigens. In the peripheral blood, only a negligible percentage of T cells (on the order of 1/10 000 cells or less) react with a specific antigen. In vitro tests of T-cell function are therefore performed using substances that stimulate all T cells regardless of the antigen-specific receptor. These substances are called *polyclonal activators* (e.g., phytohemagglutinin and concanavalin A).

Antibodies against the CD3 complex of the T-cell receptor can lead to cross-linkage of the CD3 molecule. This imitates physiological antigen binding, which stimulates most T cells. Cytokines (e.g., GM-CSF, IL-2, IL-4, and IFN-γ) in supernatant are then measured as parameters of T-cell activation. The intracytoplasmic calcium ion concentration is a very early parameter of activation; it can be detected within a few seconds after cross-linkage of the antigen receptor (see p. 17). Special dyes that change their fluorescence emission spectrum when they bind to calcium (e.g., Indo-1) are used to measure the increase in the intracytoplasmic potassium concentration. The shift in fluorescence can be precisely measured using a flow cytometer (see p. 74).

The expression of activation-dependent surface antigens can also be measured by flow cytometry. Molecules such as CD69 or the transferrin receptor CD71 are upregulated on the cell membrane within a few hours after activation. Others, such as CD25 or MHC molecules, are not upregulated before 1–3 days.

Cell cycle analysis (CCA) is another way to test for cell activation. CCA makes it possible to precisely count the number of dormant, activated, and proliferating cells.

B. Proliferation Test

The proliferative capacity is often used as a parameter for assessment of T-cell function (*lymphocyte stimulation test* or *transformation test*).

The cells are cultivated in 5 % CO_2 in an incubator for 72–96 hours at 37 °C in the presence of different stimuli. The process of cell division, which is associated with a doubling of the DNA content, starts after around 48 hours. Because of the addition of radioactively labeled thymidine in culture medium (an H-position of the molecule is occupied by ^{3}H, tritium), radioactive tritium is incorporated into the DNA of the dividing cells.

After further 16–24 hours of cultivation, the cells are "harvested" on automated equipment. In other words, they are rinsed out of the wells of the culture plate and passed through a glass fiber filter. The cells, that is, high-molecular-weight DNA molecules, are caught in the filter, while unbound thymidine is washed out. A beta counter is used to measure the radioactivity in the filter, which correlates with the extent of DNA replication and proliferation.

C. T Cell Function In Vivo: Mérieux Multitest

The Mérieux multitest is a commercial test comprising eight tines with tips containing various bacterial or fungal antigens dissolved in gelatin. Most individuals have been exposed to these antigens. The tines are pressed into the skin for intracutaneous delivery. The skin is checked approximately 48 hours later for delayed hypersensitivity reactions (see p. 57**A**). The test is considered positive if a skin induration of >2 mm in diameter is detected.

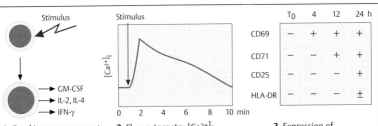

1. Cytokine measurement (ELISA)
2. Flow cytometry $[Ca^{2+}]_i$
3. Expression of activation antigens

A. Activation assays

	T_0	4	12	24 h
CD69	−	+	+	+
CD71	−	−	+	+
CD25	−	−	−	+
HLA-DR	−	−	−	±

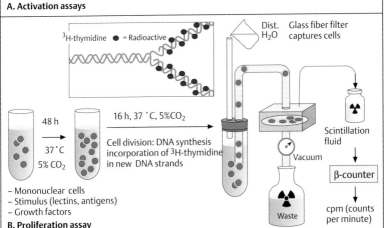

B. Proliferation assay

– Mononuclear cells
– Stimulus (lectins, antigens)
– Growth factors

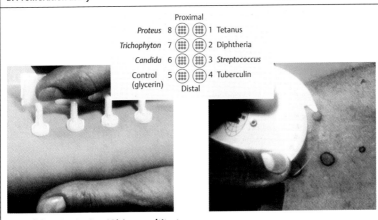

C. T-cell function in vivo: Mérieux multitest

A. Generation of Antigen-Specific T-cell Clones

Despite their low numbers in the peripheral blood (usually from 1/10 000 to 1/100 000), antigen-specific T cells can be isolated and expanded in vitro. This is done by culturing the cells in the presence of the target antigen, IL-2, and irradiated autologous mononuclear cells as feeder cells. In this case, the mononuclear cells serve as antigen-presenting cells. The antigen and antigen-presenting cells are again added around seven days later. This type of stimulation is repeated several times at weekly intervals. Under these conditions, the few antigen-specific T cells present in the starting culture do proliferate, but they are still diluted in a large majority of non-antigen-specific T cells. A *limiting dilution* is therefore performed in the cultures with macroscopically visible cell growth (some of the proliferating cells form huge cell aggregates). As a result, some of the cavities in the culture plate contain only a single T cell. Clonal expansion of the antigen-specific T cells in these wells is achieved by adding IL-2 and the target antigen.

B. Cytotoxicity Test: Chromium Release Assay

Antigen-specific cytotoxic T lymphocytes (CTL) can kill cells that present the appropriate antigen in their HLA molecules. Natural killer (NK) cells, on the other hand, kill cells that either do not express MHC molecules or express foreign or aberrant MHC molecules (see p. 36). The *chromium release assay* is the classical test of NK cell function and CTL function. The test is performed by labeling the target cells with radioactive chromium (^{51}Cr), which binds to cytoplasmic proteins. Only a small fraction of the radioactivity is spontaneously released by the cells (spontaneous lysis, background lysis). Effector cells are added at various concentrations for 4–6 hours, which leads to lysis of the target cells. Rupturing of the cell membrane, which is induced by perforins and granzymes (see p. 37**D**), leads to the release of radioactive chromium, which can be measured in the supernatant. This type of lysis is also referred to as "killing." The more effective the lysis, the higher the amount of chromium released. Maximal chromium release is achieved by lysing all of the cells in a suitable detergent (e.g., Triton). The efficacy of cell lysis is partially dependent on the ratio of effector cells to target cells and can be determined using a simple formula. The disadvantage is that cells that die due to apoptosis are not correctly measured in the test (see below).

C. Cytotoxicity Test: Jam Test

The chromium release assay often underestimates the killing efficacy of effector cells. Some of the cells are killed not by lysis but by apoptosis. The assay does not detect cells killed by apoptosis because apoptotic vesicles have an intact cell membrane and, thus, do not release ^{51}Cr.

In the so-called *jam test*, the target cells are first cultured in the presence of tritium-labeled thymidine, which is incorporated into the DNA of the cells. When cells die due to apoptosis (see p. 65), their DNA is fragmented into tiny pieces. The cultured cells are then processed on an automated cell harvester. The high-molecular-weight DNA of intact cells is caught in the filter, whereas the low-molecular-weight DNA of apoptotic cells is removed with the washing fluid. The rate of lysis can be calculated using an appropriate formula.

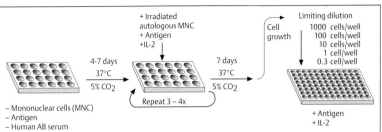

+ Irradiated
autologous MNC
+ Antigen
+IL-2

4-7 days
37°C
5% CO$_2$

Repeat 3 – 4x

Cell
growth

7 days
37°C
5% CO$_2$

Limiting dilution
1000 cells/well
100 cells/well
10 cells/well
1 cell/well
0.3 cell/well

– Mononuclear cells (MNC)
– Antigen
– Human AB serum

+ Antigen
+ IL-2

A. Generatiion of antigen-specific T cell clones

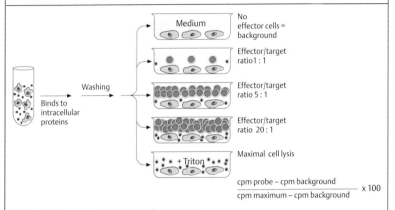

Binds to
intracellular
proteins

Washing

Medium

No
effector cells =
background

Effector/target
ratio1 : 1

Effector/target
ratio 5 : 1

Effector/target
ratio 20 : 1

+ Triton

Maximal cell lysis

$$\frac{cpm\ probe\ -\ cpm\ background}{cpm\ maximum\ -\ cpm\ background} \times 100$$

B. Cytotoxicity assay: Chromium release assay

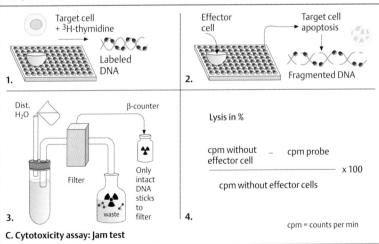

Target cell
+ ^{3}H-thymidine

Labeled
DNA

1.

Effector
cell

Target cell
apoptosis

Fragmented DNA

2.

Dist.
H$_2$O

β-counter

Filter

Only
intact
DNA
sticks
to
filter

waste

3.

Lysis in %

$$\frac{cpm\ without\ effector\ cell\ -\ cpm\ probe}{cpm\ without\ effector\ cells} \times 100$$

4.

cpm = counts per min

C. Cytotoxicity assay: Jam test

Laboratory Applications

A. IFN-γ ELISPOT

The ELISPOT (enzyme-linked immunosorbent spot assay) is used to determine the frequency of antigen-specific T cells in cell cultures. Antigen-stimulated cytokine production is measured to determine the degree of antigen specificity. The antigen, antigen-presenting cells, and T cells are placed together in a well (of a membrane-coated microtiter plate) coated with antibodies against the target cytokine (e.g., IFN-γ) and incubated for 24 to 48 hours. Cells stimulated by the antigen produce IFN-γ, which is bound on the spot by the membrane-bound antibodies. After incubation, the cells are removed by careful washing and incubated with a biotin-conjugated second antibody against IFN-γ. In the third step, streptavidin binds to the antibody-bound biotin. The enzyme attached to streptavidin activates a chromogenic substrate that stains the spots where the stimulated T cells produced IFN-γ. The number of spots indicates the frequency of cytokine-producing cells, which is expressed as the number of spot-forming cells (SFC) per 100 000 cells.

B. Intracellular Cytokine Staining

Unlike the ELISPOT assay, which can only determine the frequency of cytokine-producing T cells, the intracellular staining technique can also precisely identify the type of activated T cells. Once stimulated with the antigen, the cell culture is incubated with Brefeldin A to inhibit the extrusion of intracellular cytokine. This results in the accumulation of large quantities of the secreted cytokine within the cells. Surface staining of the cells is performed (e.g., for CD4 and CD8) followed by fixation with paraformaldehyde. Subsequent treatment with the detergent saponin permeabilizes the cell membranes to allow the antibodies that bind intracellular cytokines to pass through the membranes. Use of two labeled antibodies (FITC-labeled IFN-γ antibodies and PE-labeled IL-4 antibodies) permits differentiation between cells that produce IFN-γ or IL-4. Labeling of surface markers is achieved using multiple red emitting fluorochromes with wavelengths that can be differentiated in a dual laser FACS sorter, for example, using PerCP (peridine chlorophyll protein, 675 nm) for CD4 and APC (allophycocyanin, 660 nm) for CD8. This permits the simultaneous identification of all four fluorescences and makes it possible to identify CD4+ or CD8+ T cells and their cytokine patterns.

C. Cytokine Secretion Assay

A bispecific antibody (catch reagent, Miltenyi) makes it possible to bind cytokines secreted by activated T cells directly on the cell surface. The antibody initially binds to CD45, a ubiquitous surface marker. The secreted cytokine (e.g., IFN-γ) is bound to the cell surface, where it is recognized by a second fluorescence-labeled antibody. T cells stained in the process can then be isolated in a FACS sorter or in a magnetic field (MACS) with the aid of iron-conjugated antibodies. The advantage over intracellular cytokine staining is that the cells remain intact and can be further analyzed by functional assays.

D. Tetramer Staining

Tetramer staining is used for direct staining of antigen-specific T cells. First, the heavy chains of MHC class I molecules (e.g., HLA-A2) are bound to a tetramer labeled with a fluorochrome (PE). The binding pockets of the MHC class I molecule are then loaded with a (synthetic) peptide. This procedure can be used to stain only those T cells (CD8+) that recognize the respective peptide in conjunction with HLA-A2. The labeled cells can subsequently be run through a FACS sorter to generate antigen-specific T-cell lines.

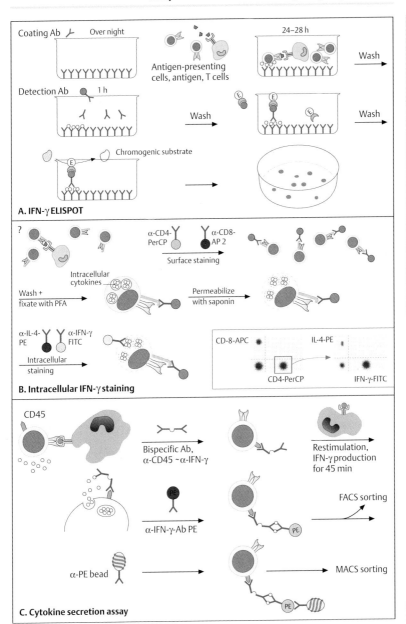

Coating Ab Over night

Antigen-presenting cells, antigen, T cells

24–28 h

Wash

Detection Ab 1 h

Wash

Wash

Chromogenic substrate

A. IFN-γ ELISPOT

?

α-CD4-PerCP α-CD8-AP 2

Surface staining

Wash + fixate with PFA

Intracellular cytokines

Permeabilize with saponin

α-IL-4-PE α-IFN-γ FITC

Intracellular staining

CD-8-APC IL-4-PE

CD4-PerCP IFN-γ-FITC

B. Intracellular IFN-γ staining

CD45

Bispecific Ab, α-CD45 ~ α-IFN-γ

Restimulation, IFN-γ production for 45 min

α-IFN-γ-Ab PE

FACS sorting

α-PE bead

MACS sorting

C. Cytokine secretion assay

A. B-Cell Activation

The quantitative immunoglobulin assay is a good parameter of in vivo B-cell function. However, if antibody deficiencies exist, functional tests must be performed.

Antibodies directed against surface immunoglobulins lead to cross-linkage of the immunoglobulin molecules, thereby imitating physiological stimulation due to antigens. Since the binding of immunoglobulins to Fc receptors has an inhibitory effect, Fab fragments from anti-IgM antibodies are used. Lyophilized *Staphylococcus aureus* bacteria of the Cowan C (SAC) group are very potent inductors of cross-linkage. As in T cells, antigen binding leads to a measurable increase in the intracytoplasmic calcium concentration within a few seconds, and to an overexpression of the antigens CD69 and CD71 (transferrin receptor) within a few hours. CD25 and CD23 antigens on the cell membrane are upregulated within 2–3 days.

B. B-Cell Proliferation

Once they have been activated due to immunoglobulin cross-linkage, B cells require a second stimulus in order to proliferate. They can be stimulated by cytokines, such as IL-2, IL-6, IL-14 (B-cell growth factor), by soluble receptors (e.g., by a soluble cleavage product of the surface antigen CD23), or by binding of the CD40 ligand to the CD40 antigen. Similarly to the process in T cells, the incorporation of tritium-labeled thymidine into B cells, as measured in 72-hour cultures, is used as a parameter of proliferation (see p. 81**B**).

When the cross-linkage of immunoglobulins is particularly effective (e.g., when SAC bacteria are used), the B cells sometimes produce autocrine growth factors, making the use of further exogenous stimuli unnecessary.

C. B-Cell Differentiation: Antibody Secretion

B cells can differentiate into plasma cells after 5–7 days of cell culture. The ELISA or RIA can be used to quantitate the number of antibodies in the supernatant, but not the actual number of B cells that produce antibodies. Various hemolytic plaque-forming cell (PFC) tests can be used to obtain this figure.

1 *Reverse hemolytic PFC assay.* Sheep red blood cells (SRBC) are conjugated with anti-human sheep or rabbit immunoglobulins and cultured with B cells on agarose gel. Terminally differentiated B cells secrete immunoglobulin molecules, which diffuse into the gel and form immune complexes with the anti-human immunoglobulin antibodies on the surface of the nearby RBCs. Complement is added, and the RBCs that are in close proximity to the antibody-secreting cells are lysed. The number of hemolytic plaques corresponds to the number of terminally differentiated B cells.

This method can also be used to study subpopulations of antibody-producing cells. The use of anti-IgM-bearing sheep red blood cells ensures that only those B cells that secrete IgM will be visualized. By allowing the antigen to bind to the SRBCs, it is possible to measure B cells that form antibodies against a specific antigen.

2 *ELISPOT test.* In this test, the B cells are spread onto culture dishes coated with an appropriate antigen. Specific antibodies produced by the B cells bind to the antigen. Free antibodies and cells are removed by washing. Enzyme-bound antibodies against immunoglobulins are added before the addition of a gel containing the corresponding chromogen. A specific color reaction takes place only where the specific antibodies are bound. This produces colored spots that can be counted to determine the number of antibody-producing cells.

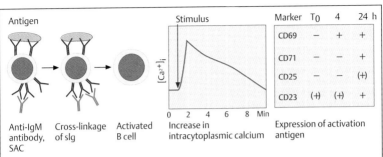

Marker	T$_0$	4	24 h
CD69	−	+	+
CD71	−	−	+
CD25	−	−	(+)
CD23	(+)	(+)	+

Antigen

Anti-IgM antibody, SAC — Cross-linkage of sIg — Activated B cell

Increase in intracytoplasmic calcium

Expression of activation antigen

A. B-cell activation

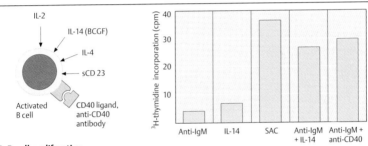

IL-2
IL-14 (BCGF)
IL-4
sCD 23

Activated B cell

CD40 ligand, anti-CD40 antibody

^{3}H-thymidine incorporation (cpm)

Anti-IgM · IL-14 · SAC · Anti-IgM + IL-14 · Anti-IgM + anti-CD40

B. B-cell proliferation

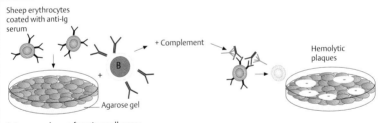

Sheep erythrocytes coated with anti-Ig serum

+ Complement

Hemolytic plaques

Agarose gel

1. Inverse plaque-forming cell assay

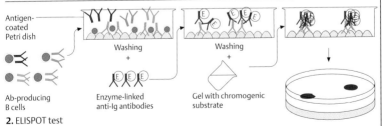

Antigen-coated Petri dish

Washing +

Washing +

Ab-producing B cells

Enzyme-linked anti-Ig antibodies

Gel with chromogenic substrate

2. ELISPOT test

C. B-cell differentiation: Antibody secretion

A. Southern Blotting

In Southern blotting, DNA fragments are separated by gel electrophoresis using capillary or electrophoretic forces and are transferred onto an immobilizing membrane. The fragments are then hybridized using specific probes. DNA fragments of interest can be generated from genomic DNA by means of restrictive enzymatic digestion or by means of a polymerase chain reaction (see **C**). The DNA fragments are detected using (radioactively or nonradioactively) labeled hybridization probes that bind to complement sequences via hydrogen bonds. Specific detection of the labeled probes is achieved by autoradiography or chromogens.

B. Northern Blotting

Northern blotting is used for hybridization of RNA (RNA fragments). In this method, the size and number of specific mRNA molecules are determined after the preparation of total RNA or poly(A) RNA. RNA molecules are separated by gel electrophoresis and transferred onto an immobilizing membrane. The RNA sequence of interest is then detected by hybridization with labeled probes.

C. Polymerase Chain Reaction (PCR)

The polymerase chain reaction is a technique for enzymatic amplification of the specific nucleic acid sequences prior to their detection. The procedure is based on the repetition of a specific reaction sequence, the individual steps of which are performed at a precisely defined temperature.

The double strands of the DNA of interest (or cDNA of interest after reverse transcription of RNA) is first denatured into single strands. *Primers* (oligonucleotides specific for the nucleic acid sequence of interest) now settle on the single strands of DNA in a process known as *annealing.* In the next step, the 3' ends of the primers are extended by addition of a thermostable polymerase (e.g., *Taq* polymerase) complementary to the matrix in a process referred to as *elongation.* The cycle of denaturation, annealing, and elongation is repeated approximately 30 times. The nucleic acid sequence of interest is amplified exponentially because each nucleic acid strand synthesized by the polymerase can function as a new matrix in the subsequent reaction. The products of PCR (amplificates) can be separated by gel electrophoresis and visualized by ethidium bromide intercalation under UV light.

D. DNA Sequencing

The most common method of sequencing DNA fragments is enzymatic synthesis of the fragments in a method based on a *chain-terminating reaction.* There are now a number of automated sequencing systems using *primers* or *terminators* (so-called chain-terminating dideoxynucleotides) labeled with fluorescent dyes. These systems use four dyes that fluoresce at different wavelengths. The detectors of an argon laser register the dye-specific signals as the samples migrate through gel. The data are analyzed using a chromogram.

One of the more recent methods is single-strand sequencing using biotinylated primers. In illustration **D**, the specific sequence is located in an insert of a phage (λ.-gt II). The biotinylated primer (*forward primer*) contains the specific sequence (sequence of interest) and a 5' sequence identical with the universal sequencing primer. The nonbiotinylated primer (*reverse primer*) contains a 3' sequence and a 5' sequence complementary to the reverse universal primer. After amplification by means of PCR with proportionate use of terminators, the specific biotinylated amplificates can then be bound to streptavidin-coated paramagnetic beads and eluted in an alkaline environment. The beads can then be used for solid-phase sequencing.

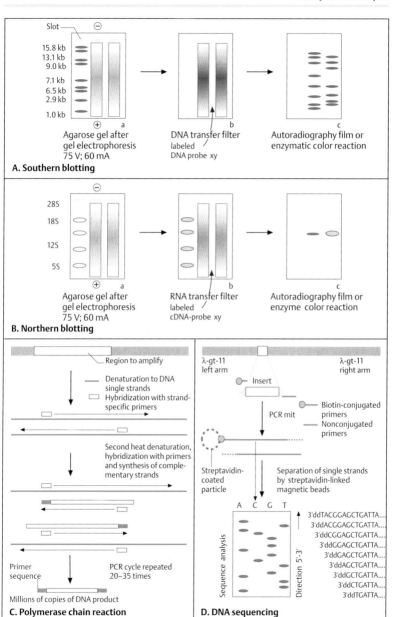

A. Southern blotting

Slot ⊖

15.8 kb
13.1 kb
9.0 kb
7.1 kb
6.5 kb
2.9 kb
1.0 kb

⊕ a

Agarose gel after
gel electrophoresis
75 V; 60 mA

b
DNA transfer filter
labeled
DNA probe xy

c
Autoradiography film or
enzymatic color reaction

B. Northern blotting

⊖

28S
18S
12S
5S

⊕ a

Agarose gel after
gel electrophoresis
75 V; 60 mA

b
RNA transfer filter
labeled
cDNA-probe xy

c
Autoradiography film or
enzyme color reaction

C. Polymerase chain reaction

Region to amplify

Denaturation to DNA
single strands
Hybridization with strand-
specific primers

Second heat denaturation,
hybridization with primers
and synthesis of comple-
mentary strands

Primer
sequence

PCR cycle repeated
20–35 times

Millions of copies of DNA product

D. DNA sequencing

λ-gt-11
left arm

λ-gt-11
right arm

Insert

PCR mit

Biotin-conjugated
primers
Nonconjugated
primers

Streptavidin-
coated
particle

Separation of single strands
by streptavidin-linked
magnetic beads

A C G T

Sequence analysis

Direction 5'-3'

3'ddTACGGAGCTGATTA....
3'ddACGGAGCTGATTA....
3'ddCGGAGCTGATTA....
3'ddGGAGCTGATTA....
3'ddGAGCTGATTA....
3'ddAGCTGATTA....
3'ddGCTGATTA....
3'ddCTGATTA....
3'ddTGATTA....

Laboratory Applications

99

A. X-linked Agammaglobulinemia

X-linked agammaglobulinemia, also referred to as Bruton's agammaglobulinemia, is an X-linked recessive chromosome defect caused by genetic mutation of a B-cell-specific tyrosine kinase. The defect leads to a B-cell maturation disorder characterized by arrested B-cell development at the pre-B cell stage. Recurrent respiratory tract infections are the most common clinical manifestations of the resulting IgG deficiency. Meningitis, pyoderma, and sepsis may also occur. These infections are typically caused by capsule-forming pyogenic bacteria, such as staphylococci, pneumococci, and streptococci. One-third of these cases are associated with seronegative oligoarthritis. Patients with X-linked agammaglobulinemia usually respond well to intravenous IgG replacement.

B. Dysgammaglobulinemia

Selective IgA deficiency. An abnormally low concentration of IgA in bodily secretions is, by far, one of the most common forms of humoral immunodeficiency. The incidence of the defect may be sporadic or familial. Selective IgA deficiency is commonly associated with an atopic disposition (elevated IgE) and HLA types B8 and DR3. Around 50% of the patients remain asymptomatic. IgA deficiency is mainly associated with recurrent respiratory tract infections, but may also occur in autoimmune diseases like systemic lupus erythematosus (SLE) and sprue.

Selective IgG subclass deficiencies (**B.1**). Depending on their specific properties, deficiencies of certain IgG subclasses can lead to variable degrees of humoral immunodeficiency. IgG2 deficiency can lead to severe infections by pathogens such as *Haemophilus influenzae*, *Meningococcus*, and *Pneumococcus*. A quantitative analysis of IgG subclasses should be performed in patients who develop recurrent respiratory tract infections of unknown cause.

Selective antibody deficiency with normal serum immunoglobulin levels. In some individuals, the immunoglobulin concentrations remain normal despite the development of recurrent infections by certain pathogens. The immune system fails to recognize a particular antigen and is therefore defenseless against it. The patients can be treated with a vaccine containing the antigen in question, which is usually administered with an adjuvant (see pp. 236–239).

Hyper-IgM syndrome (**B.2**): Hyper-IgM syndrome is characterized by the arrested development of B cells at the IgM level (*switching defect*). There is an abundance of circulating μ^+ and δ^+ B cells, but hardly any γ^+ or α^+ B cells. The defect is X-chromosome-linked and recessively inherited. Since it is based on mutations in the gene of the CD40-ligand, CD40 is no longer able to mediate class switching in B cells. Recurrent respiratory tract infections are the main clinical features of IgG and IgA deficiencies. Besides the characteristic B cell pattern, thrombopenia and neutropenia may also be observed. IgG and antibiotic administration is the treatment of choice.

C. Common Variable Immunodeficiency

Common variable immunodeficiency (CVID) is a heterogeneous group of diseases all associated with inadequate immunoglobulin production. Similar to SLE, CVID is often associated with HLA A1, B8, and DR3 antigens. Some of the most common causes of immunoglobulin underproduction are listed below:

- Arrested B-cell development at the pre-B cell stage, thus preventing the formation of plasma cells,
- Disturbance of B-cell regulation by T-helper cells,
- Recognition of maturing B cells by autoantibodies,
- Blockage of immuniglobulin secretion due to defective glycosylation.

CVID is usually detected at a late stage when recurrent bronchopulmonary infections have already led to bronchiectasis.

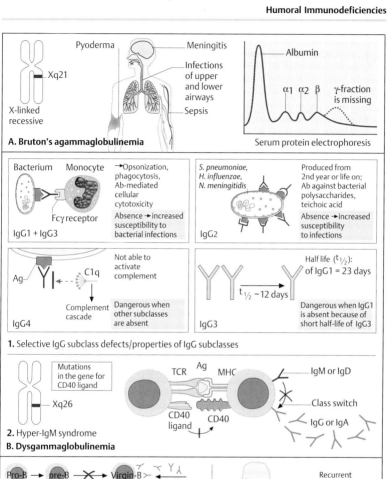

A. Bruton's agammaglobulinemia

Pyoderma — Meningitis — Infections of upper and lower airways — Sepsis

Xq21 X-linked recessive

Albumin

α_1 α_2 β γ-fraction is missing

Serum protein electrophoresis

Bacterium Monocyte → Opsonization, phagocytosis, Ab-mediated cellular cytotoxicity

Fcγ receptor Absence → increased susceptibility to bacterial infections

IgG1 + IgG3

S. pneumoniae, H. influenzae, N. meningitidis

Produced from 2nd year or life on; Ab against bacterial polysaccharides, teichoic acid

Absence → increased susceptibility to infections

IgG2

Ag C1q Not able to activate complement

Complement cascade Dangerous when other subclasses are absent

IgG4

Half life ($t_{1/2}$): of IgG1 = 23 days

$t_{1/2} \sim 12$ days

Dangerous when IgG1 is absent because of short half-life of IgG3

IgG3

1. Selective IgG subclass defects/properties of IgG subclasses

Mutations in the gene for CD40 ligand

Xq26

TCR Ag MHC

IgM or IgD

Class switch

CD40 ligand CD40

IgG or IgA

2. Hyper-IgM syndrome
B. Dysgammaglobulinemia

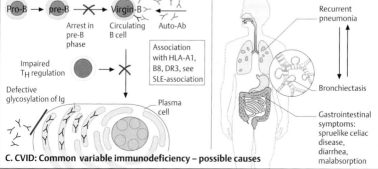

Pro-B → pre-B —✗→ Virgin-B

Arrest in pre-B phase Circulating B cell Auto-Ab

Impaired T$_H$ regulation

Association with HLA-A1, B8, DR3, see SLE-association

Defective glycosylation of Ig

Plasma cell

Recurrent pneumonia

Bronchiectasis

Gastrointestinal symptoms: spruelike celiac disease, diarrhea, malabsorption

C. CVID: Common variable immunodeficiency – possible causes

A. Severe Combined Immunodeficiency

Severe combined immunodeficiency syndrome (SCID) is a heterogeneous group of T-cell defects. Children affected by the defect start to develop symptoms at 3–6 months of age once the antibody protection from the mother starts to diminish. The main signs of SCID in a baby are failure to thrive and recurrent infections. Respiratory tract infections (mainly caused by *Pneumocystis carinii* and *Candida*) and gastrointestinal infections (*rotavirus*) are the most common manifestations. Eczema is also typical. The thymus, lymph nodes and tonsils are usually absent, and CD3-positive cells cannot be detected in the blood.

SCID syndrome has various causes, e.g.,

- an autosomal recessive defect of the recombinase gene that prevents the proper linkage of the V, D, and J genes for TCR and immunoglobulins; and
- point mutation of the gene for the γ chain of the IL-2 receptor, leading to inhibition of receptor activity.

SCID can also be induced by various purine metabolism disorders, e.g.,

- defective cell division, especially of T cells, due to the inhibition of thymidylate synthetase because of an increase in desoxyadenosine in the absence of adenosine deaminase (ADA); and
- T cell damage resulting from the formation of toxic inosine metabolites due to the defective degradation of inosine to hypoxanthine in the absence of purine nucleoside phosphorylase.

Allogeneic bone marrow transplantation is now considered to be the treatment of choice. Because of the defect, no rejection response can be induced by endogenous T cells.

B. Di George Syndrome

Di George syndrome is caused by malformation of the 3rd and 4th pharyngeal pouches during fetal development. All organs that arise from these structures are severely dysfunctional. Primary hypoparathyroidism manifests as hypocalcemic tetany. In around 20% of cases, hypoplasia of the thymus is accompanied by recurrent infections due to T-cell deficiencies. Facial dysmorphism, malformation of the aortic arch, hypothyroidism, and esophageal atresia are also observed in patients with Di George syndrome. Therapy is mainly symptomatic and consists of the administration of Ca^{2+} and vitamin D supplements.

C. Ataxia Teleangiectasia

Ataxia telangiectasia, or *Louis-Bar syndrome*, is characterized by a clinical triad of symptoms, namely progressive immunodeficiency, cerebellar ataxia, and oculocutaneous telangiectasia. This syndrome is a heterogeneous group of hereditary disorders transmitted as autosomal recessive defects all of which have chromosomal instability in common. Breakage and translocation of chromosomes, especially chromosome 14, lead to defects in the gene loci for TCR and immunoglobulins. Since DNA repair is also greatly impaired, the patients are extremely sensitive to ionizing radiation. Hence, radiographic examinations should not be performed in these patients unless the benefits clearly outweigh the risks. Apart from the typical clinical symptoms, the disorder is also characterized by elevated alpha-fetoprotein levels and greatly reduced levels of IgA and IgE. This progressive immunodeficiency leads to severe bouts of sinusitis and lung infection (so-called *sinopulmonary syndrome*). Therapy is symptomatic.

D. Wiskott–Aldrich Syndrome

Wiskott–Aldrich syndrome (WAS) is a hereditary disease characterized by thrombocytopenic purpura, recurrent infections, and eczema. The disease is transmitted as an X-linked recessive chromosome defect. Wiskott–Aldrich syndrome is caused by altered expression of CD43, a glycoprotein that forms an important part of the cytoskeleton. Defective actin bundle formation in T cells and thrombocytes can be visualized by electron microscopy.

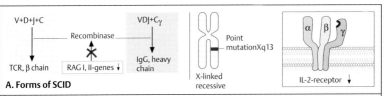

A. Forms of SCID

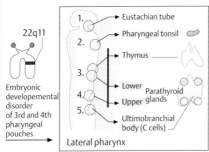

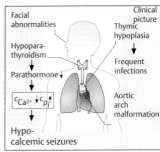

B. Di George syndrome

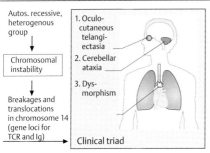

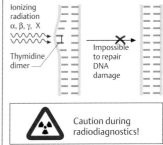

C. Ataxia telangiectasia

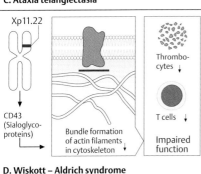

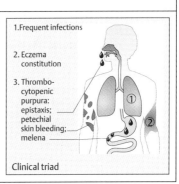

D. Wiskott – Aldrich syndrome

Clinical Immunology

A. Infantile Septic Granulocytosis

Infantile septic granulocytosis (ISG) is characterized by the intracellular killing of bacteria by microbicidal oxygen radicals in the presence of normal bacterial binding and phagocytosis. The defect is caused by a lack of cytochrome b_{558} in the phagosomal membrane of granulocytes. NADPH is unable to transport the electrons required for the formation of oxygen radicals through the membrane and transfer them to O_2 molecules. Cytochrome b_{558} deficiency is an X-linked recessive chromosome defect. NADPH oxidase plays a key role in this redox reaction. Glucose-6-phosphate dehydrogenase makes NADPH available in the cytoplasm after removing it from the hexose monophosphate pathway. An NADPH oxidase defect and a lack of glucose-6-phosphate dehydrogenase also make granulocytes incapable of killing phagocytosed bacteria. The clinical manifestations of the granulocyte defect are lymphadenitis, oronasal pyoderma, and colonization of septic bacteria in the lungs, intestines, bone, and liver. The most common pathogens are *Staphylococcus*, *Serratia*, *Klebsiella*, and *Aspergillus* strains. Catalase-negative strains such as *Streptococcus* and *Haemophilus influenzae* can be killed intracellularly because they form H_2O_2, which the granulocytes can use as a bactericide.

Therapy consists of symptomatic treatment with antibiotics and surgical removal of the septic foci of infection.

B. Chediak–Higashi Syndrome

This disease is an autosomal recessive defect that occurs in a disproportionate number of individuals of Jewish origin. Defective chemotaxis and defective intracellular killing of bacteria can be observed. Abnormal, giant granules can be observed upon microscopy. The absence of degranulation is attributed to microtubular dysfunction. In addition to the granulocyte activity, impairment of natural killer cells and a reduction in antibody-dependent cellular cytotoxicity (ADCC) can also be observed. The main clinical manifestations of Chediak–Higashi syndrome are partial oculocutaneous albinism associated with photophobia and various neurological symptoms. Patients with this defect are particularly susceptible to infections caused by catalase-negative bacteria. Cholinergic agents are therapeutically effective because they promote microtubular repair by increasing the intracellular levels of cGMP.

C. Leukocyte Adhesion Protein Defects

There are two types of leukocyte adhesion protein defects (LAPD). In type 1, adhesion, chemotaxis, and phagocytosis are impaired due to reduced expression of CD18, the β chain of the adhesion surface protein LFA-1, complement receptor 3, and the C3dg receptor. Type 2 is characterized by impaired interaction between granulocytes and endothelial cells which, in turn, inhibits the granulocytes from rolling on the vessel walls and migrating to the foci of infection. This type of interaction is normally mediated by selectins and their receptor molecules. Sialoglycoprotein Sgp50 is the receptor for L-selectin in leukocytes, and sialyl-Lewis^x-oligosaccharide is the receptor for E-selectin in endothelial cells. Each has carbohydrate chains with fucose molecules that were not derived from mannose due to an enzyme defect.

D. Myeloperoxidase Deficiency

Myeloperoxidase (MPO) converts H_2O_2 and chloride ions to OCl⁻, which is stored in specific granules. MPO deficiency is caused by a significant reduction in the number of granules in granulocytes and monocytes. As a result, intracellular bactericidal action is reduced, though not entirely absent. None the less, *Candida albicans* cannot be killed without myeloperoxidase.

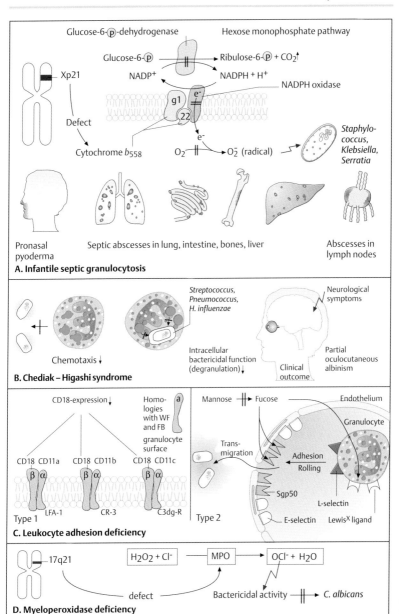

Glucose-6-$\textcircled{p}$-dehydrogenase Hexose monophosphate pathway

Glucose-6-$\textcircled{p}$ → Ribulose-6-$\textcircled{p}$ + $CO_2\uparrow$

$NADP^+$ $NADPH + H^+$ ← NADPH oxidase

Xp21

Defect

Cytochrome b_{558}

O_2 → O_2^- (radical) → *Staphylococcus, Klebsiella, Serratia*

Pronasal pyoderma   Septic abscesses in lung, intestine, bones, liver   Abscesses in lymph nodes

A. Infantile septic granulocytosis

Streptococcus, Pneumococcus, H. influenzae

Chemotaxis ↓

Intracellular bactericidal function (degranulation)↓

Neurological symptoms

Partial oculocutaneous albinism

Clinical outcome

B. Chediak – Higashi syndrome

CD18-expression ↓

Homologies with WF and FB granulocyte surface

CD18 CD11a   CD18 CD11b   CD18 CD11c
β α   β α   β α
LFA-1   CR-3   C3dg-R

Type 1

Mannose ⊣→ Fucose   Endothelium

Granulocyte

Transmigration

Adhesion
Rolling

Sgp50

L-selectin

E-selectin   Lewis^X ligand

Type 2

C. Leukocyte adhesion deficiency

17q21

$H_2O_2 + Cl^-$ → MPO → $OCl^- + H_2O$

defect

Bactericidal activity ⊣→ *C. albicans*

D. Myeloperoxidase deficiency

The lack of properly functioning complement proteins has effects similar to those of immunoglobulin deficiency. The patients have an increased frequency of severe bacterial infections. These infections are generally controlled by opsonization and complement lysis in individuals with a healthy immune system. A second type has signs and symptoms similar to those of SLE and various vasculitides (see table).

A. C1 Inhibitor Deficiency

Low serum concentrations of C1 inhibitor result in recurrent angioedematous swelling of the skin and mucosae. If localized in the oropharyngeal region, acute obstruction of the upper airways may also occur. There are two types of C1 inhibitor deficiency: autosomal dominant and acquired. In both cases, the C1 inhibitor is degraded more rapidly than it is produced. Uncontrolled protease activity leads to the release of inflammation mediators that increase local vessel permeability, thereby making the tissues susceptible to edema formation. Treatment is with androgen derivatives. Danazol, for example, increases C1 inhibitor production using the preserved and functional gene in the liver of patients with the hereditary form of the disease.

B. Paroxysmal Nocturnal Hemoglobinuria (PNH)

Paroxysmal nocturnal hemoglobinuria (PNH) is caused by a defect of complement-regulating surface proteins. The mechanism involves surface molecules anchored to the membrane by glycosylated phosphatidylinositol (GPI). Decay-accelerating factor (DAF), erythrocytic acetylcholinesterase, and LFA-3 are prime examples. PNH is characterized by the proliferation of hematopoietic stem cell clones with membrane-bound protein deficiencies. The increased receptivity of their erythrocytes to homologous C3b triggers the alternative pathway of complement activation. Lysis occurs more rapidly and more frequently after the formation of membrane attack complex (MAC). Patients with PNH therefore suffer from recurrent attacks of intravascular and extravascular hemolysis, the clinical manifestation of which is hemoglobinuria.

C. Positive Feedback Loop Dysfunction

Inhibitory factors H and I effectively control C3 activation in healthy individuals. When a deficiency of these regulatory proteins exists, the positive feedback loop around the C3bBb-C3 convertase enzyme consumes all available native C3 unproductively. A certain autoantibody also binds to the C3bBb complex. This prevents the molecule from dissociating into C3b and Bb fragments, a process mediated by factor H. As in primary C3 deficiency, both of these regulatory dysfunctions manifest clinically as diffuse subcutaneous lipodystrophy and mesangiocapillary glomerulonephritis. Recurrent pyogenic infections are also observed because opsonization and cell lysis are reduced due to the absence of C3.

Complement Receptor Deficiency

Neutrophil-mediated adhesion, chemotaxis, and phagocytosis of foreign substances opsonized by iC3b is severely impaired in this rare hereditary disease. Virtually no neutrophils infiltrate the sites of inflammation. The patients develop life-threatening sepsis. The severity of the disease is dependent on the degree of impaired surface expression of complement receptors CR3 and CR4 and LFA-1. Other clinical features of this immunodeficiency syndrome are described in the table below.

Complement Deficiencies	
Complement proteins	**Deficiency-associated manifestations**
C1–C4	SLE, pyogenic infections (e.g., pneumococcal sepsis)
C3, FH, FI	Pyogenic infections, glomerulonephritis
C8	Infections, especially by *Neisseria* spp. (gonococci, meningococci); sclerodactyly
CR3, CR4, LFA-1	Gingivitis, delayed deciduation of the umbilical cord, recurrent sepsis

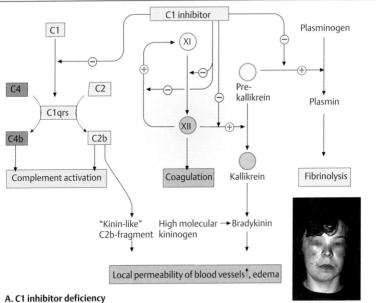

A. C1 inhibitor deficiency

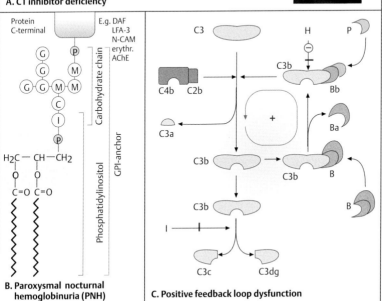

B. Paroxysmal nocturnal hemoglobinuria (PNH)

C. Positive feedback loop dysfunction

Clinical Immunology

A previously unknown immunodeficiency syndrome that predominantly affected homosexual males was first described in 1981. The syndrome was associated with life-threatening *Pneumocystis carinii* pneumonia and Kaposi's sarcoma—two conditions that had been rare until then. Similar cases of acquired immunodeficiency syndrome (AIDS) were later observed in hemophiliacs who had received clotting factor VIII transfusions and in other recipients of blood or blood products. It was therefore assumed that the agent responsible for AIDS was transmitted by infectious, sexual, and hematogenic routes. A frantic search for the causative agent led to the discovery of the new virus by a group headed by Luc Montagnier in 1983. The virus was later named the human immunodeficiency virus (HIV).

A. Structure of the Genome and Virion

HIV is a member of the lentivirus subfamily of retroviruses. All retroviruses contain *reverse transcriptase*, an enzyme that transcribes single-stranded genomic RNA into DNA. The HIV genome comprises approximately 10 kb. The protein-encoding genes *gag* (group-specific antigen), *pol* (reverse transcriptase and other enzymes), and *env* (integral membrane proteins for the lipid membrane envelope) are three additional features that HIV shares with other retroviruses (e.g., HT-LV). The HIV genome also contains other regulatory genes for the transcription or organization of the late replication cycle: *vif* (virion infectivity factor), *rev* (regulator of expression of virion proteins), and *nef* (negative regulatory factor). The genes overlap, that is, they are located on the same segment of the RNA molecule. Differential transcription by the protein synthesis mechanism of the host cell yields the various gene products.

The HIV virion is about 100 nm in diameter. Its outer lipid envelope is studded with 72 spikes derived from glycoprotein gp120. The spikes are anchored in the membrane by transmembrane protein gp41. The lipid membrane makes HIV especially vulnerable to attack by lipophilic detergents, such as alcohol.

B. Binding to the Host Cell

The attachment of the viral particle to the surface of the host cell involves two steps: binding of gp120 to the second domain of the CD4 molecule, and secondary binding to a chemokine receptor after a conformational change.

C. Replication Cycle in the Host Cell

After the two lipid membranes fuse, the contents of the virion are released into the cytoplasm. Immediately afterward, the reverse transcriptase starts to transcribe the RNA in double-stranded DNA. The LTR (long terminal repeats) on both ends of the retrovirus, together with the enzyme integrase, permit the integration of the genome into the host-cell genome, where it exists as a provirus. Production of the viral protein, which is supplied by cell's protein synthesis mechanism, can now be initiated by regulatory sequences of the LTR and by the genes *rev*, *tat*, and *vpr*.

D. Cells Susceptible to HIV Infection

HIV attacks CD4$^+$ T cells and other cells of the immune system. This includes cells of the monocytic system, such as monocytes, tissue macrophages, and Langerhans cell. It is still unclear whether HIV can infect pluripotent stem cells. Cells of the gastrointestinal tract and central nervous system can be infected. Microglia (macrophages), astrocytes, oligodendrocytes, and the endothelial cells of the cerebral blood vessels are the CNS cells most commonly infected by HIV. It is unclear whether neurons can also be infected.

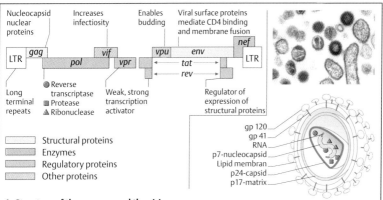

A. Structure of the genome and the virion

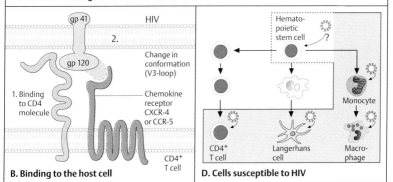

B. Binding to the host cell

D. Cells susceptible to HIV

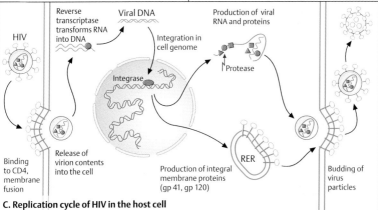

C. Replication cycle of HIV in the host cell

A. Course of HIV infection

The latency from HIV infection to the onset of severe symptoms of immunodeficiency (AIDS) is a mean 10 years. The immune system manages to keep the HIV infection under control during the latency period. In the initial phase of infection, the virus is able to proliferate with virtually no resistance. The number of free viral particles increases dramatically. The infected T-helper cells and macrophages produce thousands of new virions by budding before they die. Only around 30% of all HIV-infected individuals develop symptoms (e.g., fever, chills, lymphadenopathy) at this stage.

B. Response of the Immune System

Together with class I MHC molecules, the infected cells present viral epitopes, thereby activating the cellular cytotoxic immune response. Class II MHC-restringent T-cell activation leads to the release of interleukins, the activation of B cells, and antibody production. The antibodies bind free viral particles and make them digestible for macrophages. The overall virus population decreases sharply. Under this strong selective pressure, new mutations continuously develop during the process of HIV replication. Mistakes in retroviral reverse transcription, which occur once in approximately every 2000 nucleotides, speed up the process. These new mutants can proliferate unchecked until the immune system has adapted to the new epitope. The constant production of new viral mutants makes the HIV population so genetically diverse that the immune system ultimately becomes "confused" and unable to control the infection effectively. It becomes impossible to mount a coordinated attack against the virus. At a production and destruction rate of around 10^9 virions per day, each HIV particle generation spans approximately 2.6 days. Hence, around 140 viral generations are produced within the course of one year. Towards the end of latency, the immune system is confronted with the production of around 10 million HIV variants per day. The exact mechanism responsible for the destruction of the immune system is still largely unknown.

C. AIDS

Persistent generalized lymphadenopathy (PGL) develops prior to the onset of full-blown AIDS. Lymphadenopathy syndrome (LAS) usually persists for more than three months and is characterized by the involvement of atypically located lymph nodes.

The collapse of the immune system leads to the manifestation of numerous symptoms. The number of T-helper cells in serum falls below the critical limit of $400/\mu L$. Furthermore, the serum IgG concentration is elevated, but mainly contains ineffective "nonsense globulins" due to the stimulation of nonspecific polyclonal B cells. Other clinical features include weight loss, fever, and night sweats. These are referred to as the *AIDS-related complex* (ARC) of symptoms.

AIDS is defined by the occurrence of opportunistic infections, such as *Pneumocystis carinii* pneumonia, *Candida* esophagitis, and oral hairy leukoplakia (EBV). AIDS is also characterized by the occurrence of certain malignant neoplasms. Kaposi's sarcoma, for example, is caused by the chronic overproduction of inflammatory and angiogenic growth factors. Co-infection with human herpesvirus 8 (HHV-8) is also a decisive factor. Malignant lymphomas occur in 10% of all individuals infected by HIV. CNS manifestations occur in the late stages of HIV infection. A distinction is made between primary encephalopathies caused by neurotropic HIV and secondary encephalopathies, such as cerebral toxoplasmosis, CMV encephalitis, and meningitides of various origins.

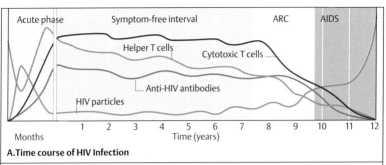

A. Time course of HIV Infection

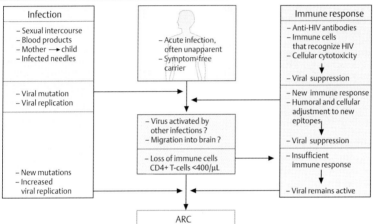

B. Immune response

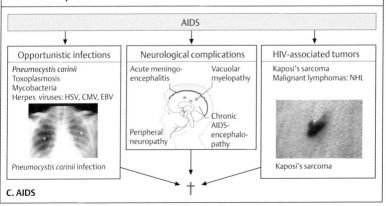

C. AIDS

A. Diagnosis of HIV Infection

The diagnosis of HIV infection is usually established by indirect detection of specific serum antibodies to HIV by enzyme-linked immunosorbent assay (ELISA). The test is performed in three steps:

1 HIV antibodies bind to HIV antigen in the coating of the test vessel.
2 The bound antibodies are labeled using an enzyme-conjugated anti-human immunoglobulin.
3 The enzyme forms a colored reaction product in the presence of HIV antibodies.

A positive ELISA test should always be confirmed by at least one other test, such as a Western blot or a specific immunofluorescence test (see pp. 82–85).

Viral culture is a rather expensive technique and, thus, is not used for routine HIV diagnosis. Gene amplification techniques, such as *polymerase chain reaction* (PCR) and *reverse transcriptase PCR* (RT-PCR), are currently being tested as HIV screening tests. The PCR is used to detect HIV's proviral DNA, and RT-PCR is used to detect the viral RNA (see p. 99**C**).

B. Treatment Strategies

Antiviral drugs (**1**): Nucleoside analogues (modified nucleosides) inhibit reverse transcriptase and lead to chain termination when incorporated into the viral DNA. Azidothymidine (AZT) was the first reverse transcriptase inhibitor developed for HIV infection, but the virus becomes resistant to AZT very quickly (**b**). The incorporation of false nucleosides also blocks cellular polymerase, which leads to side effects similar to those observed with cytostatic drugs.

Another group of compounds binds to the catalytic center of reverse transcriptase, thereby inactivating the enzyme (**a**). More recently developed compounds of this group remain effective after multiple *pol* gene mutations. The efficacy of these drugs, which is measured as the reduction in viral load, can be enhanced by administering them in combination with other virustatics. They are especially effective when combined with the new group of *protease inhibitors* (**c**). Protease inhibitors are structurally similar to the precursor protein sequence recognized by the viral protease.

Vaccines (**2**): The use of the attenuated live virus is too risky because the immunity observed in the animal model (monkeys) cannot be extended to humans. The development of hybrid viruses has opened new possibilities. The HIV gene for gp120 can be transferred to harmless viruses, such as cowpox. This may permit the use of functionally weakened but still highly immunogenic viruses as a live vaccine. Another approach is to use purified DNA as the vaccine. Because the injected DNA is incorporated in the cell genome, it can imitate the events of a viral infection without the virulence.

Interleukins (**3**): Activated CD8+ T cells produce interleukin (IL-)16 (lymphocyte chemotactic factor, LCF), which inhibits the replication of the virus. At the same time, it also induces the cross-linkage of CD4 molecules on the surface of CD4+ T cells. The viral production of infected CD4+ cells is reduced by one-tenth. The chemokines RANTES, MIP-1α, and MIP-1β have similar effects on the T cells due to the blockade of chemokine receptors required for HIV docking. Recombinant interferon-α (rIFN-α) and IL-12 inhibit a number of steps in the replication cycle. They are currently being used in conjunction with reverse transcriptase inhibitors for treatment of asymptomatic HIV-infected subjects in experimental combination drug therapies.

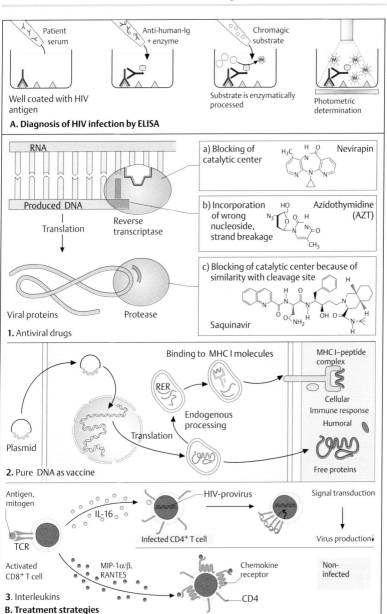

A. Diagnosis of HIV infection by ELISA

Patient serum

Anti-human-Ig + enzyme

Chromagic substrate

Well coated with HIV antigen

Substrate is enzymatically processed

Photometric determination

RNA

a) Blocking of catalytic center

Nevirapin

Produced DNA

Translation

Reverse transcriptase

b) Incorporation of wrong nucleoside, strand breakage

Azidothymidine (AZT)

Viral proteins

Protease

c) Blocking of catalytic center because of similarity with cleavage site

Saquinavir

1. Antiviral drugs

Binding to MHC I molecules

MHC I–peptide complex

RER

Endogenous processing

Cellular Immune response

Humoral

Plasmid

Translation

Free proteins

2. Pure DNA as vaccine

Antigen, mitogen

IL-16

HIV-provirus

Signal transduction

Infected CD4+ T cell

Virus production

TCR

Activated CD8+ T cell

MIP-1α/β, RANTES

Chemokine receptor

Non-infected

CD4

3. Interleukins

B. Treatment strategies

Clinical Immunology

113

A. ABO System of Blood Typing

The ABO system discovered by Karl Landsteiner in 1901 is the most important system for blood typing. It is based on the occurrence of *natural antibodies* (isoagglutinins) against A and B blood group antigens expressed on red blood cells. Antibodies develop only against antigens not expressed by host RBCs. Type A individuals (around 42% of the population in Central Europe, 41% of American whites, and 27% of Americans of black or Mexican origin) have antibodies directed against the B blood group antigen. These antibodies are capable of agglutinating and lysing RBCs bearing B antigens and are called *anti-B antibodies*. If such erythrocytes are transfused to an A+ individual, they are immediately lysed. Type B individuals (ca. 14% in Europe, 20% of American blacks, 13% of Mexicans, and 25% of Asians), on the other hand, have native *anti-A antibodies*. In Type AB individuals (approximately 6% of the population), both A and B antigens are expressed on red blood cells, and neither anti-A nor anti-B antibodies are present in the serum. In Type O individuals (ca. 38% in Europe, 45% of American whites, 49% of American blacks, and 56% of American Mexicans), neither of the antigens is expressed on red blood cells, and both anti-A and anti-B antibodies are present in serum. A antigens are subdivided into subtypes A1 (80%) and A2 (20%). Anti-A1 antibodies seldom occur in A2-positive individuals. The A and B antigens are mainly expressed on red blood cells, but are also weakly expressed on platelets and endothelial cells.

B. Development of A and B Antibodies

Newborns develop anti-A and anti-B antibodies on contact with ubiquitous antigens. Bacteria and pollen, in particular, have large amounts of A and B antigens. If these antigens are expressed on the host RBCs, clones of cells that produce antibodies against them will be eliminated.

C. Development of ABO Antigens

The AB and O genes are located on the long arm of chromosome 9. They code for various glycosyltransferases that transfer various sugar molecules onto a precursor substance. L-fucose is transferred onto a precursor chain (paragloboside) by a gene product (the so-called *H gene*) that is active in 99.9% of the population. This leads to the development of *H antigen*, which is expressed on red blood cells and consists of glucose, galactose, *N*-acetylglucosamine, galactose, and fucose. An active A gene (in individuals with blood type A) codes for a specific *N*-acetylgalactosaminyltransferase. This leads to elongation of the H antigen by an *N*-acetylgalactosamine molecule, thereby forming the A antigen. If the B gene is active, a galactosyltransferase molecule is synthesized instead. In other words, a galactose molecule attaches to the H antigen in individuals with blood type B. In individuals with active A and B genes, both A and B antigen are expressed on red blood cells. Other individuals have an active O gene. This gene is a silent allele that leaves H antigen unmodified and corresponds to blood type O.

The AB and O genes are inherited according to Mendel's principles. Hence, type A individuals may have genotype AA or AO, and type B individuals may have genotype BB or BO. Type AB individuals have genotype AB, and individuals with type O blood have genotype OO. The natural anti-A and anti-B antibodies are mainly IgM-class immunoglobulins. Individuals with blood type O, however, also have IgG antibodies against A and B antigen.

Since anti-A and anti-B isoagglutinins occur naturally, severe hemolysis can occur after a single transfusion of ABO-incompatible red blood cells. After first-time exposure, new immunoglobulins are formed in addition to the preexisting natural antibodies.

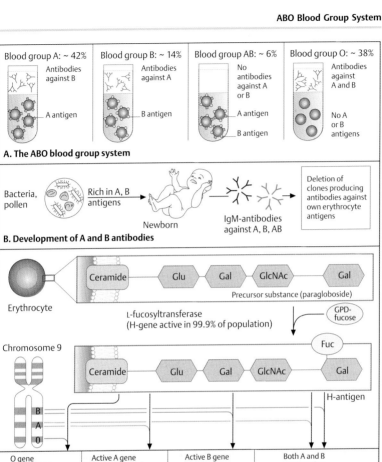

Blood group A: ~ 42%
Antibodies against B
A antigen

Blood group B: ~ 14%
Antibodies against A
B antigen

Blood group AB: ~ 6%
No antibodies against A or B
A antigen
B antigen

Blood group O: ~ 38%
Antibodies against A and B
No A or B antigens

A. The ABO blood group system

Bacteria, pollen → Rich in A, B antigens → Newborn → IgM-antibodies against A, B, AB → Deletion of clones producing antibodies against own erythrocyte antigens

B. Development of A and B antibodies

Erythrocyte

Ceramide — Glu — Gal — GlcNAc — Gal
Precursor substance (paragloboside)

L-fucosyltransferase
(H-gene active in 99.9% of population)

GPD-fucose

Chromosome 9

Ceramide — Glu — Gal — GlcNAc — Gal — Fuc

H-antigen

B
A
0

O gene (silent allele)	Active A gene (galactosaminyl-transferase)	Active B gene (galactosyl-transferase)	Both A and B genes active
Unmodified H antigen	N-Acetyl-galactosamine	Galactose	A antigen + B antigen
	A antigen	B antigen	
Blood group O	Blood group A	Blood group B	Blood group AB

C. Development of the ABO antigens

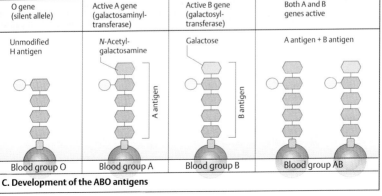

Clinical Immunology

115

More than 20 different blood group systems are present on red blood cells. The clinically most important systems are the ABO system, the rhesus system, the Kell system, and the Duffy system.

A. Rhesus System

The rhesus (Rh) system is genetically and phenotypically complex. The rhesus antigens are designated DdCcEe and are encoded by the corresponding genes. The "d" component is a silent allele that does not lead to antigen expression. According to a simplified model, they are controlled by two neighboring gene loci on chromosome 1. Either the silent *d* gene or the *D* gene that codes for the D antigen may be active on locus 1. Four alleles are located on the second, adjacent locus: *CE*, *Ce*, *cE*, and *ce*. The genes of the two loci are codominant. In other words, the gene product of the first locus is expressed together with that of the second locus. The following combinations may occur: *DCE*, *DCe*, *DcE*, *Dce*, *dCE*, *dCe*, *dcE*, *dce*. Since we all inherit one maternal and one paternal allele, the genotype potential is very diverse. All gene products in which a D gene product is expressed are said to be rhesus-positive (Rh+), and all genotypes lacking D antigen (or in which the silent *d* allele is active) are defined as rhesus-negative (Rh-). The most common genotypes are listed in (**A**). D antigen is by far the most immunogenic antigen.

B. Alloimmunization against Rh Antigens

Alloimmunization to rhesus antigens occurs following exposure to incompatible red blood cells. This occurs, for example, when Rh-negative patients receive a transfusion of Rh-positive RBCs. Rh-positive blood volumes as small as 1 ml lead to the formation of IgM class anti-D antibodies in 15% of cases, and 80% of all Rh-negative individuals develop anti-D antibodies after receiving 250 ml of Rh-positive erythrocytes. Reexposure to even small quantities of Rh-positive erythrocytes can induce the prompt formation of IgG antibodies to D antigen. *Hemolytic disease of the newborn* (HDN) is an important clinical example (**2**). In an Rh-negative mother with an Rh-positive fetus, for example, the mother forms anti-D IgM antibodies during the passage of fetal Rh+ red blood cells (usually during delivery). If a second pregnancy occurs, contact with even small quantities of fetal RBCs activates the production of IgG antibo-

dies that cross the placenta. The fetus may die in utero as a consequence of the resulting severe hemolytic anemia (erythroblastosis fetalis). Hemoglobin cleavage products may be deposited in the brain, particularly in the brainstem (kernicterus). To prevent anti-D immunization, Rh-negative women should receive anti-D immunoglobulins within 72 hours after delivery, amniocentesis, spontaneous abortion, or interruption of pregnancy. The administration of these antibodies can immediately eliminate any fetal red blood cells that may have been transferred and prevent stimulation of the maternal immune system and antibody formation.

C. Other Red Cell Antigens

The Kell blood group system is important due to the powerful immunogenicity of K antigen (roughly corresponds to the rhesus D antigen). K antigen occurs in only 9% of the population. The transmission of K-positive red blood cells during pregnancy or blood transfusion leads to the formation of anti-K antibodies, which must be considered in subsequent transfusions. Bacterial antigens can also induce the formation of anti-K antibodies.

Since *Duffy antigens* (Fy[a] and Fy[b]) are only weakly immunogenic, anti-Fy antibodies are rare. Both antigens are absent in 68% of all African-Americans. This is attributed to natural selection since the Fy glycoprotein serves as the receptor for the malaria pathogen *Plasmodium vivax*. Hence, the absence of Fy antigens results in resistance to malaria. New findings indicate that the Duffy antigen is a chemokine receptor (Duffy Antigen Receptor for Chemokines, DARC) that is also present on endothelial cells and postcapillary venules. It is a receptor for many different CXC and CC chemokines (see Tab. 9).

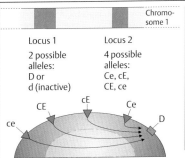

Most common genotypes	Frequency	Phenotype
DCe/DCe	18%	
DCe/dce	35%	
DCe/DcE	13%	Rh+
DcE/dce	12%	
DcE/DcE	2%	
Dce/dce	2%	
dce/dce	15%	Rh-

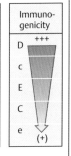

Immunogenicity: D +++, c, E, C, e (+)

A. Rhesus system

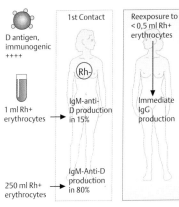
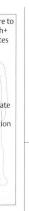

1. Anti-D immune response

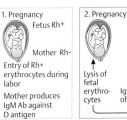

2. Hemolytic disease of the newborn

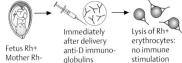

3. Prophylaxis by Rh immunization

B. Alloimmunization against Rh antigens

Kell system = K and k	
Phenotype	Frequency
K- k+	91%
K+ k+	8.8%
K+ k-	0.2%

K immunogenic after
– pregnancy
– infection
– transfusion

Duffy system = Fya and Fyb	Frequency (USA)	
Phenotype	Whites	Blacks
Fya+b-	17%	9%
Fya+b+	49%	1%
Fya-b+	34%	22%
Fya-b-	<1%	68%

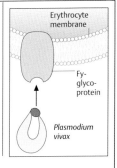

C. Other erythrocyte antigens

Clinical Immunology

117

Anti-red cell antibodies can induce lysis of the erythrocytes, regardless of whether they are induced physiologically after the transfusion of incompatible red blood cells (RBCs) or due to immune dysregulation (autoimmune hemolysis).

A. Mechanisms of Hemolysis

Hemolysis is characterized as intravascular or extravascular. The adherence of IgM antibodies to RBCs can lead to complement binding in the bloodstream and pore formation after activation of the lytic sequence (**1**). This type of intravascular hemolysis leads to the release of large quantities of hemoglobin, which is bound by a *hemoglobin-binding protein* (haptoglobin) in serum. When the protein's binding capacity is exhausted, free hemoglobin is excreted by the kidney (hemoglobinuria). Since hemoglobin molecules precipitate in an acidic environment, damage to the renal tubules occurs. The process is aggravated by the precipitation of immune complexes of antibodies and antigens from the membrane of the damaged RBCs. The immune complexes and free hemoglobin additionally activate the coagulation cascade. This results in *disseminated intravascular coagulation* (DIC) associated with microthrombosis in the kidneys, lungs, brain, and liver.

Extravascular hemolysis occurs when there is no direct complement binding by the antibodies, that is, when the lytic complement sequence (C5–C9) is not activated in the circulation. By way of Fc receptors and receptors for complement cleavage products (C3b), the erythrocytes undergo phagocytosis in the reticuloendothelial (RE) system and intracellular digestion (**2**). The course of extravascular hemolysis is less dramatic than that of intravascular hemolysis.

B. Antiglobulin Test (Coombs Test)

Coombs serum is a polyspecific serum used to detect RBC antibodies to human IgG, IgM, and complement (**1**). Because anti-IgA antibodies are usually absent in Coombs reagents, IgA autoantibodies are often not detected.

The *direct Coombs test* is used to detect erythrocyte-bound or complement-bound antibodies. If these are present, Coombs serum causes cross-linkage of the antibodies and agglutination of the cells (**2**).

The *indirect Coombs test* is used to detect the presence of anti-erythrocyte antibodies in the serum (**3**). The patient's serum is incubated with different test erythrocytes that have a known antigen profile. If the serum contains antibodies to one of the test antigens, the antibodies bind to the RBCs, which will agglutinate on addition of Coombs serum. The Coombs test is used to detect antibodies to erythrocyte antigens before blood transfusions and if hemolysis is suspected during pregnancy.

C. Detection of Complete and Incomplete RBC-Bound Antibodies

IgM antibodies agglutinate RBCs in isotonic saline solution; hence, they are called *complete antibodies*. IgG antibodies, on the other hand, are monovalent molecules that are unable to span the distance between two RBCs. Although IgG may be bound to RBCs, agglutination of the cells does not occur. IgG antibodies are therefore referred to as *incomplete antibodies*. The presence of incomplete antibodies and complement cleavage products on the surface of RBCs is detected by addition of Coombs serum.

D. Hemolysis and Antibody Affinity

Lysis of aging RBCs (after a lifespan of around 120 days) is one of the tasks of the RE system. The severity of hemolysis usually correlates with the number of antibody molecules bound to each RBC. In rare cases, severe hemolysis may be induced by small concentrations of high-affinity antibodies. The lifespan of a red blood cell can be reduced to three days by as few as 10 anti-Rh antibodies. In this case, the Coombs test may be negative or only weakly positive since the lower limit of detection of most Coombs reagents is 300–500 antibodies per RBC. Complement components, such as C3b, can significantly increase the rate of hemolysis.

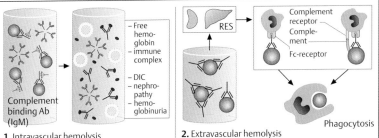

1. Intravascular hemolysis

- Free hemoglobin
- immune complex
- DIC
- nephropathy
- hemoglobinuria

Complement binding Ab (IgM)

RES

Complement receptor
Complement
Fc-receptor

Phagocytosis

2. Extravascular hemolysis

A. Mechanisms of hemolysis

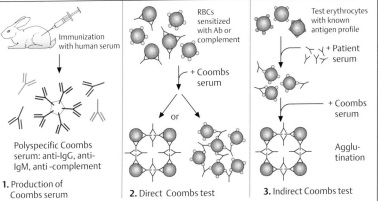

Immunization with human serum

Polyspecific Coombs serum: anti-IgG, anti-IgM, anti-complement

1. Production of Coombs serum

RBCs sensitized with Ab or complement

+ Coombs serum

or

2. Direct Coombs test

Test erythrocytes with known antigen profile

+ Patient serum

+ Coombs serum

Agglutination

3. Indirect Coombs test

B. Detection of erythrocyte antibodies: Antiglobulin test (Coombs test)

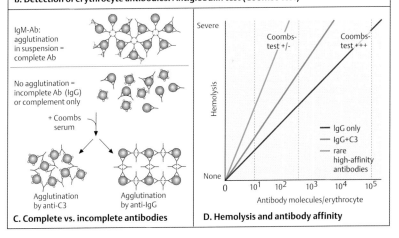

IgM-Ab: agglutination in suspension = complete Ab

No agglutination = incomplete Ab (IgG) or complement only

+ Coombs serum

Agglutination by anti-C3

Agglutination by anti-IgG

C. Complete vs. incomplete antibodies

Severe

Coombs-test +/-

Coombs-test +++

Hemolysis

None

IgG only
IgG+C3
rare high-affinity antibodies

$0 \quad 10^1 \quad 10^2 \quad 10^3 \quad 10^4 \quad 10^5$

Antibody molecules/erythrocyte

D. Hemolysis and antibody affinity

Clinical Immunology

119

A. Pathogenesis of Autoimmune Hemolytic Anemias

The origin of autoimmune hemolytic anemia (AIHA) is unknown (idiopathic hemolysis) in around 50% of cases. The other 50% of cases are caused by various etiologies, such as infections that induce the formation of autoantibodies due to the cross-reaction of bacterial or viral antigens with red cell antigens. Connective tissue diseases, especially systemic lupus erythematosus (see pp. 172–175), are characterized by increased T-helper activity in addition to the increased autoantibody production. T- and B-cell lymphoproliferative diseases and thymomas can interfere with regulatory T-cell function, thereby leading to the overproduction of autoantibodies. Hematological disorders, such as Hodgkin's disease, non-Hodgkin's lymphoma, and chronic lymphocytic leukemia, may develop due to the malignant transformation of autoreactive B cells that produce autoantibodies or may disrupt inhibitory mechanisms that normally prevent autoantibody formation. Another important type of autoimmune hemolysis is caused by certain drugs (see p. 124).

B. Warm Antibodies

Hemolytic anemias are classified according to the thermic activity of the autoantibodies involved. *Cold antibodies* bind more efficiently to RBCs at 4 °C, whereas *warm antibodies* bind more efficiently at 37 °C. Approximately 70% of patients with AIHA have warm antibodies, 15–20% have cold antibodies, and the rest have a mixture of the two. The warm antibodies are usually class IgG immunoglobulins. Complement fixation by these antibodies is suboptimal because the C1 complement molecule must undergo conformational changes in order to become activated. This happens only when C1 binds to two closely adjacent immunoglobulin molecules. This is always the case with polyvalent IgM antibodies that naturally occur as pentamers, but occurs with IgG antibodies only when the antigen density on the cell membrane of the RBCs is very high. Lysis of IgG-bearing RBCs by macrophages is mainly extravascular. The hemolytic process is relatively inefficient because circulating immunoglobulins block the Fc receptors. The only site where the process is efficient is in the spleen, where the circulation of RBCs is extremely slow. This reduces the concentration of serum immuno-globulins with respect to the number of erythrocytes. The rate of hemolysis increases when C3b is bound to the RBC membrane.

C. Clinical Signs of Hemolysis

Autoimmune hemolysis manifests as a decreasing hemoglobin concentration in conjunction with marked anisocytosis. With warm antibodies, erythrocyte lysis takes place mainly in the RE system; the serum concentration of the hemoglobin-binding protein haptoglobin decreases only if there is severe hemolysis. Hepatosplenomegaly occurs due to the increased rate of hemolysis in the spleen and liver. Intracellular enzymes, such as lactate dehydrogenase (LDH), are released. Erythropoiesis is stimulated in the bone marrow, and reticulocytes are increased. The freed hemoglobin is reduced to bilirubin, which binds to glucuronate in the liver and is excreted in the bile. Hyperbilirubinemia, which leads to yellowish discoloration of the sclera and skin (jaundice), is frequently seen. Urobilinogen, another degradation product, causes dark discoloration of the urine.

D. Management of Warm Antibody Autoimmune Hemolysis

In most cases, these patients are initially treated with corticosteroids. These drugs suppress antibody production, but may also reduce the efficacy and number of Fc and C3 receptors on the macrophages. High-dose immunoglobulins also block Fc receptors. Corticosteroids and immunoglobulins usually do not achieve long-term cures. Splenectomy or splenic radiotherapy is often performed because the sequestration of agglutinin-coated RBCs mainly occurs in the spleen. Large quantities of IgG are also produced in the spleen. Immunosuppressants, such as cyclophosphamide, azathioprine, or cyclosporine, can also be used as a last resort. Recently, good results have been obtained with an anti-CD20 monoclonal antibody (Rituxan®). This antibody eliminates B lymphocytes, which are the source of autoantibodies.

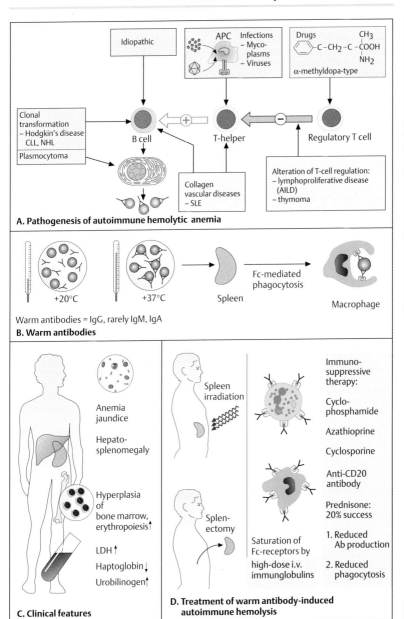

A. Pathogenesis of autoimmune hemolytic anemia

Warm antibodies = IgG, rarely IgM, IgA
B. Warm antibodies

C. Clinical features

D. Treatment of warm antibody-induced autoimmune hemolysis

Clinical Immunology

A. Cold Antibody Autoimmune Hemolysis

Cold antibodies are usually IgM and only occasionally IgG. Accordingly, they can cause agglutination of erythrocytes and are therefore called agglutinins. They are most commonly observed following infections, especially by *Mycoplasma*, Epstein–Barr virus, or cytomegalovirus, and rarely after bacterial diseases. These infections usually lead to the formation of polyclonal cold-reactive antibodies that bind to erythrocytes most efficiently at low temperatures. In most cases, cold antibodies are directed against I antigen, which is mainly expressed on mature RBCs, but also on some pathogens. Some malignant lymphatic diseases may lead to secretion of monoclonal agglutinins (see p. 142). Monoclonal agglutinins may be directed against both I and i antigen (immature fetal erythrocytes). Monoclonal cold agglutinins also induce **chronic idiopathic cold hemagglutinin disease** (peak incidence between 70 and 80 years of age).

The severity of cold agglutinin-induced hemolysis is dependent on the thermic amplitude of the antibody, which is defined as the amount of antibody binding to the RBC at a given temperature. As the temperature decreases, antibody binding increases, but the lytic activity of complement decreases. Hemolysis therefore occurs only in an overlap zone, which usually ranges from 10 °C to 30 °C (**2**). If the thermic amplitude of the antibody is very large (over 30 °C), hemolysis occurs at temperatures that are easily achieved in the skin. Cold agglutinins are often discovered incidentally due to the agglutination of RBCs in routine RBC counts (**3**). Electronic blood cell counters detect the clumped cells as large individual cells. This results in a falsely high mean corpuscular volume (MCV) and a falsely low red cell count in patients with a normal hemoglobin concentration.

Since the temperature in the capillaries of the skin can drop below 30 °C, the cold agglutinins cause the erythrocytes to clump together. This intravascular agglutination process leads to capillary obstruction, which manifests as acrocyanosis (bluish discoloration of the fingers, ears, and tip of the nose) or livedo reticularis (reddish/bluish reticular pattern of the skin). Trophic lesions (ulcers, necrosis) may occur in severe forms.

B. Mechanism of Hemolysis

Cold antibodies bind to erythrocytes most efficiently at +4 °C and bind poorly or hardly at 37 °C. The degree of binding at room temperature varies. Since cold agglutinins are usually IgM antibodies, complement activation can mediate direct intravascular hemolysis with a dramatic clinical picture including hemoglobinuria, renal failure, and disseminated intravascular coagulation (see also p. 118). Fortunately, this happens rarely. Hemolysis develops gradually in most cases. The C3b molecule bound to the RBC surface mediates binding to complement receptors on Kupffer cells in the liver. Since phagocytes do not have Fc receptors for IgM, Fc-mediated phagocytosis does not take place (in contrast to warm antibody hemolysis). Hence, the prospects of successful management of cold antibody hemolysis by splenectomy, high-dose immunoglobulins, or steroids are not good.

C. Management

Low levels of cold agglutinins are often detected in laboratory tests. However, this finding generally is not clinically relevant since cold agglutinins usually have a low thermic amplitude. Also, many patients with cold hemagglutinin disease have only slight, gradually progressive hemolysis that does not require treatment. In some cases, however, severe hemolytic crises may occur upon exposure to the cold. Blood transfusions should not be administered unless vital for survival. The blood should be warmed to 37 °C during the transfusion. There is no specific treatment. The most important preventive measure is to wear warm clothing. If the symptoms are extremely severe, relocation to a warmer climate is the only solution. Excision or radiotherapy of the spleen is usually ineffective. Cytostatics or immunosuppressants are potentially useful only when there is an underlying lymphoproliferative disease. Recent publications suggest that treatment with a monoclonal antibody directed against CD20 (Rituxan®) may result in control of hemolysis.

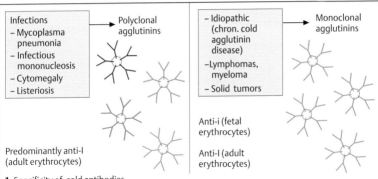

Infections
- Mycoplasma pneumonia
- Infectious mononucleosis
- Cytomegaly
- Listeriosis

→ Polyclonal agglutinins

- Idiopathic (chron. cold agglutinin disease)
- Lymphomas, myeloma
- Solid tumors

→ Monoclonal agglutinins

Anti-i (fetal erythrocytes)

Anti-I (adult erythrocytes)

Predominantly anti-I (adult erythrocytes)

1. Specificity of cold antibodies

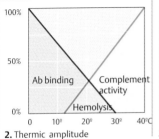

2. Thermic amplitude

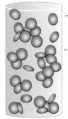

- Falsely high MCV
- Falsely low erythrocyte count

3. Changes in blood chemistry

- Anemia
- Acrocyanosis
- Livedo reticularis
- Trophic disorders

4. Clinical symptoms

A. Autoimmune hemolysis by cold antibodies

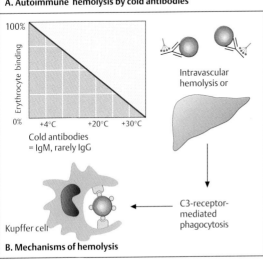

Erythrocyte binding

Cold antibodies = IgM, rarely IgG

Intravascular hemolysis or

C3-receptor-mediated phagocytosis

Kupffer cell

B. Mechanisms of hemolysis

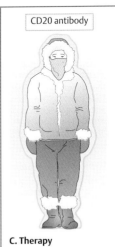

CD20 antibody

C. Therapy

Clinical Immunology

123

Clinical Immunology

A. Drug-Induced Autoimmune Hemolysis

Drugs may cause hemolysis by a number of immune mechanisms.

1 In penicillin-induced hemolysis, the drug acts as a **hapten**. In this case, the antibodies are specifically directed against the antibiotic. Strictly speaking, this does not qualify them as true autoantibodies. Hemolysis occurs if the drug firmly attaches to the cell membrane of RBCs. Penicillin can even form covalent bonds with proteins on the RBC membrane. High antibody titers are most commonly observed in patients receiving high-dose penicillin. The antibodies in question are usually IgG warm antibodies, and hemolysis occurs due to Fc-mediated phagocytosis. Patients treated with cefalosporins frequently develop positive Coombs tests, but hemolysis occurs rarely.

2 Other drugs, such as quinidine or stibophen, first form immune complexes with IgG or IgM antibodies directed against the drug. These immune complexes then bind to the surface of the red blood cells. This activates the complement cascade, thereby leading to lysis of uninvolved RBCs. This is sometimes referred to as the "**innocent bystander**" mechanism of hemolysis. Today, many workers believe that at least some of the antibodies are directed against red-cell antigens and that the drugs causing this type of hemolysis act as haptens. In other words, they must be bound to carrier proteins in order to generate an immune response.

3 Certain drugs, such as α-**methyldopa**, induce the specific inhibition of regulatory T cells, thereby causing the uncontrolled production of autoantibodies. This is a true form of autoimmune hemolytic anemia. The antibodies react mostly with rhesus antigen components. Approximately 15% of patients on α-methyldopa develop antibodies (positive Coombs' test), but only around 1% will develop hemolysis.

B. Transfusion Reactions

Adverse events may develop after a blood transfusion. Severe hemolytic reactions are usually attributable to the mistaken transfusion of incompatible blood. A1, Kell, and Duffy antigens are most commonly involved. Although strongly immunogenic, rhesus antigens are rarely the cause of transfusion reactions because rhesus incompatibility is easier to detect.

Febrile, nonhemolytic reactions occur in about 1% of all transfusions. This type of post-transfusion reaction is an allergic reaction induced by allergens or IgE immunoglobulins in the serum of the donor. The allergens lead to the release of IL-1 and histamine. The use of washed blood or premedication with antihistamines should reduce this problem.

Alloimmunization against foreign HLA antigens (contaminated leukocytes in the blood product), or against red-cell E, D, C antigens, may occur after blood transfusion in multiply transfused or multiparous patients. The processes of alloimmunization are physiological immune reactions that can be minimized by leukocyte filtering and careful donor screening.

Graft-versus-host (GVH) reaction (see p. 158) is a rare complication of blood transfusion. GVH reactions are caused by viable lymphocytes in the transfusion product that attack normal tissue in an immunocompromised transfusion recipient. This problem can be prevented by using leukocyte filters or by irradiating the blood product prior to use.

The use of contaminated blood products is rarely the cause of infection transmission. The most frequently transmitted pathogens are hepatitis, cytomegalovirus, and HIV. Malaria, Chagas' disease, and filarial diseases can be transmitted in endemic regions. Bacteria, such as *Pseudomonas*, *E. coli*, and *Yersinia*, are rarely transmitted in blood donations.

Patients with IgA deficiency (1/600 individuals) may also develop anaphylactic reactions after blood transfusions. The reason is that the transfusion products often contain small quantities of serum immunoglobulins. These patients should therefore receive only carefully washed blood products.

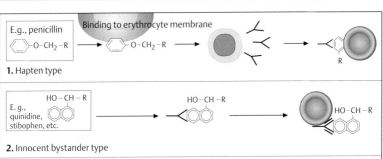

A. Drug-induced autoimmune hemolysis

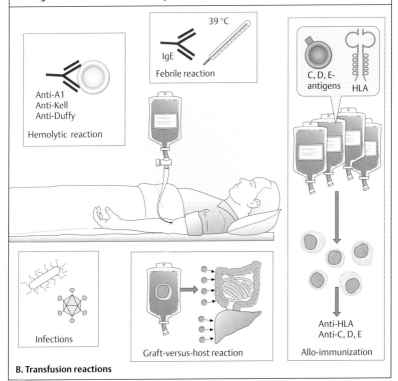

B. Transfusion reactions

Clinical Immunology

A. Autoimmune Neutropenia

Neutropenia may be caused by antibodies, cytokines, or the direct cytotoxic effects of T cells and NK cells. Autoantibodies against NA1 and NA2 granulocyte antigens are frequently observed in autoimmune idiopathic neutropenias (AIN). These antigens also play a role in maternofetal immunization (newborn neutropenia). Autoantibodies may also be formed in the course of systemic lupus erythematosus (SLE) and Felty's syndrome, a special type of rheumatoid arthritis. *Large granular lymphocyte (LGL) leukemia* of T-cell type is associated with the clonal development of T cells with cytotoxic activity against neutrophilic granulocytes. Patients with this disease have a high incidence of autoimmune disorders, including thrombocytopenia, pure red cell aplasia (PRCA), thyroiditis, SLE, and systemic scleroderma. A third of the patients have rheumatoid arthritis.

Tumors of the thymus (thymomas) may lead to the development of *pure white cell aplasia*, a condition in which large quantities of T-suppressor cells (regulator cells) are generated. These cells exclusively inhibit the development of granulocytes. In HIV-infected individuals, neutropenia usually results from the inhibition of neutrophil production in bone marrow due to direct injury by HIV, opportunistic infections of the bone marrow, or the toxic side effects of therapy. Rarely, anti-neutrophil antibodies play a role.

B. Aplastic Anemia

In aplastic anemia, the entire process of hematopoiesis is failing. Blood tests reveal pancytopenia, that is, the co-occurrence of anemia, leukocytopenia, and thrombocytopenia. Clinical signs are paleness and fatigue, increased susceptibility to infections, and bleeding tendency. The disease can be caused by infections, toxic damage, or autoimmunity. Autoimmune pathogenesis should be suspected when increased numbers of lymphatic cells are detected within the bone marrow. These cells are T-regulatory cells that inhibit pluripotent stem cells either directly or via stromal cells. γ-interferon, tumor necrosis factor-α, and interleukin-2 seem to be involved. CD34$^+$ cells are killed via Fas-induced apoptosis. These patients can be successfully managed by immunosuppression (steroids, cyclosporine, bone marrow transplantation).

C. Pure Red Cell Aplasia

Pure red cell aplasia is a disease that exclusively affects erythropoiesis without disturbing leukocyte or platelet formation. The disease is frequently associated with thymomas and parvovirus B19 infections. T-regulatory cells that selectively inhibit erythropoiesis are presumably activated. Antibodies against erythrocytic precursors have also been observed.

D. Immune Thrombocytopenia

Immune thrombocytopenia is associated with the formation of anti-platelet antibodies (usually IgG). This disease can occur in connective tissue disease (especially SLE), after the use of certain medications, or following viral infections. A prior viral infection is the suspected cause in many cases of unknown etiology (idiopathic thrombocytopenic purpura, ITP). The antibodies shorten the lifespan of thrombocytes. Despite proliferation of megakaryocytes within the bone marrow, the number of platelets in the blood decreases. Patients with severe disease have a tendency to develop hemorrhages. The bleeding usually occurs as petechial hemorrhage. Life-threatening cerebral hemorrhages are infrequent events, even in patients with platelet counts below 30 000/ml. The immune reaction targets glycoprotein (gp) platelet antigens gpIIIa, gpIIb (gpIIIa/gpIIb complex), and gpIb. The antibodies are detected as platelet-associated immunoglobulins (PAIgG). Antigen–antibody complexes that attach to platelets via Fc receptors form in the presence of heparin. Platelets that are "innocent bystanders" can then be lysed or phagocytosed by macrophages. ITP in childhood is usually an acute form associated with a high rate of spontaneous remission. In adults, the course of disease tends to be chronic and refractory to treatment. The established treatment alternatives include corticosteroids, immunosuppressants, high-dose intravenous immunoglobulins, and splenectomy. Recently, good results have been achieved with an anti-CD20 monoclonal antibody (Rituxan®).

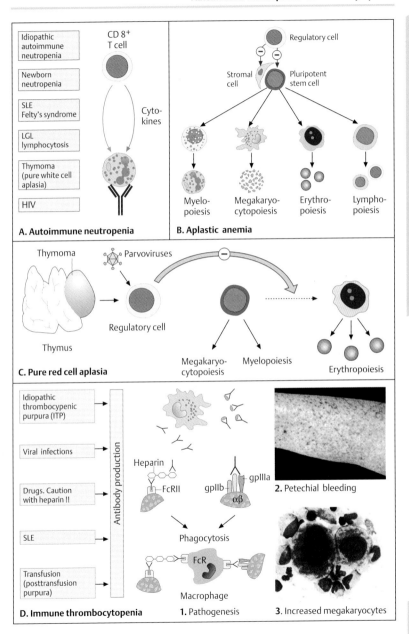

A. Autoimmune neutropenia

- Idiopathic autoimmune neutropenia
- Newborn neutropenia
- SLE Felty's syndrome
- LGL lymphocytosis
- Thymoma (pure white cell aplasia)
- HIV

CD 8+ T cell

Cytokines

B. Aplastic anemia

Regulatory cell

Stromal cell

Pluripotent stem cell

Myelopoiesis   Megakaryocytopoiesis   Erythropoiesis   Lymphopoiesis

C. Pure red cell aplasia

Thymoma

Parvoviruses

Thymus

Regulatory cell

Megakaryocytopoiesis   Myelopoiesis

Erythropoiesis

D. Immune thrombocytopenia

- Idiopathic thrombocypenic purpura (ITP)
- Viral infections
- Drugs. Caution with heparin !!
- SLE
- Transfusion (posttransfusion purpura)

Antibody production

Heparin

FcRII   gpIIb   gpIIIa   αβ

Phagocytosis

FcR

Macrophage

1. Pathogenesis

2. Petechial bleeding

3. Increased megakaryocytes

Clinical Immunology

127

Acute leukemias are neoplastic diseases in which precursor cells of the bone marrow become unable to differentiate and have high proliferative activity. The uncontrolled growth of neoplastic cells suppresses the normal hematopoiesis. If left untreated, acute leukemia leads to death within a few weeks.

A. Hematopoiesis and the Origin of Leukemia

Many leukemias develop from pluripotent stem cells. This type of undifferentiated leukemia is difficult to classify morphologically. Other types arise from myeloblasts and exhibit the corresponding morphology. Myelomonocytic leukemias develop from common precursors of the granulocytic and monocytic lineage. According to the French-American-British (FAB) classification system, acute myeloid leukemias (AML) are divided into eight subgroups (M0 to M7) using morphological criteria and cytochemical staining techniques (e.g., the detection of specific enzymes, such as myeloperoxidase, MPO).

B. Phenotypic Features of Acute Myeloid Leukemias

Lymphoid and myeloid leukemias are managed differently. Immunological typing is most important in cases where it is not possible to determine the lineage using morphological criteria. "Immature" leukemias, such as M0 leukemia, are characterized by the expression of only a few antigens (e.g., CD117 and CD34) or the weak expression of early myeloid antigens (CD13 and CD33). It is usually easy to distinguish AML types M1, M2, and M3 by light microscopy. There is no correlation with the expression of specific antigens. In myelomonocytic leukemia (AML-M4) and monocytic leukemia (AML-M5), the patients test positive for CD14 and CD64. M6 leukemias express glycophorin-A, an antigen of the erythrocytic lineage. M7 leukemias are positive for CD61, an integrin found on platelets and megakaryocytes.

C. Phenotypic Features of Acute Lymphatic Leukemias

Undifferentiated leukemias that do not express lineage-specific antigens are rare. In this case, the enzyme terminal deoxynucleotidyltransferase (Tdt) is usually detectable. Several subtypes of lymphoblastic leukemia can be distinguished. Most leukemias arise from neoplastic proliferation at the early stages of B-cell maturation (pro-B and pre-B leukemia). In children, the expression of CD10 (common ALL antigen) defines a subgroup of leukemias with a good prognosis. However, CD10 is of little predictive value in adults. In mature-cell B-cell leukemias, immunoglobulins are expressed on the cell membrane (sIg), while in pro-B and pre-B ALL the immunoglobulin-associated α-chain is expressed. Mature B-type leukemias have a poor prognosis and must be treated aggressively. Leukemias of T-cell lineage express CD3 either in the cytoplasm or on the cell surface. The expression of CD1a and CD2 identifies various subtypes of leukemia (pro-T, pre-T, cortical thymocyte type, and mature T-ALL) but is of little clinical relevance.

D. Cytogenetic Features of Acute Myeloid and Lymphatic Leukemias

Mutations, chromosome deletions (del), and chromosome translocations (t) that cause the dysfunction or inhibition of a gene product important for cell differentiation or division are the most common causes of leukemia. These biological features are of great prognostic importance, but they seldom correlate with specific morphological criteria. M3 promyelocytic leukemia, which develops due to 15:17 chromosome translocation, is morphologically characterized by large quantities of azurophilic granules. Leukemias with chromosome 16 inversion or deletion are associated with eosinophilia (M4Eo). Translocations involving chromosomes 8 and 21 are often observed in M2 myeloid leukemia. These three types of leukemia have a better prognosis than most other types, especially those with complex genetic anomalies. Translocations or other abnormalities of band q23 of chromosome 11 are frequently found in myelomonocytic leukemias and particularly in secondary leukemias that develop after exposure to certain drugs. In the future, prognostically significant classifications of leukemia will be based on genetic features. The most common anomalies are listed in (D).

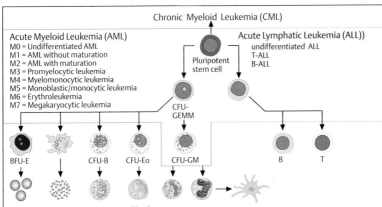

Chronic Myeloid Leukemia (CML)

Acute Myeloid Leukemia (AML)
M0 = Undifferentiated AML
M1 = AML without maturation
M2 = AML with maturation
M3 = Promyelocytic leukemia
M4 = Myelomonocytic leukemia
M5 = Monoblastic/monocytic leukemia
M6 = Erythroleukemia
M7 = Megakaryocytic leukemia

Pluripotent stem cell

Acute Lymphatic Leukemia (ALL))
undifferentiated ALL
T-ALL
B-ALL

CFU-GEMM

BFU-E   CFU-B   CFU-Eo   CFU-GM   B   T

A. Hematopoiesis and origin of leukemia

	MPO	HLA-DR	CD34	CD117	CD13	CD14	CD15	CD33	CD61	CD64
M0	+/-	+/-	+/-	+	+/-	-	-	+/-	-	-
M1	+	+/-	+/-	+/-	+/-	-	-	+/-	-	-
M2	+	+	+/-	+/-	+	-	+/-	+/-	-	-
M3	+	-	-	-	-/+	+	+	+	-	+/-
M4	+	+	-/+	+/-	+	+/-	+/-	+	-	+
M5	-	+	-/+	-/+	+	+/-	+	+	-	+
M7	-	+/-			+/-	-	-	+/-	+	
M6	= positive for glycophorin -A									

B. Immunophenotypic features of acute myeloid leukemias

	TdT	CD1a	CD2	cyCD3	mCD3	CD10	CD19	CD79α	cyIg	sIg
Pro-T-ALL	+	-	-	+		+/-	-	-	-	-
Pre-T-ALL	+	-	+	+		+/-	-	-	-	-
Cortical-ALL	+	+	+	+/-	+/-	+/-	-	-	-	-
Mature T-ALL	+/-	-	+	-	+	-	-	-	-	-
Pro-B-ALL	+	-	-	-		-	+	+	-	-
Pre-B-ALL	+	-	-	-		+/-	+	+	+	-
Mature B-ALL	-	-	-	-		+/-	+	+	-	+

C. Immunophenotypic features of acute lymphatic leukemias

Myeloid leukemias		Lymphatic leukemias	
t(8;21)	M2	t(9;22)	Ph'+-ALL
inv(16), del(16q)	M4Eo	t(4;11)	newborn -ALL or biphenotypic ALL
t(15;17)	M3	t(8;14), (2;8), (8;22)	B-ALL
t(11;17)	M3-like	t(11;14), (1;14)	T-ALL
del(11)(q22-23)	M5, M4	t(1;19)	pre-B-ALL
t(9;11), t(11;19)	M5, M4	t(5;14)	B-ALL
monosomy/del 7 & 5	M1, M2, M5	del 9, t(9;n..)	hyperleuk., extramedull. manifestations

D. Cytogenetic features of acute myeloid and lymphocytic leukemias

Overview of Lymphoma Classifications

Malignant lymphomas are proliferative diseases that arise from the lymph nodes or extranodal lymphatic tissue. In accordance with the variety of stages involved in the maturation and differentiation of lymphatic cells, a number of different types of lymphomas exist.

Hodgkin's disease was viewed as a separate entity because of its distinctive morphological and clinical features. The cell of origin of Hodgkin's lymphoma was a matter of discussion for many years; the strict distinction between Hodgkin's lymphoma and other lymphomas collectively defined as "non-Hodgkin's lymphomas" may be dropped in the future.

The *Kiel classification* was established on the European continent in the past few decades. It attempted to relate the various lymphoma entities to immunologically defined cells of origin. This was based not only on morphological criteria, but also and most importantly on the immunophenotypic features of lymphoma cells as determined by immunohistochemical staining techniques. Centrocytic and centroblastic lymphomas, for example, were characterized according to the normal physiology of the germinal center, and differences between T-cell and B-cell lymphomas were defined. By differentiating between low-grade and high-grade malignant lymphomas, the Kiel system also attempted to describe the clinical relevance of the lymphomas.

The Kiel classification did not gain acceptance on the American continent. The Revised European-American Lymphoma Classification (REAL) was therefore established by an international panel in 1994. The REAL classification did not attempt to be a "biologically correct" lymphoma classification, but merely provided a list of well-defined entities based on the latest morphological, immunological, molecular biological, and genetic techniques. Some lymphoma categories were provisionally defined.

The REAL classification of malignant lymphomas is presented in (A). The lymphoma entities of the Kiel classification are also listed for comparison. Hodgkin's disease will be discussed on p. 132, and other lymphomas (non-Hodgkin's lymphomas) will be discussed on pp. 134–141.

Kiel Classification of Malignant Non-Hodgkin's Lymphomas

B-Cell Lymphomas	T-Cell Lymphomas
Low-grade Malignant Lymphomas	
• Lymphocytic: B-CLL, B-PLL, hairy cell leukemia	• T-CLL, T-prolymphocytic leukemia (PLL)
• Lymphocytic/plasmacytoid lymphoma (immunocytoma)	• Large granular lymphocyte lymphocytosis
• Plasmacytoid lymphoma, plasmacytoma	• Mycosis fungoides, Sézary syndrome
• Centroblastic/centrocytic lymphoma (follicular, follicular + diffuse, diffuse) T-zone lymphoma	• Lymphoepithelioid lymphoma
• Angioimmunoblastic lymphoma (AILD, LgX)	• Pleomorphic small-cell lymphoma
Intermediate-grade Malignant Lymphomas	
• Centrocytic lymphoma	
High-grade malignant lymphomas	
• Centroblastic lymphoma	• Pleomorphic medium to large-cell T-cell lymphoma
• Immunoblastic lymphoma Burkitt's lymphoma	• T-immunoblastic lymphoma
• Large-cell anaplastic CD30⁺ B-cell lymphoma	• T-lymphoblastic lymphoma
	• Large-cell anaplastic CD30⁺ T-cell lymphoma

B-Cell Lymphomas

I. Precursor B-cell neoplasia

Precursor-B-lymphoblastic lymphomas/leukemias — B-lymphoblastic lymphoma

II. Peripheral B-cell neoplasia

	1. REAL classification	2. Kiel classification
1.	CLL, PLL, small-cell lymphocytic lymphomas	B-lymphocytic lymphoma
2.	Lymphoplasmacytoid lymphoma (immunocyt.)	Lymphoplasmacytic immunocytoma
3.	Mantle cell lymphoma	Centrocytic lymphoma Centrocytoid subtype of centroblastic lymphoma
4.	Follicular center lymphoma, follicular, grade I – III diffuse (predominantly small cell) (preliminary)	Centroblastic-centrocytic lymphoma Follicular, diffuse
5.	Marginal zone-B-cell lymphoma, extranodal (MALT-type, +/- monocytoid B cells), nodal (+/- monocytoid B cells)	Monocytoid lymphoma, including marginal zone lymphoma
6.	Marginal zone lymphoma of the spleen (preliminary)	
7.	Hairy cell leukemia	Hairy cell leukemia
8.	Plasmocytoma/myeloma	Plasmocytic lymphoma
9.	Diffuse large cell B-cell lymphoma (subtype: primary mediastinal large cell B-cell lymphoma)	Centroblastic lymphoma, B-immunoblastic Lymphoma, large cell anaplastic Ki1+ lymphoma
10.	Burkitt's lymphoma	Burkitt's-lymphoma
11.	High-malignancy B-cell lymphoma, Burkitt-like	Centroblastic, immunoblastic lymphoma

T-Cell and Natural Killer-Cell Lymphomas

I. Precursor T-cell neoplasias

Precursor T-lymphoblastic lymphoma /leukemia — T-lymphoblastic lymphoma

II. Peripheral T-cell and NK-cell neoplasias

1.	T-CLL /T-PLL (prolymphocytic leukemia)	T-lymphocytic lymphoma, CLL-type, PLL-type
2.	Large cell granular lymphocyte leukemia a) T-cell type; b) NK-cell type	T-lymphocytic lymphoma, CLL-type
3.	Mycosis fungoides/Sézary syndrome	Mycosis fungoides, Sézary syndrome
4.	Peripheral T-cell lymphomas, subcutanous panniculitic lymphoma (preliminary), hepatosplenic γ-δ-lymphoma (preliminary)	T-zone lymphoma, lymphoepitelioid lymphoma, Pleomorphic small/large cell lymphoma, T-immunoblastic lymphoma
5.	Angioimmunoblastic T-cell lymphoma	Angioimmunoblastic lymphoma (AILD, LgX)
6.	Angiocentric lymphoma	
7.	Intestinal T-cell lymphoma (+/- enteropathy)	
8.	Adult T-cell lymphoma/leukemia, HTLV1+	Pleomorphic HTLV1+ lymphoma
9.	Anaplastic large cell lymphoma (T and null)	Anaplastic large cell T-cell lymphoma (Ki1+)

Hodgkin's Lymphoma

I.	Lymphocyte-predominante type	
II.	Nodular-sclerosis type	Nodular sclerosis type
III.	Mixed cellularity type	Mixed cellularity type
IV.	Lymphocyte depletion type	Lymphocyte-depletion type
V.	Lymphocyte-rich classic type	Lymphocyte-predominante type

1. REAL classification **2.** Kiel classification

A. Lymphoma entities: REAL classification vs. Kiel classification

Clinical Immunology

A. Pathogenetic Model

Some 160 years after it was first described, the pathogenesis of Hodgkin's disease still has not been fully explained. The characteristic **R**eed–**S**ternberg (RS) cells or **H**odgkin's **d**isease (HD) cells (binuclear or polynuclear cells with large nucleoli and a broad, bright cytoplasm) comprise only 1–2% of the total cell population of an affected lymph node. The rest is a variegated infiltrate consisting of lymphocytes, histiocytes, eosinophils, plasma cells, and fibroblasts. Clonal translocation of genes for heavy immunoglobulin chains was found in a number of RS cells. This finding indicates that the cells are of B lymphocyte origin. The Epstein–Barr viral genome can be detected in the RS cells in 50% of cases, and strong expression of B-cell antigens can also be observed. It is therefore undisputed that the lymphocyte-predominant type (B.1) corresponds to a B-cell lymphoma. Nonetheless, some rare HD/RS cells exhibit features of activated T cells, whereas other express antigens typical of dendritic cells, e.g., CD83 and p55. RS cells also possess all molecules required for antigen presentation: class I and II MHC molecules, co-stimulatory antigens CD80 and CD86, and adhesion molecules CD54 and CD58. CD30 interacts with CD30L, an antigen expressed by T lymphocytes, monocytes, and macrophages. This, in turn, induces the secretion of cytokines by RS cells. IL-5, and particularly eotaxin, are responsible for eosinophilic infiltration. IL-1, IL-6, and IL-9 act as autocrine and paracrine growth factors. Abnormal upregulation of the transcription factor NFκB is a typical hallmark of the disease and contributes to the upregulation of cytokine production. Fibrosis, a typical feature of Hodgkin's disease, is caused by IL-1 and TGF-β.

B. Histological Classification

Nodular sclerosis is the most common subtype of Hodgkin's disease and is characterized by collagen bands with various degrees of sclerosis. Nodular sclerosis HD has a good prognosis. In lymphocyte-predominant subtypes (*paragranulomas*), only a few RS cells are present. This subtype is clearly of B-cell origin, it shows a slow growth tendency and has an excellent prognosis. Lymphocyte depletion is the least uncommon subtype. This form of Hodgkin's disease is morphologically similar to a different entity, the large-cell anaplastic lymphoma (see p. 135). Any variant not matching one of these three types is defined as mixed cellularity Hodgkin's disease.

C. Symptoms

Painless enlargement of the lymph nodes is common in Hodgkin's disease. The presenting symptoms are recurrent fever, night sweats, and weight loss ("B symptoms") in 10–50% of patients, depending on the stage of the disease. In advanced stages, the manifestations of Hodgkin's disease become more and more pronounced in extralymphatic organs, such as the liver, bone marrow, bone, lungs, and skin.

D. Laboratory Findings

The typical signs of inflammation in Hodgkin's disease include a high erythrocyte sedimentation rate (ESR), anemia, iron deficiency, and elevated α_2-globulin, ferritin, and copper levels. Neutrophilia or monocytosis is common. Eosinophilia is rare but can be extreme. Lymphocytopenia occurs in more than 30% of patients. A soluble form of CD30 antigen (sCD30) is occasionally present in serum. Elevated sCD30 levels correlate with the stage of disease. This finding is a negative prognostic factor; so is the concentration of soluble IL-2 receptor (sCD25) in serum.

E. Therapy

Most patients with Hodgkin's disease can now be cured. The prognosis depends on the degree of spread and the presence of risk factors (e.g., large mediastinal tumor, extranodal involvement, massive splenic involvement, elevated ESR). When started in early stages, radiotherapy leads to remission in ca. 80% of patients without risk factors. Both the affected and the adjacent lymph node regions are often irradiated in the so-called "upper mantle field" and "inverted Y field" protocols (**1**). Polychemotherapy is performed in advanced disease or in high-risk patients. High-dose chemotherapy with autologous stem cell transplantation may be indicated if relapse occurs. Experimental treatment strategies are now being tested. One of these is based on *bispecific antibodies* that bring cytotoxic T cells to CD30$^+$ Hodgkin's cells (targeting) (**3**).

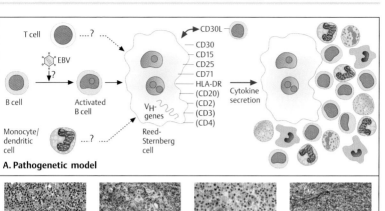

A. Pathogenetic model

T cell ....?

EBV

B cell → Activated B cell → Reed-Sternberg cell

Monocyte/dendritic cell ....?

V_H-genes

CD30L
CD30
CD15
CD25
CD71
HLA-DR
(CD20)
(CD2)
(CD3)
(CD4)

Cytokine secretion

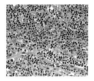
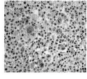

Lymphocyte predominant type ca.12%

Nodular sclerosis type ca. 46%

Mixed cellularity type ca. 31%

Lymphocyte-depletion type ca. 10%

B. Histological classification

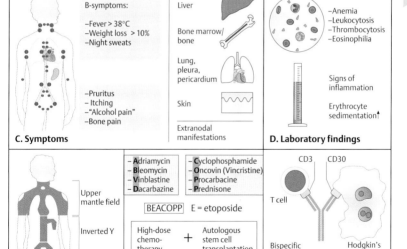

B-symptoms:

−Fever > 38°C
−Weight loss > 10%
−Night sweats

−Pruritus
− Itching
– "Alcohol pain"
−Bone pain

Liver

Bone marrow/bone

Lung, pleura, pericardium

Skin

Extranodal manifestations

C. Symptoms

−Anemia
−Leukocytosis
−Thrombocytosis
−Eosinophilia

Signs of inflammation

Erythrocyte sedimentation↑

D. Laboratory findings

Upper mantle field

Inverted Y

− **A**driamycin
− **B**leomycin
− **V**inblastine
− **D**acarbazine

− **C**yclophosphamide
− **O**ncovin (Vincristine)
− **P**rocarbacine
− **P**rednisone

BEACOPP E = etoposide

High-dose chemo-therapy + Autologous stem cell transplantation

CD3   CD30

T cell

Bispecific antibody

Hodgkin's cell

1. Radiotherapy

2. Polychemotherapy

3. Experimental approaches

E. Therapy

A. Precursor T-Lymphoblastic Lymphoma/Leukemia (T-LBL)

Lymphoblastic lymphomas primarily arise from the lymph nodes and later colonize the bone marrow, whereas lymphoblastic leukemias primarily arise from the bone marrow and later infiltrate the lymph nodes. Since it is often difficult to distinguish between the two, leukemia is diagnosed when lymph cells comprise more than 25% of the cell population within the bone marrow. T-cell lymphoblastic lymphomas comprise around 40% of all lymphoma cases in children. In adults, on the other hand, they comprise only around 2% of all non-Hodgkin's lymphomas (NHL) and around 15% of all acute lymphatic leukemias. Young men are most commonly affected. They present with rapidly growing mediastinal masses (arising from the thymus) and/or peripheral lymphadenopathy. If left untreated, the lymphoma cell contents are released from the lymph nodes and the disease rapidly progresses to death. Lymphoblasts arise from thymocytes; they have round nuclei with small quantities of cytoplasm. The tumor cells express CD7 and CD3 in the cytoplasm or on the cell surface. The expression of other T-cell markers, such as CD2 and CD5, is variable. The enzyme terminal deoxynucleotidyl transferase (Tdt) is typically expressed in the nucleus. Aggressive chemotherapy can cure this otherwise fatal disease.

B. Peripheral T-Cell Neoplasms

1 T-cell chronic lymphocytic leukemia (T-CLL) is a rare form of non-Hodgkin's lymphoma. In most case of T-CLL, the cells have irregular nuclei with prominent nucleoli and a relatively broad cytoplasm. They are therefore classified as prolymphocytes. The disease is indistinguishable from T-cell prolymphocytic leukemia (T-PLL). The lymphocytes usually infiltrate the bone marrow, spleen, liver, and lymph nodes, but may also infiltrate skin and mucosae. Lymphocyte counts of over 100 000/mm³ are often observed. The leukemic cells express the T-cell markers CD2, CD3, CD5, CD7 and, in most cases, CD4 (65%); the concomitant expression of CD4 and CD8 is occasionally observed. Inversion of chromosome 14 (q11:q32) is found in 75% of cases; trisomy 8 has also been reported. The prognosis is unfavorable, in fact, much worse than that of chronic B-cell lymphocytic leukemia.

2 Large granular lymphocyte (LGL) leukemia arises from circulating CD8⁺ T cells or NK cells. Moderate leukocytosis (lymphocyte counts of up to 20 000/mm³) is a typical finding that is often associated with neutropenia. Anemia and mild splenomegaly usually occur in the T-cell subtype. The course of disease is mild, with cytopenia being the most common cause of symptoms. The tumor cells have an eccentric, roundish to oval nucleus within a pale bluish cytoplasm containing azurophilic granules. The phenotype of the T-cell subtype (CD3⁺, CD8⁺, CD16⁺, TCRαβ⁺) corresponds to cytotoxic T cells. That of the NK subtype, on the other hand, is CD3⁻, TCRαβ⁻, CD56⁺/⁻, CD16⁺, and CD8⁺/⁻.

3 *Mycosis fungoides*, a cutaneous lymphoma, and *Sézary syndrome*, its generalized counterpart, arise from peripheral epidermotropic CD4⁺ T cells. The patients present with pruritic eczema, which later transforms into cutaneous plaques or nodules. Patients with Sézary syndrome develop diffuse erythroderma (*homme rouge*), which is sometimes unbearably pruritic. High numbers of lymphoma cells circulate in the blood in Sézary syndrome, but only isolated cells occur in mycosis fungoides. Anaplastic large-cell lymphoma (ALCL) may develop as the disease progresses. Histological studies reveal the presence of small lymphocytes with cerebriform nuclei in infiltrates from the skin and paracortex of lymph nodes. The tumor cells express CD2, CD3, CD5 and, in most cases, CD4.

4 *Peripheral T-cell lymphomas* can arise from peripheral T cells at various stages of maturation. These neoplasms comprise ca. 10% of all NHL. This is a heterogeneous but still provisionally defined group of lymphomas. The tumor cells often have irregular nuclei and are greatly variable in size. T-cell markers are variably pronounced. Most of the tumor cells are CD4⁺. Some have a high content of epithelioid cells (Lennert's lymphoma or lymphoepithelioid lymphoma). Hepatosplenic γ/δ lymphoma is characterized by extensive infiltration of the liver and spleen. Unlike most other lymphomas, the lymphoma cells express γ/δ T-cell receptors.

5 Other peripheral lymphomas are listed separately because they represent clinically well defined entities. *Angioimmunoblastic T-cell lymphoma* manifests with symptoms of generalized lymphadenopathy in conjunction

with fever, weight loss, skin redness, and polyclonal hypergammaglobulinemia. This disease is also referred to as *angioimmunoblastic lymphadenopathy with dysproteinemia* (AILD). The lymph node architecture is destroyed, the sinus is dilated, and the infiltrates penetrate through the capsule into the perinodal fatty tissue. Aggregates of follicular dendritic cells (FDC) surround proliferating, branching venules. The tumor cells exhibit translocation of the T-cell receptor. They express T-cell markers and are usually CD4+. High-grade malignant T-cell or B-cell lymphomas may occasionally develop.

6 *Angiocentric lymphomas* presumably arise from NK cells or T cells; they affect the nose, palate, and skin. These lymphomas may be indolent or aggressive. Infiltrates containing small lymphocytes and atypical lymphoid cells are usually found. The vascular lumen becomes sealed off, thus leading to ischemic necrosis. The tumor cells express CD2 and, in many cases, CD7 and CD5. They are sometimes CD3- and CD56+.

7 *Intestinal T-cell lymphomas* most commonly occur in patients with a history of gluten-sensitive enteropathy. The entity was formerly called "malignant intestinal histiocytosis." The patients have multifocal malignant ulcers in the jejunum that tend to perforate. The lymphomas contain a mixture of cells of different sizes. The abnormal cells are CD3+ and CD7+ and sometimes CD8+. They may also express CD103, a mucosal T-cell-associated antigen.

8 *Adult T-cell lymphoma/leukemia* is caused by HTLV1, the human T cell lymphotropic virus. This entity mainly occurs in Japan and the Caribbean, but also occurs sporadically in Europe. The course of disease is usually acute, with severe leukocytosis, hepatosplenomegaly, hypercalcemia, and osteolysis. The mean survival time is less than one year. Cells with multilobular, cloverlike nuclei are present in the peripheral blood. The tumor cells express CD3, CD2, CD4, and CD25, and are CD7-negative. A chronic form characterized by less severe leukocytosis and a lack of hepatosplenomegaly and osteolysis has a somewhat better prognosis.

9 *Anaplastic large-cell lymphomas (ALCL)* arise from CD30+ extrafollicular blasts. The disease may be primarily systemic or cutaneous, or may occur as a secondary neoplasm. The primary cutaneous subtype has a much better prognosis. The tumor cells are large, cytoplasm-rich blasts that often have horseshoe-shaped or multiple nuclei, each with multiple nucleoli. The multinucleate forms sometimes resemble Reed–Sternberg cells. The majority of these tumors have T-cell-associated markers (CD3+/-, CD25+/-); rearrangement of the T-cell receptor is observed in over 50%. Along with CD30, the tumor cells also express epithelial membrane antigen (EMA). Primary systemic ALCL is often associated with 2:5 translocation in which the nucleophosmin gene NPM, a cell cycle-regulating nucleolar protein, fuses with a kinase belonging to the family of insulin receptors (anaplastic lymphoma kinase, ALK) to give origin to the NPM-ALK fusion protein. Alterations of the kinase is assumed to play a role in the lymphoma genesis.

Clinical Immunology

135

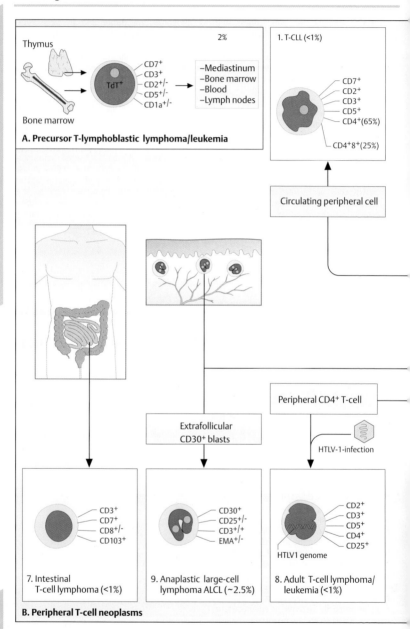

A. Precursor T-lymphoblastic lymphoma/leukemia

Thymus

Bone marrow

TdT+

CD7+
CD3+
CD2+/−
CD5+/−
CD1a+/−

2%

−Mediastinum
−Bone marrow
−Blood
−Lymph nodes

1. T-CLL (<1%)

CD7+
CD2+
CD3+
CD5+
CD4+ (65%)

CD4+8+ (25%)

Circulating peripheral cell

Peripheral CD4+ T-cell

Extrafollicular
CD30+ blasts

HTLV-1-infection

7. Intestinal
T-cell lymphoma (<1%)

CD3+
CD7+
CD8+/−
CD103+

9. Anaplastic large-cell
lymphoma ALCL (~2.5%)

CD30+
CD25+/−
CD3+/+
EMA+/−

8. Adult T-cell lymphoma/
leukemia (<1%)

CD2+
CD3+
CD5+
CD4+
CD25+

HTLV1 genome

B. Peripheral T-cell neoplasms

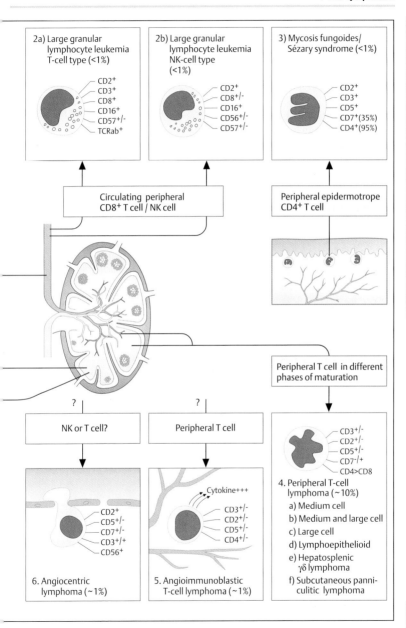

2a) Large granular lymphocyte leukemia T-cell type (<1%)

- CD2+
- CD3+
- CD8+
- CD16+
- CD57+/-
- TCRab+

2b) Large granular lymphocyte leukemia NK-cell type (<1%)

- CD2+
- CD8+/-
- CD16+
- CD56+/-
- CD57+/-

3) Mycosis fungoides/ Sézary syndrome (<1%)

- CD2+
- CD3+
- CD5+
- CD7+(35%)
- CD4+(95%)

Circulating peripheral CD8+ T cell / NK cell

Peripheral epidermotrope CD4+ T cell

Peripheral T cell in different phases of maturation

- CD3+/-
- CD2+/-
- CD5+/-
- CD7-/+
- CD4>CD8

NK or T cell?

Peripheral T cell

4. Peripheral T-cell lymphoma (~10%)
   a) Medium cell
   b) Medium and large cell
   c) Large cell
   d) Lymphoepithelioid
   e) Hepatosplenic γδ lymphoma
   f) Subcutaneous panni- culitic lymphoma

Cytokine+++

- CD3+/-
- CD2+/-
- CD5+/-
- CD4+/-

- CD2+
- CD5+/-
- CD7+/-
- CD3+/+
- CD56+

6. Angiocentric lymphoma (~1%)

5. Angioimmunoblastic T-cell lymphoma (~1%)

Clinical Immunology

137

Clinical Immunology

A. Precursor B-Cell Tumors

Neoplastic diseases involving precursor B cells can manifest with the clinical picture of acute lymphoblastic leukemia with bone marrow infiltration and leukemic blood picture. In children, the disease is frequently characterized by tumorous swelling of lymph nodes and skin infiltration, with or without bone marrow involvement. In the latter case, the leukemic course associated with bone marrow infiltration develops in the later stages. The tumor cells express B-cell-specific antigens, such as CD19, cytoplasmic CD22, and CD79a. In many cases, CD10/common ALL antigen is also positive. This corresponds to a subgroup of leukemias with a relatively favorable prognosis in children, but not in adults. The expression of surface immunoglobulins by the lymphoma/leukemia cells reflects a very poor prognosis. Translocations involving chromosomes 1 and 19 and/or chromosomes 9 and 22 or changes in chromosome 11q are also associated with a very poor prognosis.

B. Peripheral B-Cell Neoplasms

1 Around 80% of all non-Hodgkin's lymphomas are peripheral B-cell neoplasms. Diseases such as chronic lymphocytic leukemia (B-CLL) or prolymphocytic leukemia (B-PLL) usually produce large numbers of leukocytes in the peripheral blood and extensive bone marrow infiltration. The lymph nodes, spleen, and liver may be involved. Most B-CLL tumor cells are small lymphocytes with round nuclei. PLL cells are larger and have a prominent central nucleolus. Prolymphocytic leukemia is associated with severe splenomegaly and aggressive behavior, whereas chronic lymphocytic leukemia often has a slowly progressive, indolent course. CLL cells express the classical B-cell markers CD19, CD20, and CD22, but also typically express CD23 and CD5 (a T-cell-associated antigen). Surface immunoglobulins are only weakly expressed. CLL is usually diagnosed by blood smear and/or bone marrow cytology. Its histological correlative in the lymph node is lymphocytic lymphoma. Chromosome 13 deletion or trisomy 12 occurs in approximately 30% of cases. Deletion of chromosome 17p is associated with a poor prognosis.

2 *Lymphocytic plasmacytoid lymphomas* (*immunocytomas*) arise from small lymphoid cells that have begun to differentiate into plasma cells. Most cases correspond to the clinical picture of Waldenström's macroglobulinemia (see p. 143**B**). Accordingly, an IgM class monoclonal paraprotein is often found. Most tumor cells are small lymphocytes with a distinct basophilic cytoplasm, but there is a variable number of plasma cells. These lymphomas are typically associated with the presence of intracytoplasmic immunoglobulins (cyt-Ig). Deletions of chromosome 11, 13, or 17 are the most common gene rearrangements. A subset of patients has chromosomal translocation t(9;14) involving the *pax-5* gene.

3 *Mantle cell lymphoma* largely corresponds to centrocytic lymphoma as defined by the Kiel classification. The tumor cells are small to medium-sized lymphocytes with a notched nucleus and, in some cases, larger nucleoli. The cells express surface immunoglobulins and T-cell-associated antigen CD5. Overexpression of cyclin D1, a cell cycle-associated protein, occurs due to translocation of chromosomes 11 and 14. The disease mainly affects older men and is often disseminated by the time of diagnosis. The prognosis is poor, with an average survival time of 3–5 years.

4 A quarter of all NHL are *germinal center lymphomas*, which arise from germinal center B cells, centrocytes, and centroblasts. Men and women are equally affected. The content of centrocytes and centroblasts varies, but centrocytes are usually far more predominant. A diffuse growth pattern is associated with a poorer prognosis. The tumor cells are positive for surface immunoglobulins and for CD10. The anti-apoptotic gene *bcl-2* is activated by 14:18 translocation, which leads to the accumulation of long-lived centrocytes.

5 *Marginal zone lymphomas* (MZL) are broken down into two subtypes: extranodal and nodal. Extranodal MZL (**a**) consist of B cells from mucosa-associated lymphoid tissue (MALT). They comprise approximately 50% of all gastric lymphomas, ca. 40% of all orbital lymphomas, and the majority of lymphomas of the lungs, thyroid, and salivary glands. The gastric lymphomas are usually associated with *Helicobacter pylori* infection, which provides the stimulatory antigen responsible for the proliferation of mucosal lymphocytes. Antibacterial treatment can achieve lymphoma regression. Nodal marginal zone lym-

phomas (**b**) arise from monocytoid B cells in the marginal zone of the lymph nodes. The incidence of these lymphomas is increased in patients with Sjögren's syndrome (see p. 190). Nodal MZL are indolent lymphomas. The cells are phenotypically similar to those of extranodal MZL.

6 *Splenic marginal zone lymphomas* (SMZL) arise from small memory B cells that possibly undergo malignant transformation in the spleen after germinal center differentiation has taken place. These lymphomas usually infiltrate the bone marrow. The tumor cells circulate in the peripheral blood as shaggy, villous lymphocytes. Most splenic marginal zone lymphomas progress very slowly. Long-term remission can be achieved with splenectomy.

7 *Hairy cell leukemia* is characterized by the presence of cells with villous projections, an oval nucleus, and a broad margin of cytoplasm. This disease is typically characterized by splenomegaly and pancytopenia. Marked fibrosis of the bone marrow is almost invariably present, whereas lymph node involvement is rather unusual. The B cells are strongly positive for CD22 and express surface immunoglobulins. Positivity for CD103 is characteristic. This disease responds very well to purine analogues and interferon.

8 The REAL classification (see p. 130) defines plasmacytoma and multiple myeloma (see p. 145) as B-cell neoplasms because they can also arise from lymphoid tissue as solitary tumors.

9 *Diffuse large-cell lymphomas* are relatively common (ca. 30% of all NHL). They mainly affect adults, but can also occur in children. These lymphomas arise from peripheral B cells at different stages of maturation. Diffuse, large-cell lymphomas are very aggressive, but are principally curable with aggressive chemotherapy. Extranodal manifestation, e.g., in the stomach, CNS, bone, kidneys, and testicles, is common. Around 30% of cases involve translocation of the *bcl-2* gene and of the *bcl-6* gene, which codes for a transcriptional repressor gene. Translocation of c-*myc* has also been observed in some cases.

10 *Burkitt's lymphoma* arises from B lymphocytes immortalized by the genome of the Epstein–Barr virus. The tumor cells are medium-sized monomorphic cells with a round nucleus and multiple nucleoli. The cytoplasm is strongly basophilic. Infiltration with macrophages that phagocytize apoptotic tumor cells leads to the typical "starry sky" appearance observed in histology. Burkitt's lymphomas frequently occur in children. In adults, they tend to be associated with immune defects, particularly HIV infections. Burkitt's lymphoma is endemic to Africa, where mandibular involvement is typical. The disease usually involves translocation of the c-*myc* gene from chromosome 8 to the heavy chain gene region on chromosome 14. Translocation of c-*myc* to the light chain region in 2:8 or 8:22 translocation is less common.

11 Proliferating peripheral B cells may induce a high-grade malignant *Burkitt-like lymphoma*. The morphology and immunotype of these lymphomas resemble those of Burkitt's lymphoma, but c-*myc* translocation does not occur. Instead, translocation of the *bcl-2* gene occurs in 30% of cases.

Clinical Immunology

139

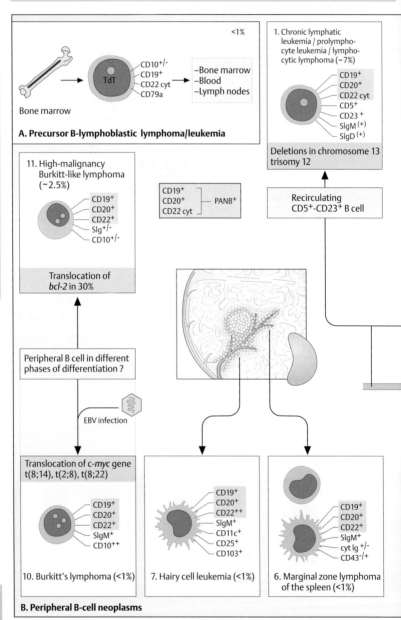

<1%

A. Precursor B-lymphoblastic lymphoma/leukemia

TdT

CD10+/−
CD19+
CD22 cyt
CD79a

Bone marrow

−Bone marrow
−Blood
−Lymph nodes

1. Chronic lymphatic leukemia / prolympho-cyte leukemia / lympho-cytic lymphoma (~7%)

CD19+
CD20+
CD22 cyt
CD5+
CD23+
SlgM (+)
SlgD (+)

Deletions in chromosome 13
trisomy 12

11. High-malignancy Burkitt-like lymphoma (~2.5%)

CD19+
CD20+
CD22+
Slg+/−
CD10+/−

Translocation of *bcl-2* in 30%

CD19+
CD20+ → PANB+
CD22 cyt

Recirculating CD5+-CD23+ B cell

Peripheral B cell in different phases of differentiation ?

EBV infection

Translocation of c-*myc* gene
t(8;14), t(2;8), t(8;22)

CD19+
CD20+
CD22+
SlgM+
CD10++

10. Burkitt's lymphoma (<1%)

CD19+
CD20+
CD22++
SlgM+
CD11c+
CD25+
CD103+

7. Hairy cell leukemia (<1%)

CD19+
CD20+
CD22+
SlgM+
cyt Ig +/−
CD43−/+

6. Marginal zone lymphoma of the spleen (<1%)

B. Peripheral B-cell neoplasms

Clinical Immunology

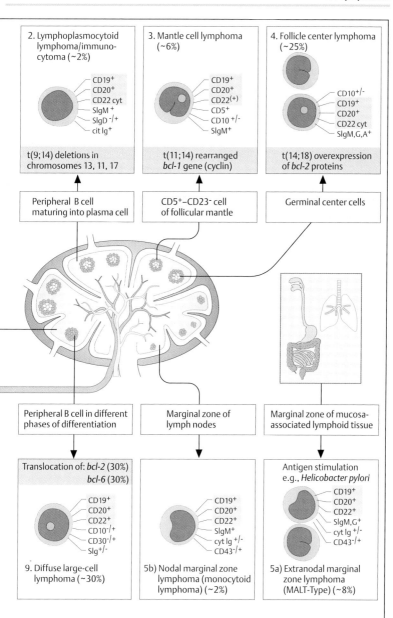

2. Lymphoplasmocytoid lymphoma/immuno-cytoma (~2%)

CD19+
CD20+
CD22 cyt
SIgM +
SIgD -/+
cit Ig+

t(9;14) deletions in chromosomes 13, 11, 17

Peripheral B cell maturing into plasma cell

3. Mantle cell lymphoma (~6%)

CD19+
CD20+
CD22(+)
CD5+
CD10 +/-
SIgM+

t(11;14) rearranged *bcl-1* gene (cyclin)

CD5+–CD23- cell of follicular mantle

4. Follicle center lymphoma (~25%)

CD10+/-
CD19+
CD20+
CD22 cyt
SIgM,G,A+

t(14;18) overexpression of *bcl-2* proteins

Germinal center cells

Peripheral B cell in different phases of differentiation

Marginal zone of lymph nodes

Marginal zone of mucosa-associated lymphoid tissue

Translocation of: *bcl-2* (30%)
                   bcl-6 (30%)

CD19+
CD20+
CD22+
CD10 -/+
CD30 -/+
SIg +/-

9. Diffuse large-cell lymphoma (~30%)

CD19+
CD20+
CD22+
SIgM+
cyt Ig +/-
CD43 -/+

5b) Nodal marginal zone lymphoma (monocytoid lymphoma) (~2%)

Antigen stimulation e.g., *Helicobacter pylori*

CD19+
CD20+
CD22+
SIgM,G+
cyt Ig +/-
CD43 -/+

5a) Extranodal marginal zone lymphoma (MALT-Type) (~8%)

Clinical Immunology

A. Polyclonal vs. Monoclonal Gamma-Globulin Proliferation

Antibody production by B lymphocytes is subject to regulation by T cells. The primary job of antibodies is to protect the body from infections by bacteria, viruses, or parasites. Since each pathogenic organism represents a mixture of different antigens, *polyclonal* B-cell stimulation always takes place. Each B-cell clone produces antibodies that target a specific antigen. Moreover, different antibodies of the various immunoglobulin classes are produced, resulting in a mixture of immunoglobulins. In protein electrophoresis, this is reflected as a broad-based increase of gamma-globulins. Malignant degeneration of B cells or defective T-cell regulation can lead to the uncontrolled proliferation of an individual B cell clone. The increased production of structurally homogeneous immunoglobulins can be identified in serum electrophoresis by the presence of so-called myeloma-associated or macroglobulinemia-associated (M) protein components, which appear as narrow-based spikes on the gamma-globulins curve (monoclonal gammopathy). Any neoplasm caused by mature B cells can theoretically lead to a monoclonal gammopathy which often remains undetected due to a low immunoglobulin content. M protein components were shown to occur in around 3% of all individuals over 70 years of age. In these patients, it is not possible to predict whether a plasma cell disorder (e.g., multiple myeloma, Waldenström's macroglobulinemia, or heavy chain disease) will develop. Hence, the diagnosis should be that of "monoclonal gammopathy of unknown significance (MGUS)" instead of the former diction "benign monoclonal gammopathy." A portion of these individuals will doubtlessly develop plasma cell dyscrasia, but many of them will die of old age before the disease becomes clinically manifest.

B. Waldenström's Macroglobulinemia

Macroglobulinemia is mainly a disease of the elderly. It is caused by the proliferation of small plasmacytoid lymphocytes with a variable fraction of more mature plasma cells. The abnormal cells initially infiltrate the bone marrow, and hepatomegaly and lymphadenopathy develop as the disease progresses. A leukemic release of the cells into peripheral blood occurs in the advanced stages of the disease. The cells secrete large quantities of monoclonal IgM molecules, which greatly increase the viscosity of the blood due to their pentameric structure. As a result, a hyperviscosity syndrome with associated circulatory disorders may develop. This may result in damage to the retina, leading to impaired vision or blindness, or may cause cerebral seizures, coma, or damage to the coronary arteries (ischemic heart disease, heart failure). The deposition of M proteins in the myelin sheath of neurons can induce polyneuropathy. Hemorrhage may also develop, especially in the skin of the lower extremities. Vasculitic changes may also occur due to the precipitation of immune complexes in the vessel walls.

C. Heavy Chain Disease

Heavy chain disease (HCD) is a rare condition characterized by the secretion of monoclonal proteins consisting of incomplete heavy chains of the immunoglobulins. *Gamma-HCD* is associated with the increased production of monoclonal γ chains of IgG. This subtype usually presents with lymphadenopathy and, infrequently, with osteolysis. *Alpha-HCD* ("Mediterranean lymphoma") is characterized by the pathological secretion of IgA by mucosal plasma cells of the intestines. This leads to the development of a malabsorption syndrome associated with diarrhea and abdominal pain. Bowel obstruction or perforation can occur during the course of the disease. This subtype mainly affects children and young adults. *Mu-HCD* occurs in conjunction with lymphoproliferative diseases, especially B-CLL. The bone marrow is typically infiltrated with vacuolated plasma cells. Light chains are also produced in many patients with μ-heavy chain disease, as is reflected by the presence of so-called Bence Jones proteins in the urine (see p. 133**A**).

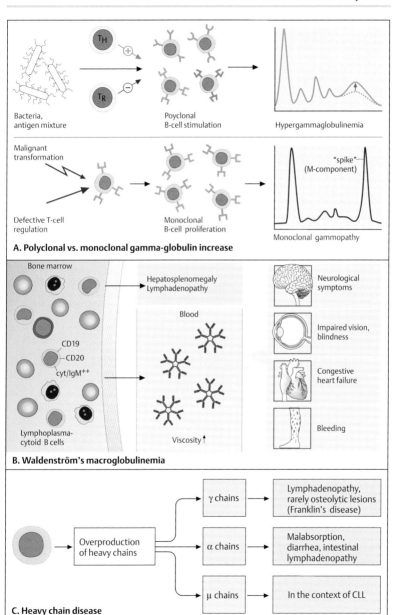

A. Polyclonal vs. monoclonal gamma-globulin increase

Bacteria, antigen mixture

Polyclonal B-cell stimulation

Hypergammaglobulinemia

Malignant transformation

Defective T-cell regulation

Monoclonal B-cell proliferation

"spike" (M-component)

Monoclonal gammopathy

B. Waldenström's macroglobulinemia

Bone marrow

Hepatosplenomegaly Lymphadenopathy

Blood

CD19
CD20
cyt/IgM++

Lymphoplasma-cytoid B cells

Viscosity ↑

Neurological symptoms

Impaired vision, blindness

Congestive heart failure

Bleeding

C. Heavy chain disease

Overproduction of heavy chains

γ chains → Lymphadenopathy, rarely osteolytic lesions (Franklin's disease)

α chains → Malabsorption, diarrhea, intestinal lymphadenopathy

μ chains → In the context of CLL

Clinical Immunology

143

Plasma cell neoplasms usually manifest as disseminated bone marrow lesions (*multiple myeloma*), but infrequently manifest as solitary extramedullary tumors classified as plasmacytomas or plasmacytoid lymphomas. Despite this difference, the terms "multiple myeloma" and "plasmacytoma" are often used synonymously. Plasma cells usually secrete IgG (ca. 60%) or IgA immunoglobulins (20%), but rarely IgD immunoglobulins (1–2%). Bence Jones plasmacytomas (15–20%) are characterized by the exclusive secretion of light chains. The complete absence of immunoglobulin synthesis or release (nonsecretory plasmacytoma) is rare (less than 1% of cases).

A. Pathogenesis and Pathomechanisms of Multiple Myeloma

IL-6 is essential for the growth of plasma cells. Autocrine production of IL-6 by myeloma cells is possible, but IL-6 and/or IL-6-like molecules can also be produced by stromal cells within the bone marrow. The potential role of Kaposi's sarcoma-associated herpes virus type 8 (HHV-8) in the development of multiple myeloma is still unclear.

Since large quantities of monoclonal protein are usually present, the viscosity of the blood can increase, thereby causing a hyperviscosity syndrome (see p. 143**B**). This most commonly occurs in IgA myelomas because IgA immunoglobulin tends to form polymers via sulfide bonds. Bence Jones plasmacytomas are characterized by exclusive light chain synthesis. In the electrophoresis, M gradients are not found since light chains are excreted with urine. However, light chains proteins (Bence Jones proteins) are also found in the urine of about 40% of patients with classical IgG or IgA plasmacytoma. They ultimately accumulate in the renal tubules as hyaline inclusion bodies, thereby causing a progressive decrease in kidney function.

There is a quantitative increase in the immunoglobulin concentration in the blood of myeloma patients, but all of the immunoglobulins have identical specificity and therefore do not contribute to immune defense. The concentration of normal immunoglobulins is usually decreased (secondary antibody deficiency) due to the disregulation of normal B cells and T cells. Cytotoxic T cells and cytokines secreted by myeloma cells inhibit erythropoiesis in the bone marrow, thereby leading to anemia. The picture of multiple myeloma is characterized by the presence of multiple osteolytic lesions that develop due to increased osteoclast activity. IL-1β and TNF-α have been identified as osteoclast-activating factors. The increasing degree of bone destruction leads to the release of calcium, resulting in hypercalcemia.

The osteolytic lesions are usually focal and occur at various sites, especially in bones with hematopoietic marrow, for example, in the ribs, sternum, vertebrae, clavicle, skull, scapula, pelvis, and proximal segments of the femur and humerus (**B**). They appear on radiographs as "hole-punch" lesions (**D**). The patients complain of bone pain, and pathological fractures frequently occur. Diffuse invasion of the vertebrae can mimic osteoporosis. Multiple myeloma is characterized by the proliferation of plasma cells within the bone marrow (**C**). The plasma cell content of the bone marrow is normally 5–10%, but can increase considerably in the presence of infections. Hence, an increase of plasma cells within the bone marrow should not be interpreted as diagnostic of multiple myeloma unless a monoclonal immunoglobulin is also detected. Plasma cell proliferation is often diffuse and can therefore be detected by bone marrow aspiration (cytology). However, a biopsy is required for diagnosis of focal bone marrow infiltration (histology). The appearance of plasma cells can vary greatly depending on the degree of maturation or malignant transformation of the cells. Large plasmablasts with nucleoli dominate the morphological picture of poorly differentiated plasma cells.

Treatment of plasmacytoma usually consists of alkylating agents (e.g., melphalan) and corticosteroids. The disease has a poor prognosis and cannot be cured by conventional chemotherapy. Younger patients may be considered for bone marrow transplantation.

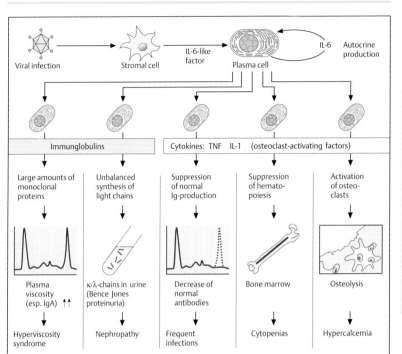

Viral infection → Stromal cell → IL-6-like factor → Plasma cell ← IL-6 Autocrine production

Immunglobulins | Cytokines: TNF IL-1 (osteoclast-activating factors)

Large amounts of monoclonal proteins

Unbalanced synthesis of light chains

Suppression of normal Ig-production

Suppression of hemato-poiesis

Activation of osteo-clasts

Plasma viscosity (esp. IgA) ↑↑

κ/λ-chains in urine (Bence Jones proteinuria)

Decrease of normal antibodies

Bone marrow

Osteolysis

Hyperviscosity syndrome

Nephropathy

Frequent infections

Cytopenias

Hypercalcemia

A. Pathogenesis and pathomechanisms of multiple myeloma

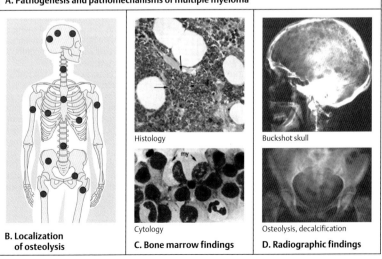

Histology

Cytology

B. Localization of osteolysis

C. Bone marrow findings

Buckshot skull

Osteolysis, decalcification

D. Radiographic findings

Clinical Immunology

145

A. Pathogenesis

Cryoglobulins are serum proteins that dissolve at 37 °C and precipitate at lower temperatures. The molecular basis of cryoprecipitation has yet to be explained. A change in the carbohydrate content, that is, a reduction in the sialic acid content, has been proposed as a possible cause.

B. Detection of Cryoglobulins

The detection of cryoglobulins in the blood requires the use of prewarmed syringes. The specimens must be immediately centrifuged at 37 °C to keep the cryoglobulins from precipitating with the cell sediment. The serum must then be promptly removed and stored at 4 °C for at least 72 hours. After subsequent centrifugation in capillary tubes, the precipitating cryoglobulins separate, forming *cryoprecipitate*.

C. Classification and Clinical Features

1 Type I cryoglobulins consist of a single monoclonal immunoglobulin component and are found in 20% of all cryoglobulinemias. They occur in multiple myeloma, Waldenström's macroglobulinemia, chronic lymphocytic leukemia (CLL), and other non-Hodgkin's lymphomas (NHL). Cryoglobulins are frequently present in multiple myeloma, whereas IgM antibodies predominate in the other diseases. In multiple myeloma and Waldenström's macroglobulinemia, around 10% and 20%, respectively, of the M proteins behave as cryoglobulins. The symptoms are primarily caused by the impaired or completely absent circulation in the capillaries of the skin: the low temperature on the skin surface leads to the intravascular precipitation of cryoglobulins and increases the serum viscosity. This may result in full vascular occlusion. Raynaud's phenomenon is a common feature (see p. 188), as are necrosis of the extremities, acrocyanosis, vascular purpura, and polyneuropathic ulcers of the ankles.

2 Type II cryoglobulins have a monoclonal immunoglobulin component (usually IgM but rarely IgA or IgG) and a polyclonal IgG component. Approximately 40% of all cryoglobulinemias correspond to this type. The monoclonal component exhibits reactivity to the F(ab)2 fragment of the polyclonal immunoglobulin (rheumatoid factor activity; see p. 172). Monoclonal immunoglobulins usually have κ light chains, but rarely λ light chains. No underlying disease can be identified in around one-third of the patients (essential mixed cryoglobulinemia). Hepatitis is common in these patients (usually chronic hepatitis C virus infection is considered to be the trigger of the disease), whereas connective tissue disease, other autoimmune disorders, and lymphoproliferative diseases are rare.

3 Type III cryoglobulins consist of polyclonal immunoglobulins, usually IgM, directed against polyclonal IgG and IgA molecules (mixed polyclonal type). About 40% of all cryoglobulins belong to this group. Type III cryoglobulins tend to arise in association with various infections and autoimmune diseases, but essential cryoglobulinemia also occurs in this group.

In mixed cryoglobulinemias, immunoglobulin-immune complexes precipitate in the vessel walls, thereby provoking an inflammatory response (vasculitis). The most prominent symptom is vascular purpura (punctiform or spot-like hemorrhages on the lower extremities). Ulcerations may develop in the region of the ankles. Motor and sensory polyneuropathies can manifest as paresis or paresthesia. Arthralgia, especially in the hands, knees, ankles, and elbows, occurs is 60–70% of patients. This can lead to redness and swelling, but joint deformity does not occur. More than 50% of these patients develop kidney disease over the course of time. The histological picture is usually one of proliferative glomerulonephritis caused by the deposition of immunoglobulins and complement (see p. 225, 227).

The prognosis of cryoglobulinemia varies in accordance with the severity of the underlying disease. Apart from avoiding the cold, the disease can be treated with corticosteroids, immunosuppressants, and interferon-α. In particular, interferon-α has been useful for the treatment of patients with hepatitis-associated cryoglobulinemia, eventually in association with antiviral substances (e.g., ribavirin). In acute crises, cryofiltration can be performed to quickly remove large quantities of cryoglobulins from the circulation.

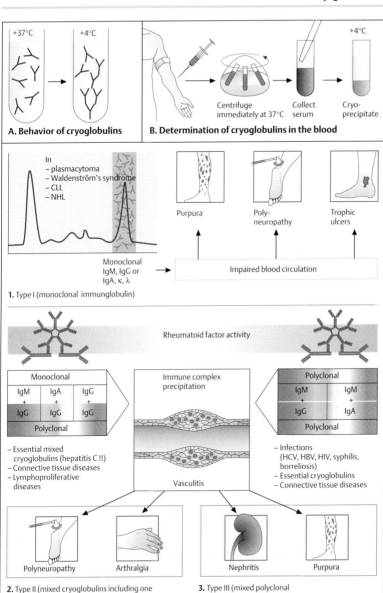

A. Behavior of cryoglobulins

B. Determination of cryoglobulins in the blood

Centrifuge immediately at 37°C — Collect serum — Cryo-precipitate

In
– plasmacytoma
– Waldenström's syndrome
– CLL
– NHL

Purpura

Poly-neuropathy

Trophic ulcers

Monoclonal IgM, IgG or IgA, κ, λ → Impaired blood circulation

1. Type I (monoclonal immunglobulin)

Rheumatoid factor activity

Monoclonal		
IgM	IgA	IgG
+	+	+
IgG	IgG	IgG
Polyclonal		

Immune complex precipitation

Polyclonal	
IgM	IgM
+	+
IgG	IgA
Polyclonal	

– Essential mixed cryoglobulins (hepatitis C !!)
– Connective tissue diseases
– Lymphoproliferative diseases

Vasculitis

– Infections (HCV, HBV, HIV, syphilis, borreliosis)
– Essential cryoglobulins
– Connective tissue diseases

Polyneuropathy

Arthralgia

Nephritis

Purpura

2. Type II (mixed cryoglobulins including one monoclonal immunglobulin)

3. Type III (mixed polyclonal cryoglobulins)

C. Classification of cryoglobulinemia

Clinical Immunology

147

A. Pathogenesis

Many disease processes are characterized by the infiltration of tissue with a homogeneous, eosinophilic material which, like starch (*amylon* = starch), is stained by iodine. These "amyloid" deposits consist of fibrillar proteins derived from polymerized peptide fragments (immunoglobulin light chains, amyloid A protein, β_2-microglobulin, transthyretin, β-protein A4, cystatin, procalcitonin, and α-natriuretic peptide). The antiparallel amyloid fibrils form twisted β-pleated sheets, which appear green under polarized light after staining with Congo red. Around 5–10% of the amyloid deposits consist of the nonfibrillary, pentagonal acute-phase protein, serum amyloid P (SAP), which is produced in hepatocytes.

B. Light Chain Amyloidosis (AL Amyloidosis)

Primary, non-hereditary light chain (AL) amyloidosis is characterized by the deposition of fibrils from fragments of immunoglobulin light chains (Bence Jones proteins; see p. 144). AL amyloidosis occurs in plasma cell dyscrasias, especially multiple myeloma or Waldenström's macroglobulinemia. Approximately 20% of all light chains tend to form amyloid, a subclass of λ chains (λ_{VI}) is often involved. Serum amyloid P produced by hepatocytes binds nonspecifically to the amyloid fibrils.

C. Amyloid A Amyloidosis (AA Amyloidosis)

Secondary or reactive systemic amyloidosis may develop as a complication of chronic infection (tuberculosis, bronchiectasis, chronic osteomyelitis), chronic inflammatory disease (rheumatoid arthritis, Crohn's disease), drug abuse, or cancer. In AA amyloidosis, the amyloid fibrils contain amyloid A, which forms after proteolytic cleavage of the acute-phase protein serum amyloid A (SAA). SAA is produced in hepatocytes or macrophages during an inflammation.

D. Hemodialysis-Associated Amyloidosis (AH Amyloidosis)

Beta-2-microglobulin (β_2m; see p. 48) is structurally similar to light chain immunoglobulin, the precursor substance of AL amyloid. Cells of the immune system and hepatocytes are the main sources of circulating β_2m. β_2m is processed by glomerular filtration and tubular reabsorption. As a result, β_2m levels in plasma are increased 40–60-fold in patients with renal failure. Since the β_2m molecule is too big to pass through most dialysis membranes, it continues to accumulate, despite hemodialysis. Newer dialysis membranes are now able to eliminate these molecules.

E. Clinical Features

Amyloidosis most commonly induces renal symptoms ranging from proteinuria to renal failure. Adrenocortical insufficiency is also common. Cardiac involvement is found in 80–90% of patients with AL amyloidosis. Amyloid deposits can lead to rigid thickening of the myocardium with cardiac insufficiency and arrhythmia. Liver function usually is not impaired despite massive hepatomegaly. Splenomegaly usually remains asymptomatic. Deposits in the carpal tunnel ligaments may compress the median nerve and cause paresthesia of the hands. Gastrointestinal involvement is observed in all forms of amyloidosis. Typical features include thickening of the tongue (macroglossia) and motility disorders associated with obstruction, malabsorption, and diarrhea. Amyloid deposits in the tracheobronchial tree may cause bronchitic symptoms.

Peripheral nervous system involvement is common in various forms of familial amyloidosis. Mutation of transthyretin, a thyroxine-binding and retinol-binding protein, is frequently observed. The clinical examination reveals sensory disorders associated with indolent ulcers or motor disorders. The accumulation of amyloid in the autonomic nervous systems manifests as dyshidrosis, incontinence, and impotence. The CNS is affected only in a form of amyloidosis called "senile amyloidosis." This entity leads to the deposition of the β-protein A4, which is coded by a gene located on chromosome 21. In some forms of Alzheimer's disease, missense mutations in the gene coding for amyloid precursor protein have been found. The abnormal peptide is prone to form plaques in the brain.

The diagnosis of amyloidosis is established by biopsy of the affected organs. Rectal biopsy and the aspiration of abdominal fat may lead to the diagnosis of systemic amyloidosis.

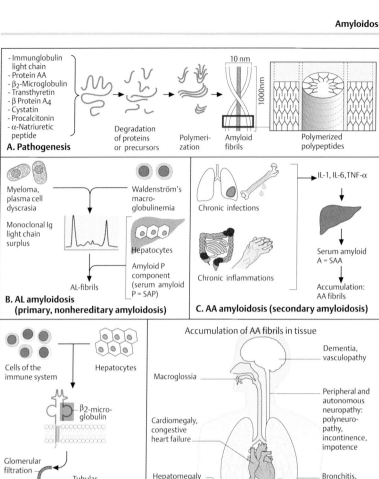

- Immunglobulin light chain
- Protein AA
- β₂-Microglobulin
- Transthyretin
- β Protein A₄
- Cystatin
- Procalcitonin
- α-Natriuretic peptide

Degradation of proteins or precursors

Polymeri-zation

Amyloid fibrils

10 nm

1000nm

Polymerized polypeptides

A. Pathogenesis

Myeloma, plasma cell dyscrasia

Waldenström's macro-globulinemia

Monoclonal Ig light chain surplus

Hepatocytes

Amyloid P component (serum amyloid P = SAP)

AL-fibrils

B. AL amyloidosis (primary, nonhereditary amyloidosis)

Chronic infections

Chronic inflammations

IL-1, IL-6, TNF-α

Serum amyloid A = SAA

Accumulation: AA fibrils

C. AA amyloidosis (secondary amyloidosis)

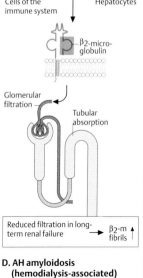

Cells of the immune system

Hepatocytes

β₂-micro-globulin

Glomerular filtration

Tubular absorption

Reduced filtration in long-term renal failure → β₂-m fibrils ↑

D. AH amyloidosis (hemodialysis-associated)

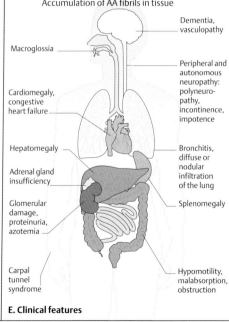

Accumulation of AA fibrils in tissue

Macroglossia

Cardiomegaly, congestive heart failure

Hepatomegaly

Adrenal gland insufficiency

Glomerular damage, proteinuria, azotemia

Carpal tunnel syndrome

Dementia, vasculopathy

Peripheral and autonomous neuropathy: polyneuro-pathy, incontinence, impotence

Bronchitis, diffuse or nodular infiltration of the lung

Splenomegaly

Hypomotility, malabsorption, obstruction

E. Clinical features

The question of whether immunosurveillance against tumors truly exists is still unsolved. Bacteria and viruses, which can be effectively recognized and controlled by the immune system, consist of a variety of foreign proteins. Tumor cells, on the other hand, differ only slightly from normal cells. Sometimes, truncated or mutated proteins are present, but otherwise the cells use normal biochemical pathways. Even if some proteins are expressed at levels higher than normal, or if fetal antigens are expressed, these are in most cases normal cellular proteins. In many cases, if mutated proteins are present, only few peptides can be potentially recognized as foreign. A number of findings indicate that immunosurveillance against tumors is not one of the primary tasks of the immune system. Patients with severe immune defects, such as HIV, have an increased incidence of virus-associated tumors, but do not exhibit an increase in the most common cancer types. Furthermore, nude mice that lack functional T cells do not develop tumors but rather die of infections. Nonetheless, the findings of experimental animal studies and clinical studies do justify hope that manipulation of the immune system will eventually result in effective immunotherapy strategies in the future.

A. Recognition of Tumor Antigens

Researchers have attempted to manufacture antibodies against tumor cells since monoclonal antibody engineering techniques were developed about 20 years ago. This involves the immunization of mice with tumor cells. After repeated application, the splenic cells are isolated and fused with myeloma cells from an "immortal" myeloma cell line by addition of polyethylene glycol (PEG). Due to an enzyme defect, unfused myeloma cells die when placed in a medium containing hypoxanthine, aminopterin, and thymidine (HAT medium) (**1**). Only those cells that inherited immortality from the myeloma cells and HAT resistance from the splenic cells will survive. Apart from HAT resistance, the fusion cells (hybridoma cells) also inherit antibody specificity from the splenic cells. Hybridoma cells that produce antibodies against tumor cells are subjected to a process known as "limiting dilution." They are then repeatedly cloned to obtain a cell line arising from a single cell that produces antibodies of a single specificity (monoclonal cell line or hybridoma).

On the other hand, T cells are potentially able to recognize tumor antigens (**2**). After intracellular degradation, such antigens (e.g., mutated proteins) can be presented to CD8+ cytotoxic T cells as MHC class I-bound peptides. The T-cell response is HLA-restricted, that is, it depends on whether the mutated tumor peptide fits in the antigen-presenting site of the HLA molecule (see p. 56). Tumor cells are not effective antigen-presenting cells because they lack important co-stimulatory molecules (see p. 36).

B. Identification of Tumor Antigens

T-cell clones that specifically lyse target cells can be isolated by cloning techniques (see p. 92). In order to identify the DNA sequence of the corresponding tumor antigen, the total DNA of the tumor cells is prepared, separated into multiple small fragments, and inserted into vectors (**1**). The fragment-bearing vectors are then transduced to cells with the same HLA restriction as the tumor cells. Only those cells containing the relevant DNA fragment present it in the MHC molecules. They can therefore be recognized and lysed by the T-cell clones.

An alternative method is the elution of peptide from tumor cells. In order to find out which of the peptides presented by a cell are tumor-specific, all peptides in the MHC molecule are first dissolved by brief acid treatment (**2**). The dissolved peptides are separated by high-performance liquid chromatography (HPLC). The individual peptide fractions are then incubated with a TAP-deficient cell line (see p. 153). The cell lines is not able to supply MHC molecules with peptides. "Empty" MHC molecules on the cell membrane are unstable and degraded quickly. The external addition of exactly matching peptides stabilizes them, and the MHC molecules are then able to present the bound peptides. If one of the peptide is tumor-specific, the corresponding presenting cell is lysed by the tumor-specific T-cell clone. Further characterization of the peptides isolated from the MHC molecules can be achieved by mass spectrometry.

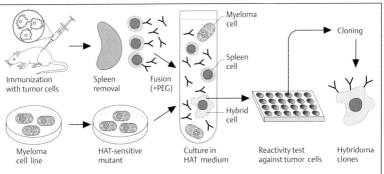

1. Production of monoclonal antibodies against tumor antigens

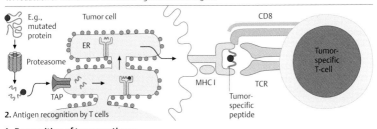

2. Antigen recognition by T cells

A. Recognition of tumor antigens

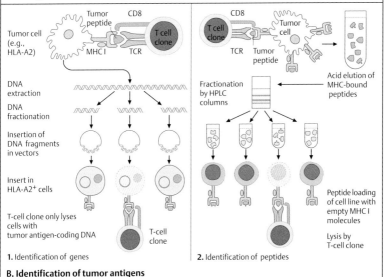

Tumor cell
(e.g., HLA-A2)

DNA extraction

DNA fractionation

Insertion of DNA fragments in vectors

Insert in HLA-A2+ cells

T-cell clone only lyses cells with tumor antigen-coding DNA

1. Identification of genes

Fractionation by HPLC columns

Acid elution of MHC-bound peptides

Peptide loading of cell line with empty MHC I molecules

Lysis by T-cell clone

2. Identification of peptides

B. Identification of tumor antigens

Clinical Immunology

151

A. Tumor Antigens

Ideally, a tumor antigen should be expressed only by tumor cells and not by normal cells in order to be recognized as foreign by the immune system. In reality, most tumor-associated antigens are overexpressed in tumor cells but are also expressed in smaller amounts in normal cells. The enzyme tyrosinase, for example, is expressed in all normal melanocytes, but much higher concentrations occur in melanoma cells. Tyrosinase-specific T cells that recognize and kill melanoma cells can be found in the blood of some melanoma patients. These T cells are indeed responsible for the depigmentation of the skin (vitiligo) in some melanoma patients. The occurrence of vitiligo frequently correlates with a response to therapy.

Oncofetal antigens, such as alpha-fetoprotein and carcinoembryonic antigen (CEA), are present in tumors of the liver and gonads and in various adenocarcinomas. These antigens are strongly expressed during fetal development, but are normally only weakly expressed in adults. Oncofetal antigens circulate as soluble proteins in the blood of tumor patients and are therefore useful as indicators of tumor progression (tumor markers).

In B-cell and T-cell lymphomas and leukemias, clone-specific determinants (idiotypes) of the immunoglobulins and of the T-cell receptor represent individual and specific tumor antigens. Hence, no reactivity with other tissues is to be expected.

Mutated proteins arising from chromosomal translocations or point mutations, on the other hand, represent completely new antigens (neoantigens). In t(9;22) BCR-ABL translocation of CML, for example, a fusion protein develops between the normal BCR and ABL genes. Peptides with sequences formed by amino acids of both of these genes can function as true tumor antigens. Point mutations, which commonly occur in tumor suppressor gene p53 and other cell cycle-regulating proteins, such as p16 and p21, also lead to the development of new tumor-specific peptides that do not occur in normal cells. However, these peptides must fit into the HLA molecules of the tumor cells in order to be recognized by the immune system. Hence, it is possible to have tumors where such tumor-specific peptides are present but not presented to the immune system by the individual MHC molecules. True viral proteins produced by HTLV1 in T-cell leukemia and Epstein–Barr virus in some malignant lymphomas are responsible for malignant transformation and are produced by tumor cells. There is clear evidence that these viral products can be successfully recognized by the immune system. In contrast to single mutated proteins, these viral proteins usually contain a large number of peptides that are potentially immunogenic, and there is a great chance that some of them will bind to the MHC molecules of the host cells.

B. Immune "Escape Mechanisms"

There are a number of reasons for the absence of an effective immune response to tumors. Each autologous protein is degraded within the cytoplasm to form peptides consisting of 9–12 amino acids. These peptides are conveyed by a transport system called "transporter associated with antigen processing (TAP)" to the endoplasmic reticulum (ER), where they are bound by class I MHC molecules and presented to CD8+ T cells on the cell surface (see p. 56).

Some tumors may not have tumor peptides that fit into the binding sites of the patient's MHC molecules (1). In tumor cells with defective antigen processing machinery (e.g., TAP deficiency), tumor peptides are not transported to the endoplasmic reticulum (3) and are not presented on the cell surface. In many cases, there is a lack of MHC class I molecules on the surface of the tumor cells due to the downregulation of MHC genes. As a consequence, the tumor antigens cannot be recognized by cytotoxic T cells (2).

Tumor cells are not professional antigen-presenting cells. They lack co-stimulatory molecules CD80 and CD86 needed for T-cell activation. Without co-stimulation, the presentation of a peptide via the MHC/TCR complex leads to T-cell anergy and tolerance (4). Some tumor cells also stop producing tumor antigen to escape an immune response (5). Alternatively, the tumor may produce immunosuppressive substances, such as IL-10 and transforming growth factor beta β (TGF-β) (6), and in some cases, MHC I-like molecules that interact with inhibitory ligands on T cells are expressed by tumor cells. Recently, regulatory T cells (CD4+ CD25+) have been shown to suppress immunoreactivity in patients with solid tumors.

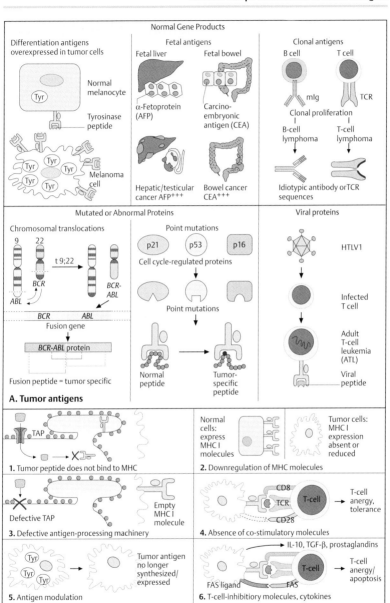

Normal Gene Products

Differentiation antigens overexpressed in tumor cells

Normal melanocyte

Tyr

Tyrosinase peptide

Tyr Tyr Tyr
Tyr Tyr

Melanoma cell

Fetal antigens

Fetal liver

α-Fetoprotein (AFP)

Hepatic/testicular cancer AFP+++

Fetal bowel

Carcino-embryonic antigen (CEA)

Bowel cancer CEA+++

Clonal antigens

B cell   T cell

mIg   TCR

Clonal proliferation

B-cell lymphoma   T-cell lymphoma

Idiotypic antibody or TCR sequences

Mutated or Abnormal Proteins

Chromosomal translocations

9   22   t 9;22

BCR   BCR-ABL

ABL

BCR   ABL

Fusion gene

BCR-ABL protein

Fusion peptide = tumor specific

Point mutations

p21   p53   p16

Cell cycle-regulated proteins

Point mutations

Normal peptide → Tumor-specific peptide

Viral proteins

HTLV1

Infected T cell

Adult T-cell leukemia (ATL)

Viral peptide

A. Tumor antigens

1. Tumor peptide does not bind to MHC

TAP

2. Downregulation of MHC molecules

Normal cells: express MHC I molecules

Tumor cells: MHC I expression absent or reduced

3. Defective antigen-processing machinery

Defective TAP

Empty MHC I molecule

4. Absence of co-stimulatory molecules

CD8
TCR   T-cell
CD28

T-cell anergy, tolerance

5. Antigen modulation

Tyr
Tyr Tyr →

Tumor antigen no longer synthesized/expressed

6. T-cell-inhibitory molecules, cytokines

IL-10, TGF-β, prostaglandins

FAS ligand   FAS   T-cell

T-cell anergy/apoptosis

B. Immune recognition escape mechanisms

Clinical Immunology

153

A. Enhancement of Nonspecific Immunity

Around the end of the 19th century, the American surgeon William Coley began to inject cancer patients with tumor cell lysates that were contaminated with bacteria due to the lack of sterile preparation techniques. Surprisingly, some tumor regression was observed. Later in the 20th century, tumor vaccination was tested again, but the use of unmodified tumor cells alone did not induce significant responses. Adjuvants were soon added in attempts to enhance the tumor-specific immune response. Attenuated mycobacterial strains, such as bacillus Calmette–Guérin (BCG) or *Corynebacterium parvum*, were primarily used. The Newcastle disease virus has also been used in more recent experiments. Some clinical studies based on this strategy are still in process. Although no sweeping successes can be expected from these trials, some positive results indicate that improved vaccination methods might be successfully developed in the future.

In the past 3–4 years, tumor cells have been modified by gene transfer to selectively induce T-cell-mediated immune responses. The goal is to stimulate the local growth of T cells or dendritic cells by the secretion of cytokines, such as IL-2, IL-4, IL-7, and GM-CSF, in the hope of activating tumor-specific T cells.

Cytokines can also be administered systemically. However, only interferon-α (IFN-α) and IL-2 have become established in a few types of tumors (**2**). In addition to its immunostimulatory effect, IFN-α also has a direct antiproliferative effect that may be responsible for some of the therapeutic effects. Renal cell carcinomas and malignant melanomas appear to respond better than other tumors to immunotherapeutic regimens, but the reason for this is still unknown. Tumor necrosis factor-α (TNF-α) is also used in patients with sarcomas and melanomas in limb perfusion together with antineoplastic drugs to enhance tumor cell damage.

B. Induction of a Specific T-Cell Response

In many patients, surgical excision can successfully eliminate the primary tumor at the time of diagnosis. However, a proportion of these patients will later develop distant metastases or local recurrences. This is why *adjuvant therapy* is performed in patients with certain risk factors (tumor type, degree of malignancy, depth of tumor invasion, lymph node involvement, etc.). Nonetheless, in most cases, it still is not possible to induce a specific T-cell response to the tumor by administering irradiated autologous tumor cells or tumor cell lysates (**1**). Even under ideal conditions where the tumor cells present tumor antigen to the T cells, a sufficient antitumor immune response is not observed because the tumor cells lack the required co-stimulatory molecules, such as B7 (CD80/86) (see pp. 36 and 153). A number of trials is being performed in which tumor cells are genetically modified to express the B7 antigen in order to increase their immunogenicity (**2**). Another way to induce an immune response to poorly immunogenic tumor cells is to allow professional antigen-presenting cells (APC) to present the tumor antigens (**3**). The professional APCs express all important stimulatory molecules needed to induce an effective T-cell response. Accordingly, dendritic cells generated ex vivo can therefore be loaded (*pulsed*) with tumor cell lysates, purified tumor antigens, or specific tumor peptides. The results of preliminary clinical trials are promising.

The local instillation of Calmette–Guérin bacillus after local resection of carcinoma of the bladder is a special form of immunotherapy. BCG treatment prevents the development of recurrences in a high percentage of cases. Instillation of the bacillus may trigger inflammatory processes in which activated antigen-presenting cells are able to capture antigens from remaining tumor cells and effectively present them to the immune system.

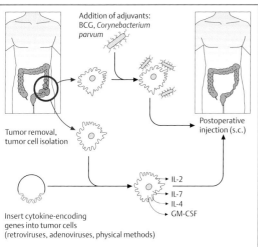

Addition of adjuvants:
BCG, *Corynebacterium parvum*

Tumor removal, tumor cell isolation

Postoperative injection (s.c.)

Insert cytokine-encoding genes into tumor cells (retroviruses, adenoviruses, physical methods)

IL-2
IL-7
IL-4
GM-CSF

1. Vaccination with adjuvants, cytokine-producing cells

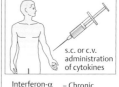

s.c. or c.v. administration of cytokines

Interferon-α – Chronic myelocytic leukemia
– Plasmocytoma
– Lymphoma
– Melanoma
– Renal cell carcinoma

Interleukin-2 – Renal cell carcinoma
– Melanoma
– Leukemias

TNF-α – local perfusion of sarcomas/melanomas

2. Cytokine therapy

A. Enhancement of nonspecific immunity

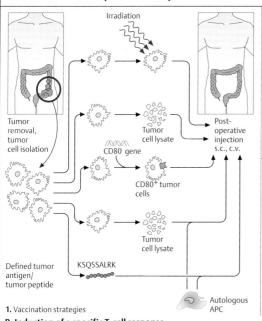

Irradiation

Tumor removal, tumor cell isolation

Tumor cell lysate

Post-operative injection s.c., c.v.

CD80 gene

CD80⁺ tumor cells

Tumor cell lysate

Defined tumor antigen/ tumor peptide

KSQSSALRK

Autologous APC

1. Vaccination strategies

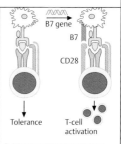

B7 gene

B7

CD28

Tolerance   T-cell activation

2. Direct antigen presentation

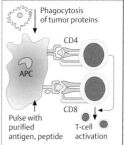

Phagocytosis of tumor proteins

CD4

APC

Pulse with purified antigen, peptide

CD8

T-cell activation

3. Indirect antigen presentation

B. Induction of a specific T-cell response

A. Production of Engineered Tumor-specific TCRs

Many tumors are extensively infiltrated by lymphocytes. Tumor-infiltrating lymphocytes (TIL) used to be removed from surgical specimens, especially from melanomas and renal cell carcinomas, then isolated and retransfused after proliferation. However, the results were rather disappointing. It is now possible to identify the DNA sequences on the variable domains of the α and β chains of the T-cell receptors of TIL. Using viral vectors, genetically engineered T lymphocytes that specifically react with the tumor can be produced. Adoptive therapy could then be performed by administering such ex vivo expanded T cells. Currently, one of the major limitations is the difficulty of gene transfer in normal T cells, but improved methods are being generated. Also, endogenous TCR must be downregulated.

B. Antibody Therapies

Monoclonal antibodies (MAb) have been used in cancer treatment for about 20 years now. Most antibodies have been generated in mice. Treatment with murine MAb leads to the formation of human anti-murine antibodies (HAMA), which reduce the efficacy of murine MAb, therefore "humanized" monoclonal antibodies were developed (**1**). In humanized monoclonal antibodies, the greater portion of the molecule is of human origin, and only the F(ab) fragment or the variable region of F(ab) is of murine origin. Humanized monoclonal antibodies have a significantly longer half-life in the patient's blood and they activate the immune effector cells more efficiently than murine monoclonal antibodies. Two humanized monoclonal antibodies have achieved remarkable results in the past three years: the CD20 antibody Rituximab (Rituxan®) has activity against B-cell lymphomas, and the antibody trastuzumab (Herceptin®) directed against human epidermal growth factor receptor 2 (HER2) is active in breast cancer. A number of other antibodies appear promising. "Bispecific" antibodies are another new development (**2**). They are produced by fusion of two hybridomas, each of which secretes a specific monoclonal antibody. The hybridomas bind simultaneously to the epitope of the tumor cell and to T cells (CD3). The T cells are therefore brought in contact with the tumor cells and are activated by CD3. Synthetic single-chain antibodies are an improvement of this strategy (**3**). These are genetically engineered antibody derivatives that consist only of the light and heavy chain of the variable region (Fv) of the monoclonal Ab. Single chains from two different antibodies can be connected by a binding fragment (spacer). Alternatively, single-chain antibodies that recognize a tumor epitope can be linked to the ζ chain, which plays an important role in the transduction of TCR signals. T cells can be transfected with such constructs, so that they can recognize a tumor antigen in the same way as antibodies do, and the signal will be transmitted to the inside of the cell by the connected TCR ζ chain. Antibodies directed against tumor-associated antigens can also be linked to immunotoxins or radioisotopes (**B.4**). In immunotoxins, the toxic components that block the synthesis of RNA are released after internalization of the antibody. In radiolabeled immunoconjugates, a radioactive substance (usually radioactive yttrium or iodine) induces the lysis of target cells but also of adjacent cells (so-called "bystander effect").

C. Mechanisms of Monoclonal Antibody Therapy

A monoclonal antibody can imitate or block the natural ligands of a receptor. An anti-CD95 antibody can, for example, activate the Fas/APO-1 receptor (CD95), thereby triggering apoptosis (**1**). On the other hand, antibodies can activate complement and thus induce pore formation in the cell membrane (**2**). In antibody-dependent cell-mediated cytotoxicity, Fc receptor-bearing natural killer cells recognize the Fc fragment of a cell-bound antibody and thus release cytoplasmic granules containing cytotoxic perforins and granzymes (**3**, see also p. 39).

As mentioned, murine Ab can induce HAMA. Some of these anti-murine antibodies may be directed against the specific idiotypic binding region of murine Ab (**4**). In this case, the anti-idiotypic antibodies imitate tumor antigens and can serve as a tumor surrogate in vaccines. On the other hand, they can also lead to the formation of anti-anti-idiotypic monoclonal antibodies, which—like murine MAbs—recognize the tumor antigen. The effect of the murine monoclonal antibodies is enhanced by this cascade.

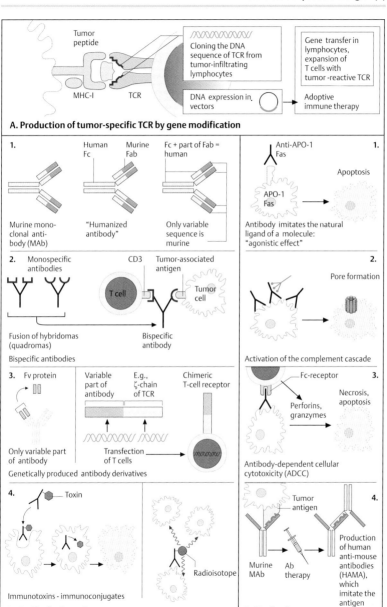

A. Production of tumor-specific TCR by gene modification

Tumor peptide

MHC-I   TCR

Cloning the DNA sequence of TCR from tumor-infiltrating lymphocytes

DNA expression in vectors

Gene transfer in lymphocytes, expansion of T cells with tumor-reactive TCR

Adoptive immune therapy

B. Antibody therapies

1.
Human Fc   Murine Fab   Fc + part of Fab = human

Murine mono-clonal anti-body (MAb)

"Humanized antibody"

Only variable sequence is murine

2. Monospecific antibodies

CD3   Tumor-associated antigen

T cell   Tumor cell

Fusion of hybridomas (quadromas)

Bispecific antibody

Bispecific antibodies

3. Fv protein

Variable part of antibody

E.g., ζ-chain of TCR

Chimeric T-cell receptor

Only variable part of antibody

Transfection of T cells

Genetically produced antibody derivatives

4.   Toxin

Radioisotope

Immunotoxins - immunoconjugates

C. Mechanisms

Anti-APO-1 Fas   1.

Apoptosis

APO-1 Fas

Antibody imitates the natural ligand of a molecule: "agonistic effect"

2.   Pore formation

Activation of the complement cascade

Fc-receptor   3.

Necrosis, apoptosis

Perforins, granzymes

Antibody-dependent cellular cytotoxicity (ADCC)

Tumor antigen   4.

Murine MAb   Ab therapy

Production of human anti-mouse antibodies (HAMA), which imitate the antigen

Clinical Immunology

157

Transplantation of Autologous Bone Marrow/Hematopoietic Stem Cells

Many tumors, especially leukemias and lymphomas, can be eliminated with sufficiently high doses of chemotherapy and radiotherapy. The toxicity of the therapy is a limiting factor because irreversible damage to the hematopoietic bone marrow (myeloablation) can occur. The transfusion of 700–800 ml of bone marrow blood from a healthy donor will suffice for reconstitution of the hematopoietic system (allogeneic bone marrow transplantation, allogeneic BMT). Bone marrow function can also be reconstituted by retransfusing autologous bone marrow removed just prior to ablative therapy (autologous BMT).

A. Stem Cell Harvesting

Bone marrow blood is harvested by repeated puncture of the iliac crest with the patient under full anesthesia. The few CD34+ stem cells present in the harvest are responsible for reconstitution of hematopoiesis. Such cells are not only present in the bone marrow, but also circulate in small quantities in the peripheral blood. The cells can therefore be extracted by leukapheresis, a process in which mononuclear cells, including stem cells, are harvested by selective centrifugation of the blood. Around 8–15 liters of blood continuously flow through the cell separator over a period of 2–5 hours. This yields approximately 350 ml of blood with enriched stem cells, which are cryopreserved for later use. The minimum requirement of CD34+ cells for successful reconstitution of the hematopoietic system is around 2×10^6 CD34+ cells/kg body weight.

B. Mobilization of Hematopoietic Stem Cells and Course of Transplantation

The number of CD34+ stem cells in the peripheral blood is low, but can be increased by administering recombinant hematopoietic growth factors, such as G-CSF or GM-CSF. Bone marrow extraction or leukapheresis is subsequently performed. The harvested transplant can be cryopreserved for as long as necessary. High-dose chemo/radiotherapy leads to bone marrow aplasia (decrease in the number of erythrocytes, granulocytes, and thrombocytes in the peripheral blood), which would be irreversible without the reinfusion of stem cells. The aplasia phase lasts only 10–15 days when cryopreserved stem cells are reinfused on completion of chemotherapy. Full reconstitution of the hematopoietic system subsequently occurs.

C. Indications

Autologous hematopoietic stem cell transplantation (AHSCT) or bone marrow transplantation is also performed in a number of hematological diseases and in isolated solid tumors, especially germinal cell tumors. The procedures are also indicated in genetic engineering of stem cells for treatment of congenital metabolic or immune defects. More recently, high-dose chemotherapy followed by stem cell reinfusion has also been performed in therapy-resistant autoimmune diseases. CD34+ cells are also able to differentiate into dendritic cells or immune effector cells in vitro. In this case, transplantation can be performed in conjunction with immunotherapy.

D. Purging the Autotransplant

In autologous transplantation, there is a risk that the transplant may contain contaminating tumor cells. The transplant material is therefore subjected to a purification procedure called *purging*. Since the CD34 antigen is not expressed on the surface of solid-tumor cells, positive selection of CD34+ cells is possible. In the presence of biotinylated anti-CD34 antibodies, the CD34+ cells are bound to a column packed with avidin and later separated. The purity of CD34+ cells harvested by this method is around 90%. Further removal of contaminating tumor cells is achieved by negative selection. This is done using iron beads coated with antibodies against tumor antigens. Cells bearing the tumor antigen are then removed by applying a magnetic field.

The contribution of contaminating tumor cells to relapse of the tumor after high-dose chemotherapy is still a matter of debate. Probably most of the relapses are due to a persistence of tumor cells in the body rather than in the transplant.

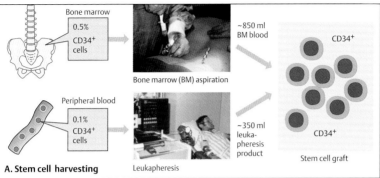

Bone marrow

0.5% CD34$^+$ cells

Bone marrow (BM) aspiration

~850 ml BM blood

Peripheral blood

0.1% CD34$^+$ cells

Leukapheresis

~350 ml leuka-pheresis product

CD34$^+$

CD34$^+$

Stem cell graft

A. Stem cell harvesting

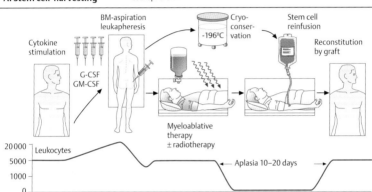

Cytokine stimulation

G-CSF GM-CSF

BM-aspiration leukapheresis

Cryo-conser-vation

-196°C

Stem cell reinfusion

Reconstitution by graft

Myeloablative therapy ± radiotherapy

Leukocytes

Aplasia 10–20 days

20000
5000
1000
0

B. Mobilization of hematopoietic stem cells and transplantation schedule

– Acute leukemias – Hodgkin's lymphoma – Non -Hodgkin's lymphoma – Breast cancer – Germ cell tumors	– Immune defects – Hemophilia – Immune therapy of cancer – Gene modification of stem cells
1. Enhancement of the chemotherapeutic effect	**2.** Genetic and experimental therapy

C. Indications

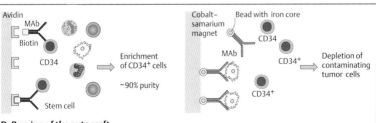

Avidin

MAb

Biotin

CD34

Stem cell

Enrichment of CD34$^+$ cells

~90% purity

Cobalt–samarium magnet

Bead with iron core

CD34

MAb

CD34$^+$

CD34$^+$

CD34$^+$

Depletion of contaminating tumor cells

D. Purging of the autograft

Clinical Immunology

A. Transplantation of Allogeneic Bone Marrow and Hematopoietic Stem Cells

A compatible donor must be available for an allogeneic transplantation. Relatives with identical HLA antigens are first sought in the immediate family. The probability of finding a fully HLA-compatible brother or sister (all HLA antigens matched) is 1:4. If there is no donor in the family, or in more distant relatives (e.g., aunts, uncles, cousins), international databases are searched for HLA-compatible donors. Bone marrow or peripheral hematopoietic stem cells are used as transplant. Cord blood can also be used; it has large quantities of CD34+ T cells and only a few mature T cells. The recipient is usually "conditioned" prior to therapy, e.g., with a combination of high-dose alkylating agents and total-body irradiation (10–14 Gy). This destroys tumor cells and produces sufficient immunosuppression to prevent the rejection of the foreign bone marrow/stem cells.

B. Indications

In malignant diseases, the transplantation is performed only during a complete remission, that is, after the majority of tumor cells have been eliminated by conventional chemotherapy. Allogeneic bone marrow transplantation is a curative treatment for chronic myeloid leukemia. In acute myeloid leukemia and acute lymphoid leukemia, transplantations are performed only in those patients with a high risk of recurrence. Other indications include severe aplastic anemias, paroxysmal nocturnal hemoglobulinuria, severe combined immune defects, and thalassemia. The role of allo-BMT in solid tumors is unclear: encouraging results are being achieved in renal cancer.

C. Complications

High-dose chemotherapy or radiotherapy causes damage to various organs (**1**). Damage to mucosal linings with ulceration and, in some cases, severe diarrhea can occur anywhere in the gastrointestinal tract. Veno-occlusive disease (VOD) is a life-threatening complication with signs ranging from mild damage to the postcapillary venules of the liver to liver failure. Interstitial pneumonia is not uncommon. Infertility is usually unavoidable, but the sperm of male patients can be frozen before therapy. Severe hemorrhagic cystitis can occur as a side effect of cyclophosphamide. Secondary neoplasms can occur as late sequelae. Infections by multiresistant staphylococci, pseudomonads, and fungi are especially dangerous during the aplasia phase (**2**). Cytomegaloviruses (CMVs), which can induce severe pulmonary and gastrointestinal infections, are the most important viral pathogens. Because platelet replacement is sometimes difficult due to transplant-related alloimmunization, there is a risk of hemorrhage.

Graft-versus-host disease (GVHD) (**3**), one of the main causes of morbidity and mortality after allogeneic transplantation, is caused by donor T lymphocytes within the transplant attacking different tissues of the recipient. In HLA-compatible transplantations, the GVHD response is directed against *minor histocompatibility antigens*. Antigen-presenting cells of the recipient presumably present the foreign tissue antigens to the donor T lymphocytes. This seems especially likely, since the activity of the APC is increased due to cytokines induced by chemo/radiotherapy, e.g., IL-1, IL-6, and TNF-α. GVHD mainly affects the skin (small-spotted exanthema), liver (cholestatic hepatitis), and bowel (diarrhea). Dryness of the mucosae and connective tissue (sicca syndrome) and myositis may also occur. GVHD prophylaxis consists of immunosuppressive therapy with cyclosporine, which can also be given in combination with methotrexate, mycofenolate mofetil, tacrolimus, and corticosteroids, if necessary.

D. T-Cell Depletion and Graft-versus-Leukemia Effect

The risk of GVHD can be reduced by depleting the T lymphocytes in the transplant. The drawback is an increased risk of transplant rejection and of tumor recurrence because the donor T lymphocytes mediate the beneficial graft versus leukemia (GVL) effect. To maintain the GVL effect while reducing the risk of GVHD, the T cells can be partially depleted from the transplant and donor T lymphocytes reinfused according to a graduated scheme.

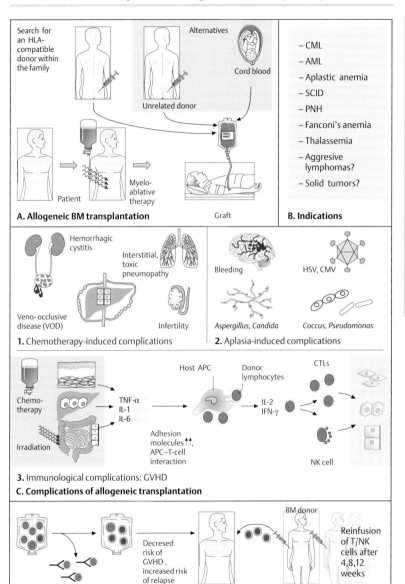

A. Allogeneic BM transplantation

Search for an HLA-compatible donor within the family

Alternatives

Cord blood

Unrelated donor

Patient

Myelo-ablative therapy

Graft

B. Indications

- CML
- AML
- Aplastic anemia
- SCID
- PNH
- Fanconi's anemia
- Thalassemia
- Aggresive lymphomas?
- Solid tumors?

Hemorrhagic cystitis

Interstitial, toxic pneumopathy

Veno-occlusive disease (VOD)

Infertility

1. Chemotherapy-induced complications

Bleeding

HSV, CMV

Aspergillus, Candida

Coccus, Pseudomonas

2. Aplasia-induced complications

Host APC

Donor lymphocytes

CTLs

Chemo-therapy

TNF-α
IL-1
IL-6

IL-2
IFN-γ

Irradiation

Adhesion molecules ↑↑, APC–T-cell interaction

NK cell

3. Immunological complications: GVHD

C. Complications of allogeneic transplantation

T-cell depletion

Decresed risk of GVHD, increased risk of relapse

BM donor

Reinfusion of T/NK cells after 4,8,12 weeks

Anti-leukemia effect

D. T-cell depletion and graft-versus-leukemia effect

Clinical Immunology

161

A. Transplantation Types

There are different types of organ transplantations. *Autologous* transplants (e.g., skin) are transferred from one site to another within the same organism. *Syngeneic* transplants are transferred between identical (monozygotic) twins. *Allogeneic* transplants are transferred between genetically different individuals, and *xenogeneic* transplants are transferred between animals of different species (e.g., monkeys to humans).

B. Criteria for Organ Removal

The main prerequisite for organ removal is dissociated brain death of the donor, which is defined as the absence of all brain waves (flat EEG), the irreversible loss of spontaneous respiration and reflexes, and the angiographically confirmed absence of cerebral blood flow. The donor and/or donor's family must consent to the donation. Once the organ or organs have been removed, the donated tissue is typed by analyzing the ABO blood group and HLA type. The presence of HIV and CMV infections must also be excluded. A recipient search is then performed by transplantation coordination centers, such as Eurotransplant. The priority of HLA compatibility is sequenced as DR–B–A–C. A *full-house match* occurs in only 20% of cases. Cross-testing of donor cells with the recipient's serum should also turn out negative.

Immunosuppressive therapy is performed after all allogeneic organ transplantations to prevent transplant rejection. *Hyperacute rejection* occurs within the first few minutes to three days after transplantation. This type of rejection reaction is due to prior host sensitization and is resistant to therapy. *Acute rejection* may occur within 4–5 days of transplantation, but most commonly occurs in the 2nd to 3rd postoperative week. Acute rejection is a critical condition, but can be managed well by drug therapy. *Chronic rejection* (develops within months to years) is characterized by the development of severe vessel changes. These rejection reactions respond poorly to high-dose immunosuppressants.

C. Examples of Organ Transplantations

Dialysis-dependent chronic renal failure is an indication for kidney transplantation (**1**). Reactivation of the primary disease within the transplant, reactivation of CMV infection, and the nephrotoxicity of some immunosuppressive drugs (cyclosporine) are major complications.

Corneal grafting (keratoplasty) can be performed as a lamellar procedure by transplanting only the epithelium and stroma, or as a perforating procedure in which the posterior endothelium is also grafted (**2**). The transplant will not be rejected as long as it is not vascularized ("sequestered antigens," see p. 63**C**).

D. Xenotransplantation

The limited supply of donor organs is still the primary problem in all transplantations. The potentials of xenotransplantation (e.g., from pigs to humans) have therefore been intensively researched. Some of the main problems in xenotransplantation are immediate rejection due to the presence of preformed antibodies and complement, the questionable efficacy of surrogate function, the possible transmission of viruses pathogenic to humans, and ethical aspects of the procedure.

In order to prevent hyperacute rejections due to complement activation, researchers are attempting to produce transgenic pigs without antigens for preformed antibodies but that, instead, express complement regulators that limit complement-induced lysis. The target complement regulators are the membrane inhibitor of reactive lysis (MIRL) CD59, the decay-accelerating factor (DAF) CD55, and the membrane cofactor (MCP) CD46. Preformed antibodies can, in part, be removed by plasmapheresis or by injecting soluble inhibitory factors.

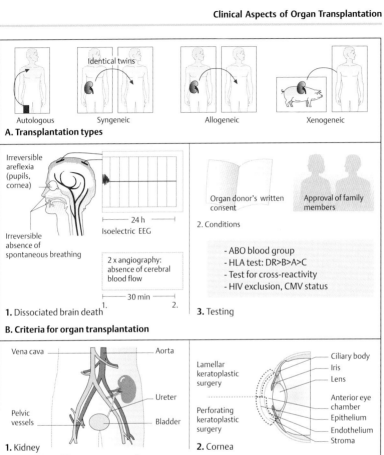

A. Transplantation types

Autologous — Syngeneic (Identical twins) — Allogeneic — Xenogeneic

Irreversible areflexia (pupils, cornea)

Irreversible absence of spontaneous breathing

Isoelectric EEG — 24 h

2 x angiography: absence of cerebral blood flow — 30 min — 1. 2.

1. Dissociated brain death

Organ donor's written consent — Approval of family members

2. Conditions

- ABO blood group
- HLA test: DR>B>A>C
- Test for cross-reactivity
- HIV exclusion, CMV status

3. Testing

B. Criteria for organ transplantation

Vena cava — Aorta — Ureter — Bladder

Pelvic vessels

1. Kidney

Lamellar keratoplastic surgery — Perforating keratoplastic surgery

Ciliary body — Iris — Lens — Anterior eye chamber — Epithelium — Endothelium — Stroma

2. Cornea

C. Transplantable organs: Examples

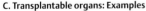

Complement regulators — Knock Out — For antigens — For preformed antibodies

DAF (CD55)
MCP (CD46)
MIRL (CD59)

Transgenic pig

Host

Plasma-pheresis

Soluble inhibitory factors of complement lysis CD35

α-Galactosyl compounds

D. Xenogeneic transplantation

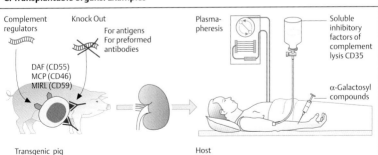

A. Immunogenicity of the Transplant

Immunogenicity reactions directed against a transplant are triggered by MHC complexes in the graft. Class I MHC molecules and the peptides presented by them may be recognized as foreign by the recipient's immune system due to genetic polymorphism. The peptides originate from cytoplasmic proteins cleaved from an enzyme complex, the proteasome. Transport-associated proteins (TAP) convey them to the endoplasmic reticulum (ER), where they bind to class I MHC molecules. Recognition of the peptide–class I MHC complex by the transplant recipient's lymphocytes triggers both cellular and humoral immune responses. Peptides originating from other cell compartments are also transported to the ER, bound to class I MHC molecules, and presented on the cell surface. These so-called "non-MHC antigens" induce a generally weaker immune response and activate only a small number of T-cell clones. The recognition of blood group antigens by the recipient as foreign is another cause of immune reactions to transplants. The ABO blood group system has preformed antibodies that may lead to a hyperacute rejection reaction.

B. Rejection Reactions

1 **Humoral rejection.** Antibody-mediated transplant rejection may become an important factor, especially in cases where prior sensitization of the recipient has occurred, e.g., during pregnancy or blood transfusion. Preformed antibodies are primarily directed against the endothelium of the transplant (donor). Their presence triggers the activation of the complement system, thereby causing complement-mediated endothelial damage, aggregation of thrombocytes, granulocytes, and monocytes, and intravascular coagulation due to the release of mediators. Antibody-dependent cell-mediated cytotoxicity (ADCC) mainly plays an important role in chronic rejection.

2 **Early phase of cellular rejection.** Early rejection reactions are mediated by professional antigen-presenting cells (APCs). APCs in the graft can migrate and directly activate host T cells, which then become specific for MHC molecules in the graft. Antigens in the transplant may also be phagocytosed and processed by host antigen-presenting cells. However, presentation on self-MHC only activates T cells that do not recognize MHC molecules in the graft.

3 **Central phase of cellular rejection.** Activated T cells infiltrate perivascular tissue and the tissue around antigen-presenting cells. The T_H1 population predominates. The release of cytokines has direct, toxic effects on the surrounding tissues. Moreover, it induces the recruitment of additional T cells as well as B cells, macrophages, and granulocytes. The activated effector cells release pro-coagulatory mediators, kinins, and eicosanoids. Under the influence of the cytokines, an increased expression of adhesion molecules and MHC molecules occurs in the surrounding tissue.

The immunomodulatory processes that occur in transplant recipients with long-term graft tolerance are complex and only partially understood. If the second signal from the co-stimulatory ligand via CD28 is absent, the activation of naive T cells will be incomplete. This condition, called *anergy*, is characterized by the absence of IL-2 and a destructive T-cell reaction. Tolerated allogeneic transplants are often infiltrated with T_H2 cells which possibly inhibit the T_H1 cells there. Furthermore, their cytokines IL-10 and TGF-β can reduce the expression of the co-stimulatory ligands CD80 and CD86.

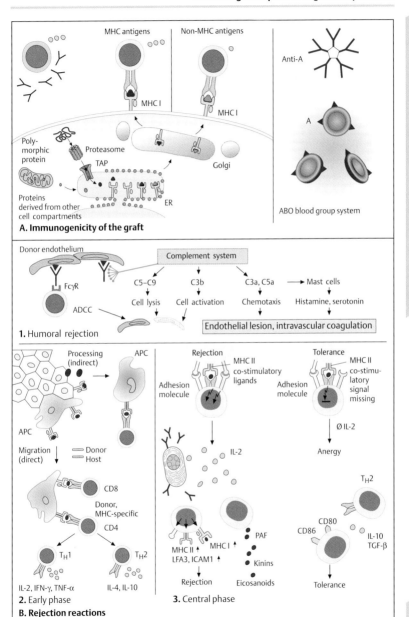

A. Immunogenicity of the graft

MHC antigens

Non-MHC antigens

Anti-A

MHC I

MHC I

Poly-morphic protein

Proteasome

TAP

Golgi

Proteins derived from other cell compartments

ER

A

ABO blood group system

Donor endothelium

Complement system

FcγR

ADCC

C5–C9 → Cell lysis

C3b → Cell activation

C3a, C5a → Mast cells

Chemotaxis

Histamine, serotonin

Endothelial lesion, intravascular coagulation

1. Humoral rejection

Processing (indirect)

APC

Rejection

MHC II co-stimulatory ligands

Tolerance

MHC II co-stimu-latory signal missing

Adhesion molecule

Adhesion molecule

APC

Ø IL-2

Migration (direct)

Donor

Host

Anergy

IL-2

CD8

Donor, MHC-specific

CD4

T$_H$1

T$_H$2

T$_H$2

MHC II ↑ LFA3, ICAM1 ↑

MHC I ↑

PAF

CD80

CD86

IL-10 TGF-β

IL-2, IFN-γ, TNF-α

IL-4, IL-10

Rejection

Kinins

Eicosanoids

Tolerance

2. Early phase

3. Central phase

B. Rejection reactions

Rheumatoid arthritis (RA; chronic polyarthritis) is the most common disease of the joints. It affects ca. 1–2% of the population. A catalog of criteria was developed by the American College of Rheumatology (ACR) to classify this disease picture. At least four out of seven criteria must be met (see Table 1 of the appendix).

A. Clinical Features of Rheumatoid Arthritis

Rheumatoid arthritis is a systemic disease that often occurs with extra-articular manifestations. RA usually begins after age 40 and predominantly affects women (ratio of 3:1). In most cases, RA begins insidiously, usually with a polyarticular and symmetrical pattern of involvement, especially of small joints in the periphery. Many patients complain of general malaise. Synovial capsular thickening and fusiform joint swelling most commonly affect the medial and proximal interphalangeal joints (PIP) of the fingers as well as the wrists and the metacarpophalangeal joints (MCP) of the toes. Nocturnal attacks of pain and morning arthralgias with persistent morning stiffness are also observed. Joint inflammation spreads in a centripetal pattern. The distal interphalangeal joints of the fingers usually remain unaffected.

Irreversible deformities that limit joint mobility occur in the advanced stages of disease, especially in the small joints. Deformities of the fingers take the form of characteristic ulnar deviations and so-called button-hole deformities and swan-neck deformities, which are caused by luxation of extensor or flexor tendons in swollen and damaged tendon sheaths. There are also destructive bone processes that begin at the insertions of the joint capsules (seen as erosions on radiographs). The terminal stage of the disease is characterized by fibrous and osseous bridges over the joint bodies. Involvement of the cervical spine is common after many years of refractory disease. This is characterized by destructive changes in the atlantodental joint and poses a risk of bone marrow compression.

Rheumatoid factors (RF) are often found when extra-articular manifestations occur. One of the main features is the formation of fibrous nodules on the extensor side of the extremities, especially on the forearm. These *rheumatoid nodules* are made of necrotic material that is surrounded in palisade-like fashion by macrophages. Visceral manifestations are attri-

butable to vasculitis with consecutive pleuritis or pericarditis (rarely clinically diagnosable). Other rare extra-articular manifestations are cutaneous vasculitis, pulmonary fibrosis, mitral valve defects, and myocarditis. Involvement of the eye, with such manifestations as scleritis or episcleritis and secondary Sjögren's syndrome (see p. 179) is characteristic of RA.

The serological features of RA include extensive changes in the general parameters of inflammation (erythrocyte sedimentation rate, ESR, and C-reactive protein, CRP). Extensive activity indicates the presence of anemia and thrombocytosis. IgM rheumatoid factors are found in around 70% of patients, and *anti-nuclear antibodies* are found in 30%.

ACR criteria for classification of RA

Criterion
1 Morning stiffness
2 Arthritis in three or more joint regions
3 Arthritis in the joints of the hand: wrists, MCPs, PIPs
4 Symmetrical swelling (arthritis)
5 Rheumatoid nodules
6 Rheumatoid factor in serum
7 Radiological changes of rheumatoid arthritis

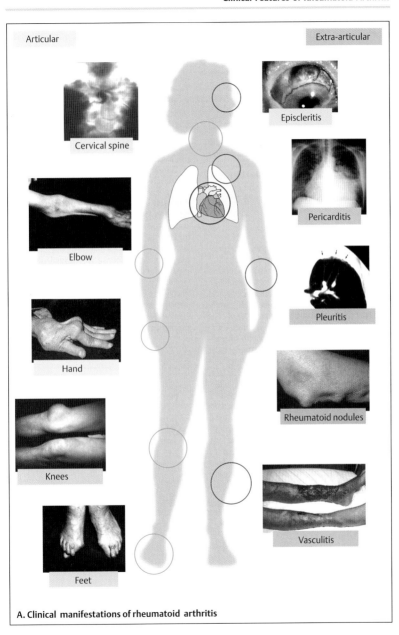

A. Clinical manifestations of rheumatoid arthritis

A. Cellular Structure of the Synovial Membrane

Broadening and villous distention of the normally smooth synovial membrane is a characteristic feature of rheumatoid arthritis. Proliferation of the lining layer of cells, which primarily consists of macrophages and activated synovial fibroblasts, can be observed. Infiltration with T lymphocytes also occurs. The CD4+ cells are predominantly found in structures resembling the lymphatic follicle. In some cases, they have characteristics similar to those of germinal centers. In contrast, CD8+ T cells diffusely infiltrate the connective tissue. The extensive vascularization of the synovial membrane is also a typical feature of the process of synovitis.

B. Cells in the Arthritic Joint

The typical patient with RA presents with synovitis-related distentson of the joint capsule and tendon sheaths (1), which can result in tendon rupture and the corresponding loss of mobility.

Extensive lymphocyte infiltration is a typical histological finding. The individual villi mainly consist of the hypertrophied lining layer of cells that contains macrophages (type A cells), fibroblasts (type B cells), and lymphocytic (round-cell) infiltrates (2). A considerable state of activation of the cells, especially macrophages and synovial fibroblasts, is observed upon electron microscopy (3). This tissue leads to the development of pannus (Latin: "a piece of cloth"), which penetrates into the bone, covers the cartilage, and ultimately destroys both structures.

Virtually all cells of immunological relevance are located in the synovial membrane (4). Hence, the synovium affected by inflammatory changes assumes the features of a lymphoid organ. The T cells are mainly of the memory cell type (CD45R0+). The germinal center-like aggregates contain activated B cells and follicular dendritic cells. There are also a number of plasma cells that produce rheumatoid factors as well as polyclonal antibodies of various specificities. The predominant cells at the cartilage–pannus boundary are activated synovial fibroblasts that produce large quantities of destructive enzymes, such as metalloproteases (collagenase and stromelysin; see table). Mononuclear cells mainly infiltrate the synovial membrane, whereas a large number of neutrophilic granulocytes infiltrate the synovial fluid.

The impact of the different cell systems on the development of rheumatoid arthritis is still controversial. The majority of researchers believe the immune system is responsible for the pathogenesis of RA (see p. 159). However, some workers hypothesize that the immunological manifestations are only secondary in nature. They propose that these manifestations may occur as a response to continual inflammatory stimuli caused mainly by unknown infections or by falsely programmed synovial fibroblasts (transformation) resulting in destructive activation processes (see p. 161**B.3**). Further research data are required for a definitive answer to these questions.

Important Proteolytic Enzymes in Rheumatoid Arthritis	
Enzyme family	**Representatives**
Matrix metalloproteinases (MMP)	MMPs 1, 2, 3, and 9
Cysteine proteinases	Cathepsins B, H, and L
Serine proteinases	Elastase, plasminogen activator, cathepsin G
Aspartic proteinases	Cathepsin D

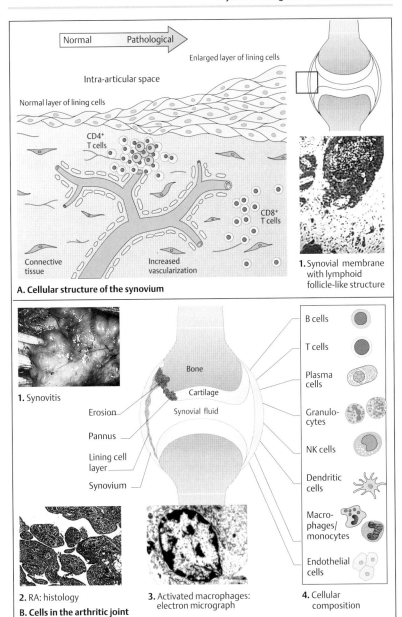

A. Cellular structure of the synovium

Normal — Pathological

Enlarged layer of lining cells

Intra-articular space

Normal layer of lining cells

CD4+ T cells

CD8+ T cells

Connective tissue

Increased vascularization

1. Synovial membrane with lymphoid follicle-like structure

B. Cells in the arthritic joint

1. Synovitis

Bone

Cartilage

Synovial fluid

Erosion

Pannus

Lining cell layer

Synovium

2. RA: histology

3. Activated macrophages: electron micrograph

4. Cellular composition

B cells

T cells

Plasma cells

Granulo-cytes

NK cells

Dendritic cells

Macro-phages/ monocytes

Endothelial cells

Clinical Immunology

A. Susceptibility to Rheumatoid Arthritis

Genetic factors play an important role in the development of rheumatoid arthritis, although the concordance of the disease is only ca. 15% in identical twins. This underlines the fact that environmental factors, presumably infectious events, also play a decisive role (cf. p. 165**B**). The HLA associations of RA were clearly elaborated when the "shared epitope hypothesis" was developed. The hypothesis states that the disease is not only associated with a certain HLA-DR specificity, but also with common epitopes on various DR molecules (especially DR4 and DR1). It was also shown that the presence of DR4 is associated with a worse course of RA with especially severe joint destruction, particularly when both chromosomes code for this molecule ("double dose" of the gene).

Pathogenetic studies suggest that the still unknown foreign antigen or autoantigen that induces the disease is bound in the pleated sheath structure of class II HLA molecules. Interaction between antigen-presenting cells and T-helper cells takes place in the third hypervariable region of the class II HLA antigen, which has a helical configuration. Here are variable amino acid groups that are coded in the region of the first domain of the HLA-DRB1 gene. The table underlines the similarity between DR4 subtypes and between DR1 and DR6Dw16, which are also associated with rheumatoid arthritis. The exchange of neutral and/or basic amino acids for the acidic amino acids Asp and Glu at positions 70, 71, and 74 of the alleles Dw10 and/or Dw13 leads to a loss of disease association. These HLA molecules are apparently unable to bind the arthritogenic peptide or peptides with sufficient affinity or are otherwise not recognized by the "right" T-cell receptor.

B. Pathogenesis of Rheumatoid Arthritis

T and B lymphocytes migrate from the postcapillary venules in the synovial membrane to the tissue through still unknown mechanisms (infection, trauma?). Synovial cells bearing aberrant class II HLA antigens and co-stimulatory molecules then present the still unknown arthritogenic peptide to the T cells. Subsequently, cytokines stimulate the activation of various cell systems. B cells are activated by polyclonal stimulation. These activated B cells produce immunoglobulins, especially rheumatoid factors, that stimulate the activation of complement through immune complexes. Moreover, proinflammatory cytokines, especially TNF-α and IL-1, lead to the increased proliferation and activation of fibroblasts. This results in synovitis with pannus formation and in consecutive bone and joint damage, which appears as erosions and deformities on radiographs.

C. Induction of Rheumatoid Arthritis

A still unknown antigen stimulates the activation of T lymphocytes that, in turn, activate synovial macrophages. The macrophages secrete the decisive cytokines, TNF-α and IL-1, which activate osteoclasts and chondrocytes. This "two-pronged attack" results in the destruction of cartilage and bone. The chondrocytes then begin to produce large quantities of fibroblast growth factor (FGF) and GM-CSF, which completes a harmful cycle that can result in reactivation of the macrophages. This may be the reason why the disease process sometimes persists for long periods of time, even after T cells have been destroyed, for example, in monoclonal antibody therapy. The new therapeutic approaches using monoclonal antibodies or similar working models are based on these concepts (see p. 261).

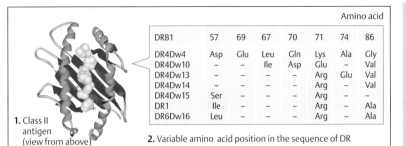

Amino acid

DRB1	57	69	67	70	71	74	86
DR4Dw4	Asp	Glu	Leu	Gln	Lys	Ala	Gly
DR4Dw10	–	–	Ile	Asp	Glu	–	Val
DR4Dw13	–	–	–	–	Arg	Glu	Val
DR4Dw14	–	–	–	–	Arg	–	Val
DR4Dw15	Ser	–	–	–	Arg	–	–
DR1	Ile	–	–	–	Arg	–	Ala
DR6Dw16	Leu	–	–	–	Arg	–	Ala

1. Class II antigen (view from above)

2. Variable amino acid position in the sequence of DR

A. Susceptibility to rheumatoid arthritis

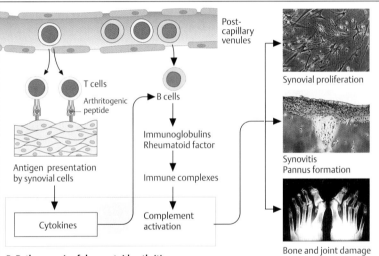

Post-capillary venules

T cells

Arthritogenic peptide

B cells

Antigen presentation by synovial cells

Immunoglobulins
Rheumatoid factor

Immune complexes

Cytokines

Complement activation

Synovial proliferation

Synovitis
Pannus formation

Bone and joint damage

B. Pathogenesis of rheumatoid arthritis

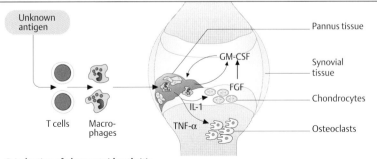

Unknown antigen

T cells

Macro-phages

GM-CSF

FGF

IL-1

TNF-α

Pannus tissue

Synovial tissue

Chondrocytes

Osteoclasts

C. Induction of rheumatoid arthritis

A. The Activated Rheumatoid Synovial Macrophage

Apart from T lymphocytes, activated rheumatoid synovial macrophages (RSM) are further central cell elements that induce destruction. Around 30% of all cells in the inflamed synovial membrane are of this cell type. RSMs bear all important molecules: the CD14 antigen, the full set of class II HLA antigens (DR, DQ, DP), Fc receptors, and the CD4 antigen. Intracellular RSMs are characterized by the presence of CD68 antigen. In addition to membrane-bound molecules, RSMs also secrete numerous mediators and cytokines, such as TNF-α and IL-1, to name a few of the most important ones. Rheumatoid synovial macrophages also produce counter-regulatory cytokines (mainly TGF-β and IL-10), but their release is probably futile to counteract the proinflammatory cytokines. In tissue cultures, the macrophages are very active and are characterized by increased phagocytosis and heightened chemotaxis.

B. Activated Cells in the Rheumatoid Synovial Membrane

Activated synovial cells are presented in the illustrations. They show (**1**), an oligodendritic, class II HLA-positive cell; (**2**), a CD14+ giant cell, which may occur in granuloma-like formations; and (**3**), a typical stellate synovial cell (*stellate cell*) that corresponds to a synovial fibroblast and bears aberrant class II HLA antigens. Stellate cells should not be confused with dendritic cells, which are also present in the synovial membrane in patients with rheumatoid arthritis.

C. Rheumatoid Factors (Antiglobulins)

Rheumatoid factors are immunoglobulins directed against the Fc region of IgG. They are the prime example of an autoimmune manifestation, since they represent an antibody directed against its own kind ("antiglobulin"). Rheumatoid factors are also present in healthy individuals in low amounts. Their significance is probably attributable to the nonspecific enhancement of antibody reactions in infections, especially in the early phases where the supply of specific immunoglobulins is not yet fully mounted. This is also the case in fierce immunological clashes, such as in endocarditis. In rheumatoid arthritis, still unknown mechanisms cause the abnormal proliferation of rheumatoid factors with affinity maturation to rheumatoid factors of the IgG class, which normally are not detectable.

Although they are found in other diseases, rheumatoid factors are still the most important humoral features of rheumatoid arthritis. IgM-RF is easy to detect. Because of its free arms, it has free reaction partners in test systems (**1**). IgG rheumatoid factors stimulate the formation of large immune complexes. In this case, the autoantibodies bind with one another, and it is difficult to separate them from these complexes. Therefore, they cannot be detected in classical rheumatoid factor tests (**2**).

D. Impaired B-Cell Regulation

Because of still unidentified disturbances at the stages of antigen presentation and regulation, B lymphocytes are stimulated to produce rheumatoid factors, which form large immune complexes. This activates the complement system and the release of chemotactic complement cleavage products, leading to substantial vasculitis. As a result, cytokines and mediators of inflammation are released in the tissue. These molecules attract granulocytes and macrophages that contribute to the process of tissue destruction. This mechanism probably plays a decisive role in the development of extra-articular vasculitis-associated lesions observed in rheumatoid arthritis.

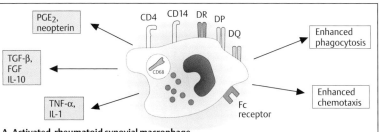

PGE₂, neopterin

TGF-β, FGF IL-10

TNF-α, IL-1

CD4 CD14 DR DP DQ

CD68

Fc receptor

Enhanced phagocytosis

Enhanced chemotaxis

A. Activated rheumatoid synovial macrophage

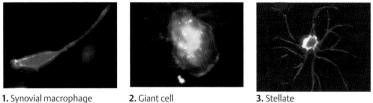

1. Synovial macrophage   **2.** Giant cell   **3.** Stellate synovial cell

B. Activated cells of the rheumatoid synovial membrane

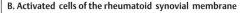

1. IgM rheumatoid factor

2. IgG rheumatoid factor (also IgA and IgE rheumatoid factor)

C. Rheumatoid factors (anti-globulins)

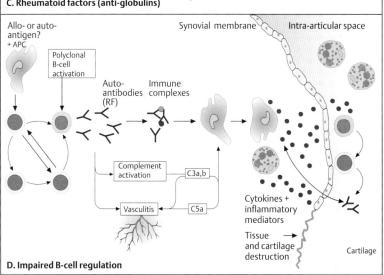

Allo- or auto-antigen? + APC

Polyclonal B-cell activation

Auto-antibodies (RF)

Immune complexes

Synovial membrane

Intra-articular space

Complement activation

C3a,b

Vasculitis

C5a

Cytokines + inflammatory mediators

Tissue and cartilage destruction

Cartilage

D. Impaired B-cell regulation

Clinical Immunology

A. Classification

There are several forms of juvenile chronic arthritis (JCA). The first is *polyarticular JCA*, a seronegative (RF-negative) form that begins in early childhood. There are significant differences between polyarticular JCA and the adult form, which occurs later and is RF-positive. *Oligoarticular JCA* is divided into early-onset pauciarticular arthritis (EOPA; type I) and late-onset pauciarticular arthritis (LOPA; type II). The early onset form is characterized by the presence of anti-nuclear antibodies, whereas the presence of histocompatibility antigen HLA-B27 is typical of the late-onset form. In addition to these forms, there is also *systemic juvenile chronic arthritis* (Still's disease), which is characterized by severe organ manifestations.

B. Systemic JCA (Still's Disease)

Still's disease presents a dramatic clinical picture with numerous manifestations. It is characterized by rashes that are often transient, high fever (up to 41 °C), polyserositis with pleural and pericardial effusions and, in many cases, hepatosplenomegaly. The disease may initially be mistaken for leukemia if the laboratory work-up reveals severe leukocytosis with left shifting in patients with frequent lymphadenopathies. Still's disease usually occurs as a symmetrical and peripheral form of polyarthritis with severe swelling and impaired joint mobility.

C. Polyarticular JCA

Seronegative polyarticular JCA usually starts between the ages of 2 and 5 years. The typical patient has mandibular joint involvement (often with micrognathia) and a symmetrical pattern of polyarthritis. Epiphyseal growth disorders with limb length differences are possible complications. Girls are predominantly affected. The laboratory tests are vague; anti-nuclear antibodies are occasionally detected. In many cases, polyarticular JCA may completely resolve after puberty.

Seropositive polyarticular JCA, which is also referred to as "early-onset rheumatoid arthritis," usually begins in children over 10 years of age. The RF-positive juvenile form is indistinguishable from seropositive adult rheumatoid arthritis. In most cases, there is a severe course of disease with symmetrical arthritic destruction. Laboratory tests reveal rheumatoid factors and anti-nuclear antibodies; the DR4 antigen is usually present.

D. Early-Onset Oligoarthritis

This disease usually affects infants. Arthritis, itself, usually is not the primary problem as the disease tends to run a mild course. Chronic iridocyclitis, which is associated with the risk of blindness, is a serious complication. This form of iridocyclitis is associated with anti-nuclear antibodies and predominantly affects girls.

E. Juvenile Spondyloarthropathy

Like the RF-positive polyarticular diseases, juvenile spondyloarthropathies are the childhood forms of adult spondyloarthropathies. Seronegative spondylarthritides usually manifest with sacroiliitis and involvement of the hip joint or of other large joints. Juvenile spondyloarthropathies usually affect boys. They are characteristically associated with the presence of HLA-B27 and the absence of rheumatoid factors and anti-nuclear antibodies. The prognosis is uncertain. The disease may either completely disappear after puberty or progress to a typical clinical picture of ankylosing spondylitis.

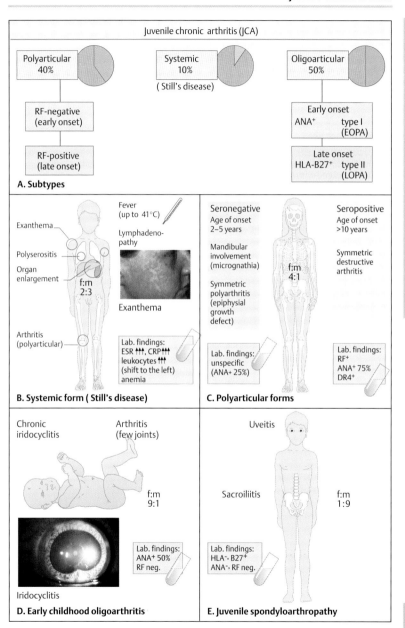

Juvenile chronic arthritis (JCA)

Polyarticular 40%

Systemic 10%
(Still's disease)

Oligoarticular 50%

RF-negative
(early onset)

RF-positive
(late onset)

Early onset
ANA⁺   type I
(EOPA)

Late onset
HLA-B27⁺   type II
(LOPA)

A. Subtypes

B. Systemic form (Still's disease)

Exanthema
Polyserositis
Organ enlargement
f:m 2:3
Arthritis (polyarticular)

Fever (up to 41°C)
Lymphadenopathy

Exanthema

Lab. findings:
ESR ↟↟↟, CRP↟↟↟
leukocytes ↟↟↟
(shift to the left)
anemia

C. Polyarticular forms

Seronegative
Age of onset 2–5 years

Mandibular involvement (micrognathia)

Symmetric polyarthritis (epiphysial growth defect)

f:m 4:1

Seropositive
Age of onset >10 years

Symmetric destructive arthritis

Lab. findings:
unspecific
(ANA+ 25%)

Lab. findings:
RF⁺
ANA⁺ 75%
DR4⁺

D. Early childhood oligoarthritis

Chronic iridocyclitis
Arthritis (few joints)

f:m 9:1

Iridocyclitis

Lab. findings:
ANA⁺ 50%
RF neg.

E. Juvenile spondyloarthropathy

Uveitis

Sacroiliitis

f:m 1:9

Lab. findings:
HLA⁻, B27⁺
ANA⁻, RF neg.

Clinical Immunology

175

These disorders have great similarities. In particular, they are linked by association with HLA-B27, the presumed immune pathogenetic factor, and typical clinical manifestations. The name "spondyloarthropathy" implies involvement of the axial skeleton. This group of disorders is classified according to the criteria of the European Spondyloarthropathy Study Group (ESSG; see table).

A. Clinical Features

This group of diseases includes ankylosing spondylitis (SpA), reactive arthritides (reA), arthritides associated with chronic inflammatory bowel disease (IBD), and psoriatic arthritis.

Ankylosing spondylitis is a systemic inflammatory disease that mainly affects the axial skeleton and joints, but sometimes the internal organs. It predominantly affects males and usually starts between the ages of 15 and 30 years. Apart from the joints, the disease also affects fibrocartilaginous structures, such as the synchondroses and intervertebral disks. Pathological changes are especially common at the sites of insertion of tendons and ligaments. The course is chronic and progressive, and the spine and sacroiliac joints are always affected. Additional involvement of the peripheral joints occurs in 25% of cases. The disease may also have extra-articular manifestations, the most common of which are anterior uveitis (iritis) and urethritis; prostatitis is common in the male patients.

Reactive arthritides are often associated with a prior bowel infection or urethritis. Oligoarthritis involving 2–4 large or small joints usually occurs after a latency of 10 to no more than 30 days. The joints of the lower extremities are almost always affected, and there is preferential involvement of the knee and ankle joints. In addition to cutaneous manifestations (keratoderma blenorrhagicum; see photograph), conjunctivitis and iridocyclitis are also common (Reiter's triad: arthritis, urethritis, conjunctivitis).

Psoriatic arthritis may arise from monoarthritis, oligoarthritis, or polyarthritis. Many patients with a long history of the disease may have polyarticular manifestations with characteristic involvement of the distal interphalangeal joints (DIJ) of the fingers and toes, the interphalangeal joints of the thumbs. The sacroiliac joints and vertebral joints may also be affected. In peripheral joint involvement, the most common problem is dactylitis, the radial inflammation of all joints of a finger or toe.

B. Pathogenesis

Spondyloarthropathies are often associated with inflammatory bowel diseases and/or urethral or cervical inflammations. The fact that large quantities of antigenic material can enter into the circulation seems to play a particularly important role in patients with inflammatory mucosal changes. If a genetic predisposition also exists, the arthritides tend to occur at a time when the triggering disease is no longer present. The promoter regions of proinflammatory cytokine genes (genetic modifiers) and the types of treatment affect the further course of disease.

C. Prevalence of HLA-B27 Antigen

The prevalence of HLA-B27 antigen is ca. 90–95% in individuals with ankylosing spondylitis, and 8–10% in the general population, depending on the ethnic composition. Some studies have concluded that up to 20% of all HLA-27-positive individuals will develop ankylosing spondylitis or undifferentiated spondyloarthropathies during their lifetime.

ESSG Classification of Spondyloarthropathies

Inflammatory spinal pain
  or
Synovitis
  asymmetric or
  predominantly in the lower limbs
and one or more of the following:
Positive family history
Psoriasis
Inflammatory bowel diseases
Urethritis, cervicitis, or acute diarrhea within
  1 month before arthritis
Buttock pain alternating between right and
  left gluteal areas
Enthesopathy
Sacroiliitis

Clinical Immunology

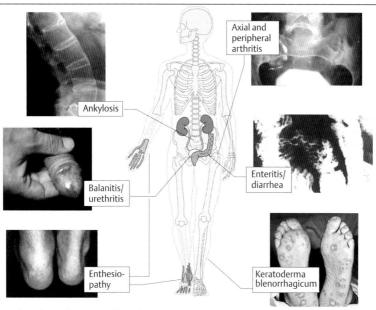

A. Clinical manifestations of spondyloarthropathies

Ankylosis

Axial and peripheral arthritis

Balanitis/ urethritis

Enteritis/ diarrhea

Enthesio-pathy

Keratoderma blenorrhagicum

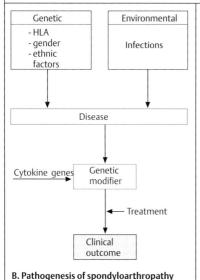

B. Pathogenesis of spondyloarthropathy

Genetic	Environmental
- HLA - gender - ethnic factors	Infections

Disease

Cytokine genes → Genetic modifier ← Treatment

Clinical outcome

C. Frequency of HLA-B27 antigen

Ankylosing spondylitis	95%
Reiter's syndrome (classic form)	80%
Undifferentiated spondyloarthropathy	70%
Arthritis with IBD	25%
Psoriatic arthritis	25%
Reactive arthritis	20–80%
Normal population	8–10%

Clinical Immunology

177

The three models described below are used to explain the question of how the HLA-B27 antigen is involved in the pathogenesis of spondyloarthropathies.

A. Molecular Mimicry

This hypothesis, like the "tolerance" theory, assumes there is great structural similarity between the polymorphic regions of the HLA-B27 antigen and bacterial pathogens. When infections occur, the bacterial antigens are recognized as foreign, and adequate T-cell-mediated and humoral responses occur. Because of the structural similarity with HLA-B27, the antigen is mistakenly identified as foreign. As a result, the immune system begins to attack endogenous tissue, which triggers a still unknown cascade that leads to the manifestations of spondyloarthropathy.

B. "Tolerance"

The tolerance model is based on similar assumptions. In this case, however, the structural similarity between HLA-B27 and the microbial antigens does not lead to an autoaggressive process, but to incorrect tolerance of the bacterial antigens. As a result, the pathogens persist in the affected joint, and they are not effectively eliminated by the immune system. The confrontation with the pathogen leads to the development of inflammatory processes that trigger arthritis.

C. The "Promiscuous" B27 Hypothesis

According to this recently developed model, HLA-B27 antigen is not directly involved in the antigen recognition of an arthritogenic peptide, but acts as an autoantigen that indirectly sets off the inflammatory cascade via CD4-mediated mechanisms. Accordingly, the HLA-B27 molecule is broken down into tiny fragments (peptides) inside the cells. The fragments enter the peptide-binding site of the HLA-DR antigen and are then presented to the actual arthritogenic CD4+ T cells. These T-helper cells set the process of arthritis in motion.

D. Induction of Spondyloarthropathy in Transgenic Rats

The direct impact of the HLA-B27 antigen was demonstrated in animal experiments with trangenic rats. Rat oocytes were transfected with human HLA-B27 combined with β_2-microglobulin and implanted in sham pregnant rats. The transgenic progeny exhibited manifestations similar to those of HLA-B27-associated spondyloarthropathies in humans. In addition to self-gene products, they also demonstrated the presence of human HLA-B27 antigen and β_2-microglobulin. The animals developed arthritis, psoriasis, nail changes, and colitis. Interestingly, the disease did not develop in animals raised in a germ-free environment. This impressively underlines the role of infections in the pathogenesis of spondyloarthropathies.

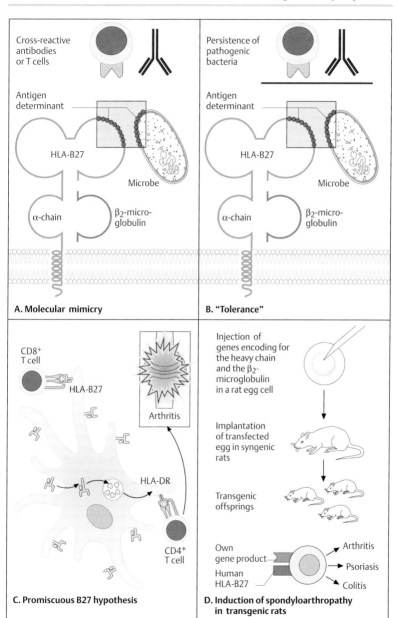

Cross-reactive antibodies or T cells

Antigen determinant

HLA-B27

Microbe

α-chain

β₂-micro-globulin

A. Molecular mimicry

Persistence of pathogenic bacteria

Antigen determinant

HLA-B27

Microbe

α-chain

β₂-micro-globulin

B. "Tolerance"

CD8⁺ T cell

HLA-B27

Arthritis

HLA-DR

CD4⁺ T cell

C. Promiscuous B27 hypothesis

Injection of genes encoding for the heavy chain and the β₂-microglobulin in a rat egg cell

Implantation of transfected egg in syngenic rats

Transgenic offsprings

Own gene product

Human HLA-B27

→ Arthritis

→ Psoriasis

→ Colitis

D. Induction of spondyloarthropathy in transgenic rats

Clinical Immunology

179

A. Gout

Primary gout results from the accumulation and deposition of uric acid due to a genetic predisposition in association with high levels of purine in the diet. Gouty crystals (monosodium urate) accumulate mainly in the joints, but also in the cartilage and connective tissue by systemic spreading.

1 Gout patients have an inherited defect in urate excretion. The condition remains asymptomatic at normal urate concentrations. However, a purine-rich diet leads to the accumulation of urate (hyperuricemia: >7 mg/dl) and, ultimately, to the precipitation of urate salts. Secondary gout is caused by increased serum urate levels due to increased cellular catabolism (e.g., in polycythemia vera, various leukemias, cytostatic therapy, and radiotherapy) or decreased excretion (e.g., tubular defects or competition from lactate, ketones, or diuretics at the tubules).

2 The precipitation of gouty crystals most commonly occurs in the joints of the lower extremities, where it triggers an inflammatory response. A gouty attack may involve the first metatarsophalangeal joint of the big toe (podagra) or the knee joint (gonagra). Granulocytes migrate into the joint and phagocytose the crystals but cannot catalyze them by lysosomal mechanisms. The crystals damage the lysosomal membrane of the granulocytes, resulting in the release of enzymes and mediators of inflammation. The gouty attack is self-propagating. In acute gouty attacks, the goal of treatment is, therefore, to disrupt the inflammatory response. These attacks can be effectively managed with colchicine, an alkaloid that arrests cell division in metaphase by disrupting the mitotic spindle. The drug also binds to the contractile elements of granulocytes, thereby preventing them from migrating to the sites of inflammation.

Chronic gout is characterized by the deposition of urate crystals in soft tissues (outer ear, heel), bone (especially proximal to the joints), and kidney (**2**). Prophylactic treatment for prevention of gouty attacks consists in reducing the urate concentration. This can be achieved through dietary measures or drug treatment. Allopurinol is a uricostatic drug that inhibits xanthine oxidase, thereby reducing urate production. Benzbromarone is a uricosuric drug that increases renal urate excretion.

B. Polychondritis

Polychondritis is an inflammation of unknown etiology that affects various cartilaginous structures, especially the ears, nose, and trachea. It often occurs in association with systemic vasculitis. The disease most commonly begins between the ages of 40 and 60 years and has an intermittent course. Inflammation and swelling of the cartilaginous structures leads to the development of deformities, such as saddle nose and cauliflower ear. Softening of the tracheal cartilage can lead to inspiratory stridor and tracheal wall collapse. The articular cartilage is affected in a pattern similar to nonerosive polyarthritis. Eye involvement that manifests as episcleritis, iritis, and uveitis is common. Vasculitis of the major blood vessels can result in aortitis and aortic insufficiency. Blood tests reveal increases in the parameters of inflammation, but there is an absence of nuclear autoantibodies. Acute episodes are managed by prednisolone therapy; severe attacks usually require azathioprine, cyclophosphamide, or cyclosporin A.

C. Behçet's Syndrome

Behçet's syndrome is a systemic inflammation of the small vessels characterized by a triad of symptoms, including aphthous ulceration of the oral mucous membranes and genitalia and uveitis. Rare manifestations include oligoarthritis of the lower extremities, vasculitis of the pulmonary vessels, and cerebrovascular symptoms. The etiology of Behçet's syndrome is unknown. An association with HLA-B52 has been found. The oral aphthous ulcerations must be differentiated from habitual oral aphthae and those associated with immune vasculitis and Crohn's disease. The patients are usually treated with local steroid therapy or systemic drugs, such as cyclosporin A and cyclophosphamide.

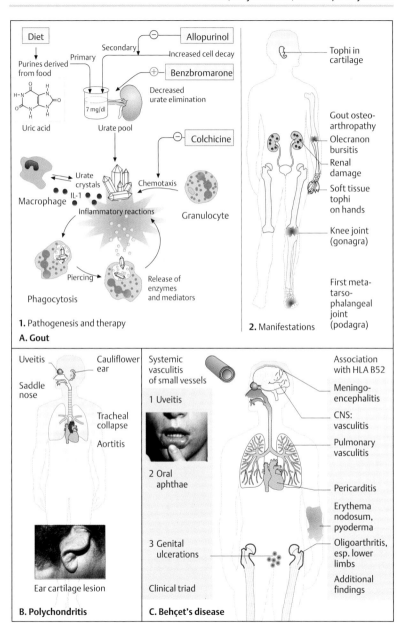

Diet

Purines derived from food

Primary

Secondary → ⊖ **Allopurinol**

Increased cell decay

⊕ **Benzbromarone**

Decreased urate elimination

Uric acid

7 mg/dl

Urate pool

⊖ **Colchicine**

Urate crystals

Macrophage

IL-1

Chemotaxis

Inflammatory reactions

Granulocyte

Piercing

Phagocytosis

Release of enzymes and mediators

1. Pathogenesis and therapy

Tophi in cartilage

Gout osteo-arthropathy

Olecranon bursitis

Renal damage

Soft tissue tophi on hands

Knee joint (gonagra)

First meta-tarso-phalangeal joint (podagra)

2. Manifestations

A. Gout

Clinical Immunology

Uveitis

Cauliflower ear

Saddle nose

Tracheal collapse

Aortitis

Ear cartilage lesion

B. Polychondritis

Systemic vasculitis of small vessels

1 Uveitis

2 Oral aphthae

3 Genital ulcerations

Clinical triad

C. Behçet's disease

Association with HLA B52

Meningo-encephalitis

CNS: vasculitis

Pulmonary vasculitis

Pericarditis

Erythema nodosum, pyoderma

Oligoarthritis, esp. lower limbs

Additional findings

A. Autoantibody Patterns

Certain autoantibodies that produce certain patterns in indirect immunofluorescence studies (see p. 75**B**) that are characteristic of systemic autoimmunopathies. In many cases, these autoantibodies allow a preliminary classification of specificity and of the diseases associated with them. Connective tissue diseases are associated with characteristic autoantibodies. They were originally called "collagen vascular diseases" because it was assumed that the collagen-containing connective tissue was the target of autoimmunity. This group of diseases includes systemic lupus erythematosus (SLE), Sjögren's syndrome, scleroderma, polymyositis/dermatomyositis, and genetic connective tissue disease (MCTD). The large majority of the target autoantigens are constituents of the cell nucleus and cytoplasm that play a role in the processing of genetic information. The patterns and disease associations are described in Table 3 "Anti-nuclear antibodies in rheumatic diseases" and Table 4 "Significance of autoantibodies in the diagnosis of autoimmune diseases" in the appendix section.

Clinical Immunology

Significance of Autoantibodies in the Diagnosis of Autoimmune Diseases

Auto-antibody	SLE	MCTD	Sclero-derma	Myo-sitis	Sjögren's syndrom	Rheuma-toid arthritis	Primary vasculitis	Anti-phospho-lipid syndrome
	Associated disease							
ANA	+++	+++	+++	+	+++	+	+	+
dsDNA	+++	-	-	-	-	-	-	-
SM	++	-	-	-	-	-	-	-
U1-RNP	+	+++	+	+	-	-	-	-
Ribosomal P	++	-	-	-	-	-	-	-
PCNA	+	-	-	-	-	-	-	-
Ro	++	+	+	-	+++	+	-	-
La	++	+	+	-	+++	+	-	-
RA33	++	++	-	-	+	++	-	-
Scl70	-	-	+++	-	-	-	-	-
Centromere	-	-	+++	-	-	-	-	-
Jo-1	-	-	-	++	-	-	-	-
PM-Scl	-	-	+	+	-	-	-	-
Cardiolipin	+++	+	+	-	+	+	-	+++
ANCA	-	-	-	-	-	-	+++	-
Rheumatoid factor	++	+	+	+	+++	+++	+	-

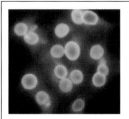

1. Rim pattern
(150x magnif; anti-DNA)

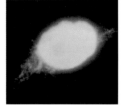

2. Homogenous pattern
(435x enlarged; anti-DNA)

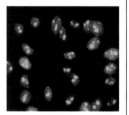

3. Nucleolar pattern
(e.g. fibrillarin)

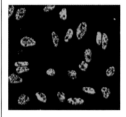

4. Coarse-speckled pattern
(U1RNP/Sm)

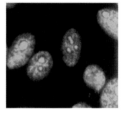

5. Fine-speckled pattern
(Ro/La)

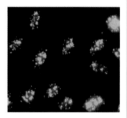

6. Anti-centromere antibody
pattern

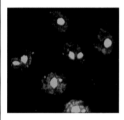

7. PM-Scl pattern

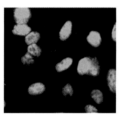

8. Anti-spindle-apparatus
antibody pattern

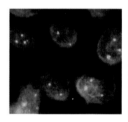

9. Anti-coilin antibody
pattern

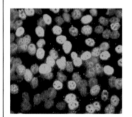

10. Anti-PCNA antibody
pattern

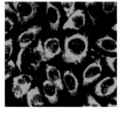

11. Anti-mitochondrial
antibody pattern

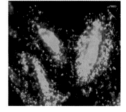

12. Anti-Jo-1 antibody
pattern

A. Autoantibody patterns

Systemic lupus erythematosus (SLE) is a chronic, intermittent autoimmune inflammatory disease that affects multiple organ systems and is characterized by the presence of anti-nuclear antibodies. The disease affects women 10 times more often than men. The age of onset is from 15 to 30 years. As for most other inflammatory rheumatoid diseases, the American College of Rheumatology (ACR) has established a catalog of criteria for classification of SLE (see Table 5 of the Appendix).

A. Clinical Features of SLE

The clinical picture of SLE varies greatly depending on the type of organ involvement. Skin manifestations are a common initial feature in 70% of these patients. Other common features include the characteristic "butterfly rash," which occurs in around 50% of patients, and discoid skin involvement, which occurs in 20% of patients; vasculitic lesions are also common. The majority of SLE patients suffer from joint pain, but only a few develop severe joint deformities (Jaccoud's arthritis, see photograph). This type of deforming arthritis is usually associated with extensive subluxation in the absence of bone destruction. Renal involvement (lupus nephritis), CNS involvement (epilepsy or stroke accompanied by secondary anti-phospholipid syndrome) and pleuropericarditis are life-threatening complications of SLE. General symptoms, such as fever and fatigue, are observed in the active phases of the disease.

Immunological diagnosis: The demonstration of anti-nuclear antibodies (ANA) is important because of their association with organ manifestations. The presence of antibodies against double-stranded DNA is a pathognomic finding.

Treatment is selected in accordance with the severity of disease and the type and severity of organ manifestations. Low-dose glucocorticoids and antimalarial agents may suffice in mild forms of the disease. These drugs are particularly effective for skin manifestations, and they reduce the frequency of attacks. Acute attacks require high-dose steroid bolus therapy. Intravenous cyclophosphamide is indicated for treatment of severe organ manifestations, such as diffuse glomerulonephritis and neuropsychiatric lupus. Azathioprine is indicated for treatment of moderate organ manifestations or subsequent to a cyclophosphamide treatment phase. Treatment modalities involving the use of monoclonal antibodies, e.g., anti-CD4, immune adsorption techniques, and autologous stem cell transplantation (see p. 159**B**) are currently in the clinical/experimental testing phase.

ACR Criteria for Classification of SLE
Malar rash
Discoid rash
Photosensitivity
Oral ulcers
Arthritis
Serositis
Renal disorder
Neurological disorder
Hematological disorder
Immunological disorder
Antinuclear antibodies

The simultaneous or serial detection of 4 or more of these 11 criteria in a patient during a given observation period is classified as diagnostic of SLE.

Clinical Immunology

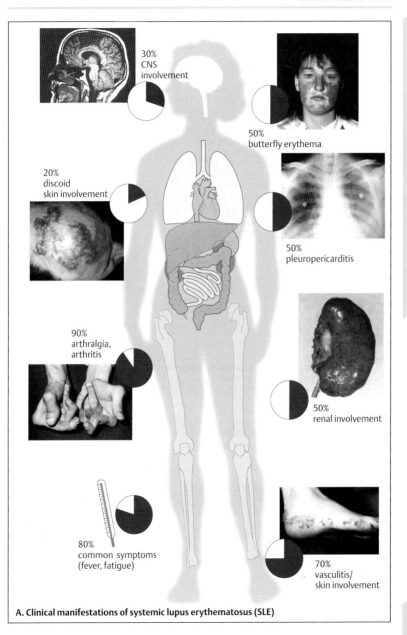

30%
CNS
involvement

50%
butterfly erythema

20%
discoid
skin involvement

50%
pleuropericarditis

90%
arthralgia,
arthritis

50%
renal involvement

80%
common symptoms
(fever, fatigue)

70%
vasculitis/
skin involvement

A. Clinical manifestations of systemic lupus erythematosus (SLE)

The theories on the pathogenesis of SLE vary as widely as the clinical manifestations of the disease. Numerous autoantibody phenomena caused by major underlying cellular autoimmunity disturbances are predominant clinical features.

A. Pathogenesis of Systemic Lupus Erythematosus

The disease-inducing mechanisms initially manifest as tissue lesions. Viral infections have been implicated as a cause, but UV radiation can also trigger the disease. Cytokines (e.g., TNF-α) released during the development of tissue lesions lead to the aberrant expression of autoantigens on the cell surface. Nuclear antigens (e.g., Ro antigen) thereby reach the surface of cells, such as keratinocytes. Apoptotic cells that were exposed to certain noxae release apoptotic blebs, which often contain antigens from the nucleus and cytoplasm. From then on, the central mechanism is the presentation of autoantigens to T-helper cells. Impairment of regulatory mechanisms and the resulting loss of peripheral tolerance presumably plays an important role in the process. B-cell help occurs, thereby allowing the B cells to present antigens to autoreactive T cells. Extension of the autoimmune response therefore occurs as "epitope spreading."

Autoantibodies against cells of the hematopoietic system are produced during the course of polyclonal B-cell activation. The most important clinical consequences of these events are leukopenia and thrombopenia. Autoantibodies against phospholipids and β_2-glycoprotein-1 develop as in secondary anti-phospholipid syndrome. This can result in complications, such as thrombosis, abortion, and cerebral stroke.

The development of immune complexes by subcellular antigens, especially native double-stranded DNA and anti-DNA antibodies is another important pathogenetic mechanism. In this case, the number of immune complexes produced is too large to be adequately phagocytosed and eliminated by the mononuclear phagocytic system (MPS).

The immune complexes accumulate in vessel walls and eventually cause vasculitis. In conjunction with complement activation, platelet aggregation, and leukocyte activation, this leads to vessel occlusion and subsequent organ damage. The accumulation of immune complexes in different regions of the glomerulus (mesangial, subendothelial, subepithelial) is responsible for the development of different types of lupus nephritis (see also p. 222 ff.).

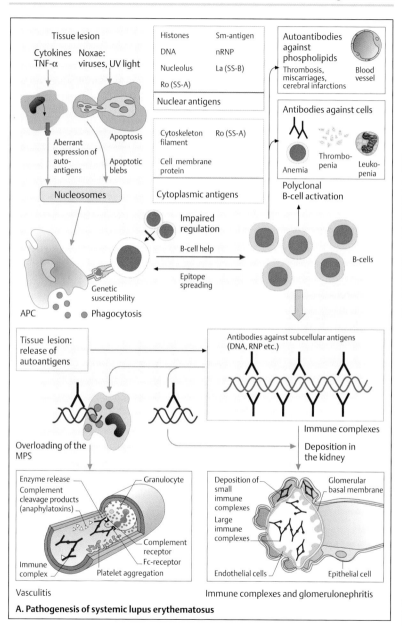

A. Pathogenesis of systemic lupus erythematosus

Clinical Immunology

A. Scleroderma

Scleroderma, or progressive systemic sclerosis (PSS), is characterized by fibrosis of the connective tissue with preferential involvement of the skin, vessels, lungs, pleura, myocardium, pericardium, esophagus, and small intestine. The cause of this multisystem disease is unknown.

1 The affected tissues exhibit an abundance of activated $CD4^+$ T cells, which trigger collagen synthesis in fibroblasts by way of IL-1 and IL-2. Increased collagen deposition in the extracellular space leads to sclerosis of the connective tissue. In vessels, the collagen deposits cause endothelial damage and occlusion due to intimal proliferation. This ultimately results in thickening and induration of the skin, dysfunction of the affected internal organs, and infarctions resulting from obliteration of the vessels.

2 Raynaud's syndrome, a circulatory disorder affecting the distal parts of the extremities, is an early symptom of scleroderma. It may precede the other symptoms by several years. In the later course of disease, initially painless edemas form in the hands (sausage-like fingers) and eventually progress to sclerodactyly (Madonna fingers) with acro-osteolysis. "Rat-bite necrosis" of the fingertips may develop due to impaired circulation. The characteristic features of scleroderma patients with facial sclerosis are a small mouth (microstomia) and pointed nose. Telangiectasias of the skin and mucosae are also common. Myocardial fibrosis and bilateral basal pulmonary fibrosis occur in 40% of all patients with scleroderma. There may be elevation of two parameters of inflammation, C-reactive protein (CRP) and the erythrocyte sedimentation rate (ESR), in addition to the detection of typical autoantibodies in the patient's serum. The demonstration of anti-centromere antibodies or antibodies against topoisomerase I (anti-Scl-70 antibodies) is a primary immunological feature. Anti-nuclear antibodies of different specificities can also be found, whereas anti-dsDNA and Sm antibodies are absent.

3 CREST syndrome is an older designation of a limited form of scleroderma. The acronym is made up of the first letters of the characteristic symptoms of the syndrome: calcinosis (C), Raynaud's syndrome (R), esophageal motility disturbance (E), sclerodactyly (S), and telangiectasia (T). Anti-centromere antibodies are a typical finding observed in 70% of all patients with CREST syndrome. The condition is often associated with primary biliary cirrhosis (PBC).

In addition to immunosuppressive therapy with steroids or basic therapeutic preparations, treatment is also symptomatic. Calcium antagonists are used to treat the circulatory disorders associated with Raynaud's syndrome; prostaglandin infusions are used for skin ulcerations. Prostacyclins have proved to be effective for angiopathy.

B. Mixed Connective Tissue Disease

Mixed connective tissue disease (MCTD), or overlap syndrome, is characterized by the overlapping of symptoms of different connective tissue diseases (SLE, scleroderma, rheumatoid arthritis, polymyositis, dermatomyositis, Sjögren's syndrome). Raynaud's phenomenon is usually the first early symptom of the disease. Other features, in decreasing order of frequency, are sclerodactyly and swelling of the hands, polyarthralgia, pulmonary symptoms, impaired esophageal motility, myositis, and skin manifestations. High titers of autoantibodies against ribonuclease P (U1-RNP) are a typical findings. Anti-nuclear antibodies and rheumatoid factors can also be detected. Autoantibodies against dsDNA, Scl-70, Sm, Ro, La, and PM are infrequently detected. The treatment of MCTD is similar to that of scleroderma or SLE. The actual regimen varies in accordance with the type and severity of the predominant symptoms.

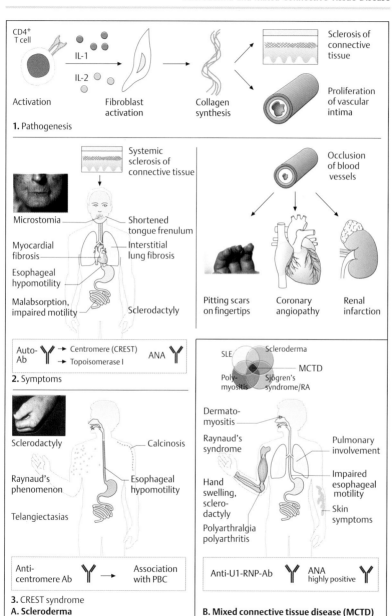

1. Pathogenesis

CD4+ T cell

IL-1

IL-2

Activation

Fibroblast activation

Collagen synthesis

Sclerosis of connective tissue

Proliferation of vascular intima

Systemic sclerosis of connective tissue

Occlusion of blood vessels

Microstomia

Shortened tongue frenulum

Myocardial fibrosis

Interstitial lung fibrosis

Esophageal hypomotility

Malabsorption, impaired motility

Sclerodactyly

Pitting scars on fingertips

Coronary angiopathy

Renal infarction

Auto-Ab → Centromere (CREST) → Topoisomerase I

ANA

2. Symptoms

SLE

Scleroderma

Poly-myositis

MCTD

Sjögren's syndrome/RA

Sclerodactyly

Calcinosis

Raynaud's phenomenon

Esophageal hypomotility

Telangiectasias

Dermato-myositis

Raynaud's syndrome

Pulmonary involvement

Hand swelling, sclero-dactyly

Impaired esophageal motility

Polyarthralgia polyarthritis

Skin symptoms

Anti-centromere Ab → Association with PBC

Anti-U1-RNP-Ab

ANA highly positive

3. CREST syndrome

A. Scleroderma

B. Mixed connective tissue disease (MCTD)

Clinical Immunology

A. Clinical Features

Distinctions are made between primary and secondary Sjögren's syndrome. The primary form is an autoimmune disease of the exocrine glands with extraglandular systemic involvement, whereas the secondary form is also associated with other autoimmune diseases, such as rheumatoid arthritis (50–60% of cases), connective tissue diseases (SLE, scleroderma, polymyositis), vasculitis (polyarteritis nodosa) and/or primary biliary cirrhosis (50% of cases), Hashimoto's autoimmune thyroiditis, and chronic active hepatitis. Second only to rheumatoid arthritis, Sjögren's syndrome is one of the most common inflammatory rheumatic diseases. Women are affected nine times more often than men. The onset is usually after 40 years of age. Dryness of the eyes (xerophthalmia) and dry mouth (xerostomia) are the most common symptoms of Sjögren's syndrome. Inflammation of the salivary and lacrimal glands followed by lymphocytic infiltration and destruction of the glandular tissue is the underlying basis of these "sicca" symptoms. Polyarthralgia (nonerosive arthritis), myalgia, Raynaud's syndrome, and lymphadenopathy are extraglandular manifestations of Sjögren's syndrome. Complications in the lungs (interstitial pneumonia), kidneys (interstitial nephritis, tubular acidosis), and liver (in PBC) are rare manifestations.

B. Pathogenesis

A number of factors play a role in the development of Sjögren's syndrome, which is associated with HLA DR3, DQ1, and DQ2 antigens. The prevalence of Sjögren's syndrome in women suggests that estrogens play at least a supporting role in its pathogenesis. The actual trigger of glandular dysfunction is assumed to be a viral infection. Epithelial cells in the infected gland present viral antigens. This attracts T cells, which infiltrate the glandular tissue and cause a local inflammatory reaction, resulting in damage to the glandular tissue. The T cells activate the glandular epithelium and, most importantly, B cells. This results in excessive, uncontrolled B-cell proliferation, which initially manifests in the peripheral blood as hypergammaglobulinemia in association with the presence of immune complexes. Increases in the ESR and CRP levels can be detected in addition to anti-nuclear antibodies (ANA), rheumatoid factors, and autoantibodies against Ro antigen (SS-A) and La antigen (SS-B). Since these autoantibodies also occur in other autoimmune diseases, their differential diagnostic value is limited. The aggressive polyclonal activation of B cells ultimately progresses to non-Hodgkin's lymphoma in 10–15% of cases.

C. Diagnosis

In addition to these hematological features, certain pathological changes are also of diagnostic importance, for example, *Schirmer's test* of tear secretion (degree of wetting of a strip of paper placed on the lower eyelid), *Saxon's test* of saliva production (the patient must chew on a compress), *sialography, salivary gland scintigraphy* for visualization of the ducts (rarefaction and luminal narrowing), and *labial biopsy* for histological diagnosis (e.g., of periductal lymphocytic infiltration). Siccalike syndromes, such as amyloidosis and AIDS, and the effects of certain drugs (e.g., antidepressants) must be considered in the differential diagnosis.

Management

Treatment is initially symptomatic and is limited to the local application of artificial tears (methylcellulose) and artificial salivary fluid. Nonsteroidal anti-inflammatory drugs and cortisone are used to treat mild joint involvement. Severe extraglandular manifestations require the use of azathioprine.

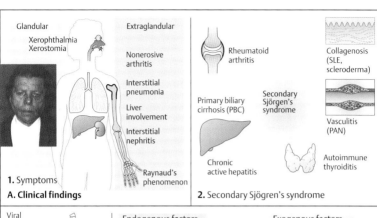

Glandular

Xerophthalmia
Xerostomia

Extraglandular

Nonerosive
arthritis

Interstitial
pneumonia

Liver
involvement

Interstitial
nephritis

Raynaud's
phenomenon

1. Symptoms
A. Clinical findings

Rheumatoid
arthritis

Collagenosis
(SLE,
scleroderma)

Primary biliary
cirrhosis (PBC)

Secondary
Sjögren's
syndrome

Vasculitis
(PAN)

Chronic
active hepatitis

Autoimmune
thyroiditis

2. Secondary Sjögren's syndrome

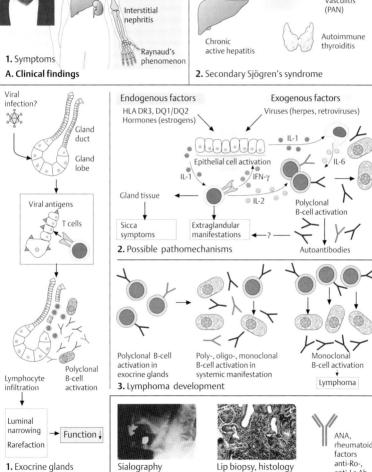

Viral
infection?

Gland
duct

Gland
lobe

Viral antigens

T cells

Lymphocyte
infiltration

Polyclonal
B-cell
activation

Luminal
narrowing → Function ↓
Rarefaction

1. Exocrine glands
B. Pathogenesis

Endogenous factors

HLA DR3, DQ1/DQ2
Hormones (estrogens)

Exogenous factors

Viruses (herpes, retroviruses)

IL-1

Epithelial cell activation

IL-6

IL-1

IFN-γ

IL-2

Gland tissue

Sicca
symptoms

Extraglandular
manifestations ← ?

Polyclonal
B-cell activation

Autoantibodies

2. Possible pathomechanisms

Polyclonal B-cell
activation in
exocrine glands

Poly-, oligo-, monoclonal
B-cell activation in
systemic manifestation

Monoclonal
B-cell activation

Lymphoma

3. Lymphoma development

Sialography

Lip biopsy, histology

ANA,
rheumatoid
factors
anti-Ro-,
anti-La Ab

C. Diagnosis

Clinical Immunology

191

A. Polymyositis, Dermatomyositis, Inclusion-Body Myositis

The clinical picture of the various forms of myositis can vary greatly. The diagnostic criteria are presented in (**4**). Polymyositis (**1**) is characterized by proximal muscle weakness, especially in the shoulders, upper arms, and thighs. The patients experience difficulties in getting up out of a chair and climbing stairs. Dermatomyositis (**2**) is additionally characterized by the occurrence of skin manifestations, especially on areas of the skin exposed to light. One of the most common manifestations is the so-called heliotrope rash (**5**). Characteristic papuloid skin changes called Gottron's sign develop on the knuckles (**6**). A concomitant tumor is often present in many dermatomyositis patients over 50 years of age. Hence, selective investigations for carcinomas must be made, especially in the region of the breasts, lungs, and gastrointestinal tract. The autoantibody findings are generally uncharacteristic; low titers of anti-nuclear antibodies are occasionally found. Conventional blood tests reveal high concentrations of creatine kinase (CK) and myoglobulin. The presence of anti-proteasome antibodies was also recently demonstrated.

Anti-synthetase syndrome (**2**) is an independent disease entity characterized by the presence of Jo-1 antibodies, which are directed against histidyl synthetase. The typical clinical features of the disease include interstitial lung disease, arthritis, Raynaud's phenomenon, skin manifestations, fever, and muscular weakness.

Inclusion-body myositis (**3**) is another distinct disease entity. Unlike the aforementioned diseases, it has a predilection for distal muscles. For the most part, this entity has no characteristic laboratory features.

B. Histology of Inflammatory Myopathies

The histological pictures of polymyositis and dermatomyositis vary greatly. In polymyositis, CD8+ T cells directly infiltrate the individual muscle cells within the muscle fibers (see also **A.7**). Dermatomyositis, on the other hand, is characterized by vasculitis with concomitant perivascular inflammation under the influence of CD4+ T cells. In this case, myocyte death occurs as a secondary effect of vessel lesions.

C. Pathogenesis

Like their histology, the pathogenesis of polymyositis (PM) and dermatomyositis (DM) also differs. Class I MHC-mediated mechanisms play a predominant role in polymyositis. In polymyositis, aberrant expression of class I HLA antigens occurs on the surface of muscle cells, which are normally HLA-negative (only a few other cells in the body are HLA-negative), due to a genetic predisposition and unknown (viral?) factors. Cytotoxic T cells then recognize the altered myocytes as "foreign" and destroy them. This is the histological basis of the aforementioned characteristic processes of cell death within the muscle bundle. Similar pathogenetic mechanisms are suspected in inclusion-body myositis (IBM). The mechanism of development of amyloid-containing cell inclusions in IBM is still unclear.

In dermatomyositis, the inflammation arises from the perimysial vessels. Hence, blood vessel damage is a central element in the pathogenesis of the disease. The resulting tissue ischemia leads to secondary death of the muscle cells, characteristically with pronounced perifascicular involvement.

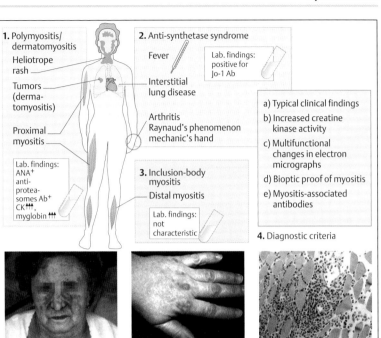

1. Polymyositis/dermatomyositis

Heliotrope rash

Tumors (dermatomyositis)

Proximal myositis

Lab. findings:
ANA⁺
anti-proteasomes Ab⁺
CK ♯♯♯,
myglobin ♯♯♯

2. Anti-synthetase syndrome

Fever

Interstitial lung disease

Arthritis
Raynaud's phenomenon
mechanic's hand

Lab. findings:
positive for
Jo-1 Ab

3. Inclusion-body myositis

Distal myositis

Lab. findings:
not characteristic

a) Typical clinical findings
b) Increased creatine kinase activity
c) Multifunctional changes in electron micrographs
d) Bioptic proof of myositis
e) Myositis-associated antibodies

4. Diagnostic criteria

5. Heliotropic exanthema

6. Gottron's sign

7. Histology of polymyositis

A. Polymyositis/dermatomyositis/inclusion body myositis

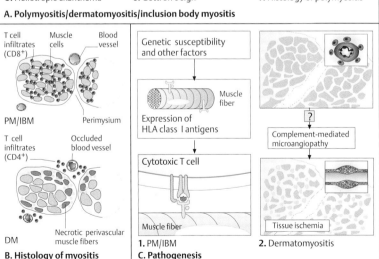

T cell infiltrates (CD8⁺)   Muscle cells   Blood vessel

PM/IBM   Perimysium

T cell infiltrates (CD4⁺)   Occluded blood vessel

DM   Necrotic perivascular muscle fibers

B. Histology of myositis

Genetic susceptibility and other factors

Muscle fiber

Expression of HLA class I antigens

Cytotoxic T cell

Muscle fiber

1. PM/IBM

?

Complement-mediated microangiopathy

Tissue ischemia

2. Dermatomyositis

C. Pathogenesis

Clinical Immunology

193

A. Chapel Hill Definition of Systemic Vasculitis

The pathological definition of vasculitis is based on the inflammatory infiltration and necrosis of the walls of blood vessels. The clinical symptoms vary greatly in accordance with the extent and location of the affected vessel segments. As a result, diagnosis of vasculitis is very complex. A number of classifications exist, but the classification based on the size of the affected vessel has proved to be useful in clinical applications. This classification is called the Chapel Hill definition after the place where the consensus conference was held (see Table 6 of the Appendix).

B. Classification of Vasculitis According to Mechanism of Development

An alternative system classifies the vasculitides according to their mechanism of development, thereby focusing on vessel lesions directly attributable to autoantibodies (ANCA- and AECA-associated vasculitis; see p. 197). The formation of circulating immune complexes plays a key role in the pathogenesis of many vasculitides. Depending on their composition, that is, the type and size of the foreign antigen or autoantigen and of involved antibodies, these immune complexes mediate the activation of inflammatory effector mechanisms (e.g., activation of complement, monocytes, lymphocytes, and thrombocytes; production of cytokines; chemotaxis of granulocytes) on the endothelium. This results in histologically demonstrable intravascular and perivascular infiltration and fibrinoid necrosis of the vessel wall.

The symptoms of vasculitis can occur in basically any infection and are common in infections by the following pathogens: *Streptococcus*, *Salmonella*, *Mycobacterium*, *Spirochaetales*, hepatitis B virus, HIV, Epstein–Barr virus, *Aspergillus*, *Leishmania*, and *Filaria*. In malignant diseases (e.g., Hodgkin's disease and hairy cell leukemia), the primary pathogens are those that affect the lymphoreticular system. A history of the use of medications, such as antibiotics, isoniazid, gold, D-penicillamine, potassium iodide, and busulfan must be considered as a potential cause.

Chapel Hill Definition of Systemic Vasculitis

Vasculitis involving large vessels
• Giant cell (temporal) arteritis
• Takayasu's arteritis
Vasculitis involving medium-sized vessels
• Polyarteritis nodosa
• Kawasaki's disease
Vasculitis involving small vessels
• Wegener's granulomatosis
• Churg–Strauss syndrome
• Microscopic polyangiitis
• Schönlein–Henoch purpura
• Essential cryoglobulinemic vasculitis
• Cutaneous leukocytoclastic angiitis

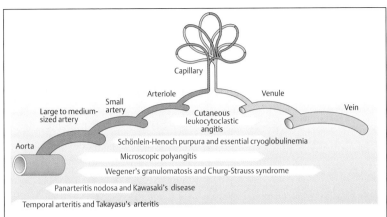

Capillary

Arteriole   Venule

Small
artery   Vein

Large to medium-   Cutaneous
sized artery   leukocytoclastic
                                    angitis

Aorta   Schönlein-Henoch purpura and essential cryoglobulinemia

             Microscopic polyangitis

             Wegener's granulomatosis and Churg-Strauss syndrome

       Panarteritis nodosa and Kawasaki's disease

Temporal arteritis and Takayasu's arteritis

A. Chapel Hill definition of systemic vasculitis

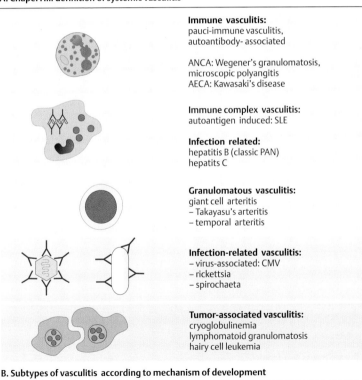

Immune vasculitis:
pauci-immune vasculitis,
autoantibody- associated

ANCA: Wegener's granulomatosis,
microscopic polyangitis
AECA: Kawasaki's disease

Immune complex vasculitis:
autoantigen induced: SLE

Infection related:
hepatitis B (classic PAN)
hepatits C

Granulomatous vasculitis:
giant cell arteritis
– Takayasu's arteritis
– temporal arteritis

Infection-related vasculitis:
– virus-associated: CMV
– rickettsia
– spirochaeta

Tumor-associated vasculitis:
cryoglobulinemia
lymphomatoid granulomatosis
hairy cell leukemia

B. Subtypes of vasculitis according to mechanism of development

A. Theory of the Development of Vasculitis Based on Wegener's Granulomatosis

Proteinase 3 (PR3), the target antigen of anti-neutrophil cytoplasmic antibodies (c-ANCA), is a central mediator in the pathogenesis of this vasculitic disease. PR3 is not accessible to the antibodies in the presence of resting polymorphonuclear neutrophil granulocytes (PMN) in the azurophilic granules (**1**). Prior activation by proinflammatory cytokines leads to the development of adhesion molecules on PMN and endothelial cells (EC) and to the translocation of intracytoplasmic PR3 on the cell membrane (**2**). The PMN then adhere to the endothelial cells (**3**). The PMN are then activated and start to degranulate due to the binding of ANCA to membrane-bound PR3. In the vicinity of endothelial cells, the PMN release toxic mediators and lysosomal proteins that are not accessible to the α-proteinase inhibitor. This results in lysis of the endothelial cells and necrotizing vasculitis (**4**).

B. Wegener's Granulomatosis

Wegener's granulomatosis usually involves the upper and lower respiratory tract and the kidneys, but additional symptoms of vasculitis may also occur in other organ systems. In most cases, the disease initially manifests as a chronic inflammation of the upper respiratory tract in conjunction with mucosal ulceration, purulent rhinitis, sinusitis or inflammation of the middle ear, and progressive destruction and deformity of the cartilaginous part of the nasal skeleton. Pulmonary manifestations include tracheobronchial erosions, pneumonia, and granulomas that may undergo cavernous degeneration. The main clinical features are coughing and hemoptysis, and the systemic features include fever and weight loss. Renal involvement (proteinuria, hematuria, progressive renal failure), arthralgia, purpura, skin ulcerations, and episcleritis are common manifestations in the generalization stage. Involvement of the heart, peripheral nerves, or gastrointestinal tract is less common. The detection of serum antibodies against PR3 (c-ANCA) is a relatively specific finding.

C. Churg–Strauss Syndrome

Churg–Strauss syndrome is a vasculitic disease closely associated with allergic diathesis (history of allergic rhinitis, bronchial asthma, chronic sinusitis, or drug allergies). Transient eosinophilic pulmonary infiltrates are often detected at the onset of the disease. As the disease progresses, organ manifestations similar to those observed in polyarteritis nodosa (PAN) develop with symptoms of arthralgia, palpable purpura, gastrointestinal pain, and hypertension. Renal involvement is uncommon. The main cause of death in these patients is cardiac failure due to cardiomyopathy. Blood tests reveal nonspecific signs of inflammation and massive eosinophilia with counts of over 1500/mm^3 (up to 80% in the differential count), high levels of total IgE, and sometimes rheumatoid factors.

D. Polyarteritis Nodosa

Polyarteritis nodosa (PAN) is a necrotizing vasculitic disease of the medium-sized (primarily visceral) arteries. The clinical picture is usually characterized by extensive yet nonspecific symptoms including general malaise, fever, weight loss, and arthralgia. Peripheral nerve involvement may manifest by way of mononeuritis multiplex (pain, parasthesia or paresis in the innervated area of the affected nerves) in the early stages due to vasculitis of the vasa nervorum. Central nervous manifestations, such as apoplectic infarctions, convulsions, or psychoses, are less common. Kidney involvement is very common, especially glomerulonephritis associated with proteinuria and hematuria. The condition can rapidly progress to renal failure. HBs antigen can be detected in up to 50% of cases.

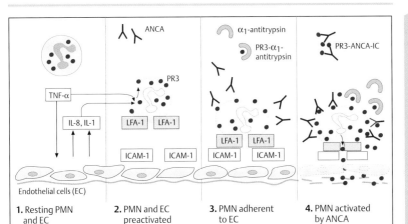

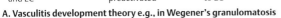

1. Resting PMN and EC

2. PMN and EC preactivated

3. PMN adherent to EC

4. PMN activated by ANCA

Endothelial cells (EC)

A. Vasculitis development theory e.g., in Wegener's granulomatosis

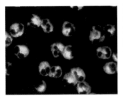

2. C-ANCA

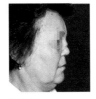

3. Saddle nose

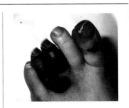

4. Vasculitis of the toes

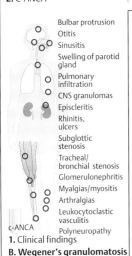

Bulbar protrusion
Otitis
Sinusitis
Swelling of parotid gland
Pulmonary infiltration
CNS granulomas
Episcleritis
Rhinitis, ulcers
Subglottic stenosis
Tracheal/bronchial stenosis
Glomerulonephritis
Myalgias/myositis
Arthralgias
Leukocytoclastic vasculitis
Polyneuropathy

c-ANCA

1. Clinical findings

B. Wegener's granulomatosis

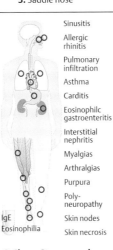

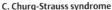

Sinusitis
Allergic rhinitis
Pulmonary infiltration
Asthma
Carditis
Eosinophilc gastroenteritis
Interstitial nephritis
Myalgias
Arthralgias
Purpura
Polyneuropathy
Skin nodes
Skin necrosis

IgE
Eosinophilia

C. Churg-Strauss syndrome

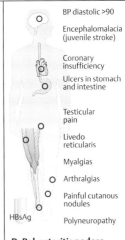

BP diastolic >90
Encephalomalacia (juvenile stroke)
Coronary insufficiency
Ulcers in stomach and intestine
Testicular pain
Livedo reticularis
Myalgias
Arthralgias
Painful cutanous nodules
Polyneuropathy

HBsAg

D. Polyarteritis nodosa

Clinical Immunology

197

There are two types of giant cell arteritis (GCA): *Takayasu's arteritis*, which affects the aorta and its branches, and *temporal arteritis*, which involves the large cranial arteries. The histological features of both types are massive thickening of the arterial wall or frank arterial stenosis (**A.6**) and the presence of polynuclear giant cells (**A.4**). The pathogenesis of these diseases is still unclear. Genetic predisposition (HLA-DR4) and T-helper cell-mediated immune mechanisms leading to granuloma formation, possibly due to still unidentified infections, are the main hypotheses on the pathogenesis of GCA.

A. Giant Cell Arteritis: Temporal Arteritis and Takayasu's Arteritis

Temporal arteritis (called also *cranial arteritis* and *Horton's arteritis*) is a relatively common disease in patients over 50 years of age; see (**3**) for diagnostic criteria. Ratio in women to men is 2:1. There is primary involvement occurs in arteries of the head region (e.g., the temporal artery, retinal artery, and cerebral arteries) but other vessel regions may also be affected. Apart from general symptoms like fever, lassitude, and weight loss, other common symptoms include headache, hyperesthesia in the head region, and palpable induration of the temporal artery (**7**). The most feared complication is sudden blindness due to retinal artery occlusion. Symptoms such as visual impairment, eye aches, or light sensitivity require intensive investigation and rapid therapeutic intervention. Fundoscopy reveals occlusion of retinal artery branches or papillary edema. Scalp ulceration due to a lack of circulation is a rare complication (**8**).

Approximately 20–30% of patients with temporal arteritis have concomitant symptoms of polymyalgia rheumatica; see (**2**) for diagnostic criteria. The predominant features are pain in the proximal shoulder and thigh muscles. There are also general symptoms, such as lassitude, fatigue, depression, and low-grade fever, which are usually extensive.

A prominent laboratory feature of both diseases is a marked increase in the erythrocyte sedimentation rate (ESR) with values often in excess of 100 mm in 1 hour. Mild anemia and leukocytosis may also be detected. Bilateral biopsy of a longer segment of the temporal artery with serial-section histology is required to establish the diagnosis of temporal arteritis. In certain cases, the diagnosis can be established by demonstrating typical echographic changes by Doppler sonography. The prognosis is good, but steroid treatment must usually be administered for one to two years before a lasting remission is achieved.

Takayasu's arteritis (aortic arch syndrome) is a vasculitic disease that predominantly affects young women. The vasculitis involves the thoracic aorta and its branches. The predominant clinical features are therefore related to vessel stenosis, e.g., claudication, pulselessness, vascular murmurs, and/or hypertension. Fever, weight loss, myalgia, and arthralgia may also be observed in the initial inflammatory phase. Headache, dizziness, visual complaints, aortic insufficiency, and aneurysm are less common. The laboratory tests reveal extensive changes in nonspecific parameters of inflammation. Takayasu's arteritis responds well to steroids. However, the prognosis is much worse when extensive vessel lesions are present at the time of diagnosis (**5**).

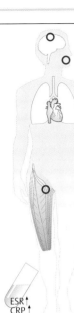

Headache

Temporal arteritis

Scalp skin necrosis

Jaw claudication

Pulmonary vasculitis (rare)

Coronary insufficiency (rare)

Cerebral infarction via extracranial vessels (rare)

Ocular findings

– Loss of vision
– Eye muscle paresis

Polymyalgia of pelvis/ shoulder (bilateral)

ESR↑
CRP↑

Aching shoulders and/ or bilateral stiffness

Disease onset within 2 weeks

Initial ESR increase of >40 mm in 1 hour

Morning stiffness >1 hour

Age over 65 years

Depression and/or weight loss

Bilateral tenderness on palpation of upper arm

2. Diagnostic criteria of polymyalgia rheumatica

Patient over 50 years at first manifestation

Newly occurrent headache

Clinical findings in temporal arteries:

tenderness on palpation, pulselessness

highly increased ESR

positive arterial biopsy

3. Diagnostic criteria of temporal arteritis

1. Clinical findings in temporal arteritis/ polymyalgia rheumatica

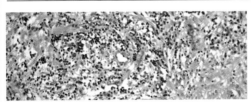

4. Histology of Takayasu's arteritis

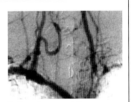

5. Branch stenosis in Takayasu's arteritis

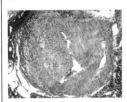

6. Histology of occluded temporal artery

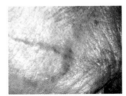

7. Temporal arteritis

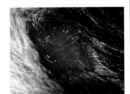

8. Head skin ulcer

A. Clinical features of giant cell arteritis: Takayasu's and temporal arteritis

Urticaria is a disease associated with wheals with pasty swelling and, in many cases, severe itching. The skin eruptions are transient and fade without scarring.

A. Pathogenesis

Cutaneous mast cells play a key role in the pathogenesis of urticaria. After a precipitating stimulus, the mast cells release preformed (histamine, heparin, enzymes) and newly formed mediators of inflammation (prostaglandins, leukotrienes) that induce dermal edema. Edemas of the skin generally subside within 24 hours and are accompanied by itching and erythema. The persistence of a single efflorescence for more than 24 hours suggests the presence of urticarial vasculitis (see **B.4**), a sign of autoimmune disease. After activation and granulation, the mast cells remain refractory for a few hours to days. Urticaria therefore cannot be induced at the same site until after a certain latency period.

B. Triggers and Types

Urticaria can be caused by many different stimuli, all of which lead to a similar clinical picture. The causes may be physical, immunological, or pseudoallergic in nature. The induction of urticaria has also been observed in infections (hepatitis or parasitic infections).

1 In *physical urticaria*, a physical stimulus leads to edema formation or mast cell degranulation in patients with a hypersensitive vascular nervous system. The reaction can be triggered by pressure, heat, cold, rewarming, light, radiation, cholinergic stimuli (sweating), adrenergic stimuli (stress), and aquagenic stimuli. In *contact urticaria*, edema formation is limited to the site of contact with the stimulus (e.g., poison ivy, insect bite, jellyfish).

2 *Acute immunological urticaria* is an allergic IgE-dependent type I reaction that can induce anaphylactic shock within a matter of minutes. Bronchospasm, glottic edema, and circulatory symptoms are typical features. Drugs, such as antibiotic and hypnotics, and certain foods are potential triggers.

3 These reactions are distinguished from *pseudoallergic reactions* to certain substances (aspirin, preservatives, radiographic contrast media) that (may) lead to urticarial and anaphylactoid reactions without a specific immunological reaction.

4 *Urticarial vasculitis* is characterized by hyperpigmented weals that persist for more than 24 hours. The basis of this disease is a type III hypersensitivity reaction and associated formation of immune complexes and complement consumption. The vasculitis leads to urticaria due to the release of vasoactive mediators.

5 *Urticaria pigmentosa* (mastocytosis) tends to be a childhood disease associated with disseminated, reddish-brown spots that form urticarial lesions when rubbed. The underlying mastocytomas usually disappear spontaneously.

C. Diagnosis and Treatment

The case history usually points to the precipitating factors. Possible mechanical causes (**B.1**) and drug triggers should also be sought. Having the patient keep a diary can be helpful. The possibility of an infectious or autoimmune primary disease must be considered in patients with chronic urticaria. In addition to avoiding the triggers, a combination of H1 and H2 antagonists can be prescribed to block the local effects of histamine.

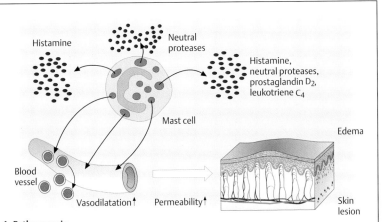

A. Pathogenesis

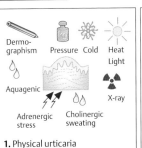

1. Physical urticaria

Dermographism Pressure Cold Heat Light

Aquagenic X-ray

Adrenergic stress Cholinergic sweating

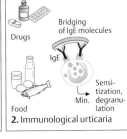

2. Immunological urticaria

Drugs

Bridging of IgE molecules

IgE

Food

Min. degranulation

Sensitization, degranulation

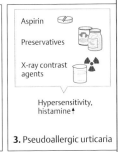

3. Pseudoallergic urticaria

Aspirin

Preservatives

X-ray contrast agents

Hypersensitivity, histamine↑

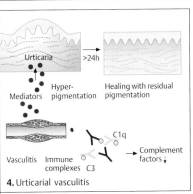

4. Urticarial vasculitis

Urticaria >24h

Mediators Hyperpigmentation Healing with residual pigmentation

Vasculitis Immune complexes C3 C1q → Complement factors↓

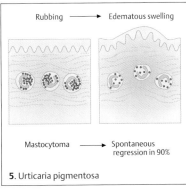

5. Urticaria pigmentosa

Rubbing → Edematous swelling

Mastocytoma → Spontaneous regression in 90%

B. Triggers and manifestations

Contact dermatitis is an inflammation of the skin caused by direct contact with an injurious agent (noxa).

A. Classification

Acute toxic dermatitis is a form of dermatitis that occurs after prior noxa-induced skin damage, for example, due to sunburn. Repeated exposure to weak irritants (e.g., by repeatedly washing and/or disinfecting the hands) can lead to cumulative skin damage (cumulative toxic dermatitis).

Unlike these two forms of dermatitis, allergic contact dermatitis is not caused by noxae but primarily by nontoxic substances that produce immunological reactions in the affected areas of the skin, resulting in inflammation. Allergic contact eczema (allergic contact dermatitis) will be described in the following.

B. Contact Allergens

Chromate in leather and nickel in clothing and jewelry are common triggers of allergic contact dermatitis. Intraepidermal edemas form at the affected sites due to the breakdown of intercellular bridges. Lymphocytes also migrate to the epidermis. Mediators of inflammation lead to vasodilatation in the dermis with subsequent edema formation.

The molecules that provoke the eczema are usually small and therefore behave as haptens. They cannot trigger an immune response without help. They must form covalent bonds with epidermal proteins or be integrated into the cell membrane to develop complete antigen efficacy when present in hapten–protein complexes. The molecules may also be present as prohaptens in the epidermis, where they are transformed into active haptens upon exposure to light (*photoallergic contact dermatitis*).

C. Pathogenesis

Langerhans cells in the epidermis play a key role in the sensitization process (**a**). Animal experiments have shown that, when the cells are removed from the skin, sensitization does not occur and tolerance to the allergen develops. Langerhans cells that act as antigen-presenting cells (APC) pick up, process, and present the allergen to T cells in the lymph nodes. The sensitized T cells are attracted by cytokines from Langerhans cells and keratinocytes and infiltrate the affected skin region.

The basis for the outbreak of allergic contact dermatitis is reexposure to the allergenic stimulus after sensitization (**b**). Keratinocyte-derived cytokines, especially TNF-α, IL-1, and chemokines, initiate the inflammatory response in the epidermis. The sensitized T cells and macrophages migrate from dermal blood vessels with endothelia that express adhesion molecules due to the induction of cytokines. Langerhans cells bearing especially large numbers of surface peptide–MHC complexes sensitize additional T cells which, in turn, release cytokines, thereby leading to the accumulation of inflammatory cells in the epidermis. The allergic contact dermatitis then becomes clinically manifest. The most effective treatment is the total avoidance of the allergenic stimulus. Hyposensitization is not effective.

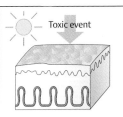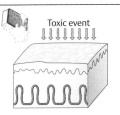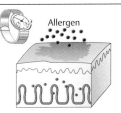

Acute toxic dermatitis

– strong event
– only once
– e. g., sunburn

Cumulative toxic dermatitis

– weak event
– repeatedly
– e. g., frequent hand washing or desinfection

Allergic contact dermatitis

– non-toxic event
– sensibilization causes type IV allergy
– e. g., nickel

A. Causes of dermatitis

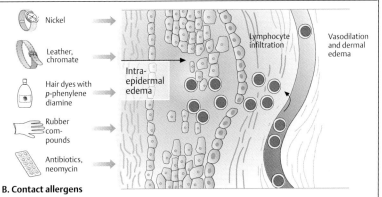

Nickel

Leather, chromate

Hair dyes with *p*-phenylene diamine

Rubber compounds

Antibiotics, neomycin

Lymphocyte infiltration

Vasodilation and dermal edema

Intra-epidermal edema

B. Contact allergens

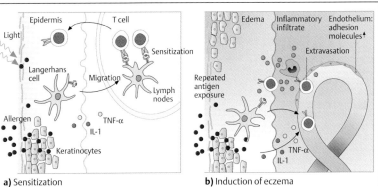

a) Sensitization

Epidermis
T cell
Light
Langerhans cell
Sensitization
Migration
Lymph nodes
Allergen
TNF-α
IL-1
Keratinocytes

b) Induction of eczema

Edema
Inflammatory infiltrate
Endothelium: adhesion molecules↑
Extravasation
Repeated antigen exposure
TNF-α
IL-1

C. Pathogenesis

Clinical Immunology

203

A. Atopic Dermatitis

Atopic dermatitis (neurodermatitis) is a chronic pruritic eczematous disease that is often accompanied by allergic asthma and allergic rhinitis. The disease occurs in intermittent attacks and mainly causes skin lesions on the face, neck, and flexural surfaces. The inflamed areas of the skin tend to become infected. The most common causes are streptococcal infection, *Streptococcus*-induced pyoderma, and eczema herpeticum due to infection with the herpes simplex virus. Genetic and environmental factors (food allergens, skin irritation, psychological factors) play a role in the appearance of the eruptions. The immune pathogenesis of atopic dermatitis is unclear. High levels of IgE and immune complexes containing IgE are often found (2). Increased expression of the receptors for IgE and FcεRI and II on monocytes and Langerhans cells can be observed. There is mainly a T_H2 response. IL-4 activates IgE production and the T_H1 response is partially suppressed, which results in an increased tendency to infection.

There is still no causal treatment for atopic eczema. The patients are treated symptomatically with topical cortisone and tar preparations to prevent inflammation and reduce itching.

B. Leukocytoclastic Vasculitis

Leukocytoclastic vasculitis (called also *allergic vasculitis* and *Schönlein–Henoch purpura*) is an inflammatory disease of the small and medium-sized cutaneous vessels. The lesions (hemorrhages, necrotic lesions, urticarial and papuloid changes) are symmetrically distributed and occur mainly on the lower extremities. Immune complexes play a critical role in the pathogenesis of the disease. The accumulation of the immune complexes in vessel walls along with the subsequent activation of complement ultimately leads to the inflammatory response. Fever, joint complaints, and gastrointestinal complaints are common general reactions; IgA nephropathy is an occasional complication. The diagnosis is established by histopathology. Mild cases respond to physical measures, but patients with systemic involvement require immunosuppressants.

The diagnosis of leukocytoclastic vasculitis is established from the findings of clinical and histological tests. Immunofluorescence microscopic techniques can also be used to demonstrate the deposition of immune complexes in the vessels. It can be extremely difficult or impossible to identify the antigen responsible for formation of immune complexes. Therefore, potential underlying diseases (infections diseases, tumor, autoimmune diseases, and particularly diseases of the collagen vascular type) should be sought.

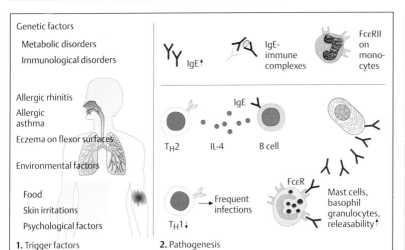

Genetic factors

Metabolic disorders

Immunological disorders

Allergic rhinitis

Allergic asthma

Eczema on flexor surfaces

Environmental factors

Food

Skin irritations

Psychological factors

1. Trigger factors

IgE↑

IgE-immune complexes

FcεRII on monocytes

T$_H$2   IL-4   B cell

IgE

Frequent infections

T$_H$1↓

FcεR

Mast cells, basophil granulocytes, releasability↑

2. Pathogenesis

A. Atopic dermatitis (neurodermatitis)

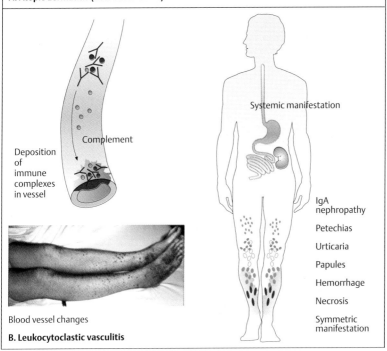

Deposition of immune complexes in vessel

Complement

Systemic manifestation

IgA nephropathy

Petechias

Urticaria

Papules

Hemorrhage

Necrosis

Symmetric manifestation

Blood vessel changes

B. Leukocytoclastic vasculitis

A. Psoriasis

Psoriasis (psoriasis vulgaris) is a hereditary dermatosis characterized by the presence of well-defined, usually circumscribed foci of inflammation covered by silvery scales. Psoriasis has an increased familial incidence and is associated with HLA-DR7, HLA-Cw6, and HLA-B13.

1 The types of psoriasis are distinguished according to their pathogenetic causes, i.e., hornification disorders (hyperkeratosis, parakeratosis) and immunological mechanisms. T cells and granulocytes migrate into the psoriatic lesions. The disease can be triggered by a number of exogenous factors (injury, UV radiation, cold) and endogenous factors (infection, HIV, medications, alcohol, hypocalcemia, stress). The duration of an attack or the chronification of the disease depends on a wide variety of epidermal and immunological factors.

2 Sites of predilection for psoriatic lesions are the extensor surfaces of the limbs, the iliosacral region, and hairy areas of the scalp. Scratching the psoriatic lesions gives the scales a typical phenomenon of waxy stains characterized by a superficial, waxy scale (**a**), or makes them exhibit a "last-pellicle" phenomenon characterized by the appearance of a silvery pellicle once all scales have been removed (**b**), or a tapering pattern characterized by punctiform bleeding after removal of the last pellicle (**c**). *Psoriasis arthropathica* (psoriatic arthritis) is a distinct entity associated with monoarthritis or polyarthritis. The joints of the fingers and toes are most commonly affected.

B. Bullous Skin Diseases

Pemphigus vulgaris is a blistering skin disease triggered by autoantibodies directed against desmoglein, a desmosomal adhesion molecule of the cadherin group. Desmogleins are glycoproteins that normally provide cell–cell contact to the desmosome by homotypic binding. Antibody-mediated activation of extracellular proteases destroys this contact. The intercellular cement of the stratum spinosum breaks down, and the individual keratinocytes become rounded (acantholysis). This results in intraepidermal splitting and subsequent blast formation and erosion. The resulting loss of fluids, proteins, and electrolytes can quickly take on life-threatening proportions.

Bullous pemphigoid is mainly a disease of the elderly. It is characterized by the presence of large, tense blisters containing clear or blood-stained fluid. The split in the basement membrane occurs in the subepidermal region. The autoantibodies that cause bullous pemphigoid (BP) are directed against basement membrane antigens (bullous pemphigoid Ag, BP-I, BP-II) located in the hemidesmosomes and lamina lucida of the basement membrane. The formation of blisters is induced by complement activation and the release of enzymes from granulocytes.

Epidermolysis bullosa acquisita is a noninflammatory dermatosis that occurs in adulthood and is characterized by subepidermal blister formation. The blisters occur on skin over the joints and are induced by trivial traumas. The disease is chronic. The blisters usually occur on the hands, feet, and the extensor surface of the lower leg, and they leave dystrophic scars and milia after they heal. The autoantibodies are directed against the type VII collagen of the lamina densa of the basement membrane.

Dermatitis herpetiformis (*Duhring's disease*) is a chronic, relapsing skin disease that is extremely pruritic. It is characterized by the development of papules and vesicles and is closely associated with gluten-sensitive enteropathy. Other characteristic features include the presence of granular IgA deposits in the dermal papillae and subepidermal blistering. There is a close association with HLA-B8, HLA-DR3, and autoantibodies to reticulin and endomysium.

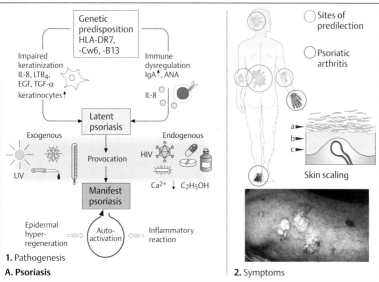

A. Psoriasis

Genetic predisposition HLA-DR7, -Cw6, -B13

Impaired keratinization
IL-8, LTB₄, EGF, TGF-α
keratinocytes↑

Immune dysregulation
IgA↑, ANA

IL-8

Latent psoriasis

Exogenous

Endogenous

Provocation

HIV

UV

Ca²⁺ ↓ C₂H₅OH

Manifest psoriasis

Epidermal hyper-regeneration

Auto-activation

Inflammatory reaction

1. Pathogenesis

Sites of predilection

Psoriatic arthritis

a
b
c

Skin scaling

2. Symptoms

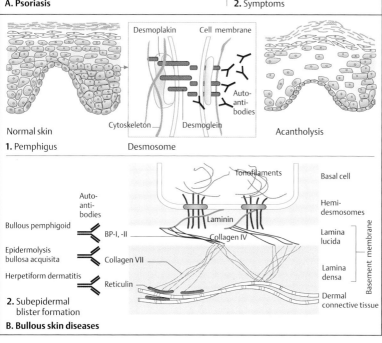

B. Bullous skin diseases

Normal skin

1. Pemphigus

Desmoplakin   Cell membrane

Cytoskeleton   Desmoglein

Auto-anti-bodies

Desmosome

Acantholysis

Tonofilaments   Basal cell

Hemi-desmosomes

Auto-anti-bodies

Bullous pemphigoid   BP-I, -II

Laminin

Collagen IV

Lamina lucida

Epidermolysis bullosa acquisita   Collagen VII

Lamina densa

Herpetiform dermatitis   Reticulin

Dermal connective tissue

Basement membrane

2. Subepidermal blister formation

Clinical Immunology

A. Chronic Atrophic Gastritis (Type A)

Chronic atrophic gastritis (type A) is an autoimmune disease associated with autoantibodies against chief cells, parietal cells, and intrinsic factor. In type A gastritis, the main changes occur in the fundus and body of the stomach, causing glandular atrophy with subsequent achlorhydria and reduced intrinsic factor production. Type A gastritis produces relatively few symptoms. It manifests late with signs of indigestion and chronic vitamin B_{12} deficiency (pernicious anemia). The hematological findings include hyperchromic macrocytic anemia and hypersegmented granulocytes. Neurological features include signs of funicular myelosis, such as reduced vibratory perception and ataxia due to impairment of the posterior funiculus of the spinal column; spastic paraparesis of the legs may occur in the late stages of disease due to degeneration of the pyramidal tract. Achlorhydria leads to fasting hypergastrinemia, and the pentagastrin test is strongly positive.

The autoantibodies against chief cells can be divided into the following groups:

- Antibodies against a microsomal antigen (PCMA), which are also associated with type I diabetes
- Antibodies against a surface antigen (PCSA), which are virtually specific for type A autoimmune gastritis

Type A gastritis occasionally occurs in conjunction with other autoimmune endocrine diseases, such as hyperthyroidism and Hashimoto's disease. It is associated with HLA-A3, -B7, -DR2, and -DR4 antigens. Treatment of pernicious anemia is with parenteral vitamin B_{12}.

B. Whipple's Disease

This disease is a chronic infection by *Tropheryma whippeli*, a Gram-positive actinomycete that survives in the phagosomes of macrophages in the intestinal flora. The pathogen is histologically characterized as a PAS-positive inclusion body. The macrophages swell and block the lymph drainage channels because they accumulate in the lymph spaces and lymph nodes. This prevents the absorption of dietary fats, resulting in malabsorption and steatorrhea. Systemic features include arthralgia and brownish hyperpigmentation. The immune defects are probably attributable to the effects of malabsorption. Whipple's disease is treated with drugs such as tetracycline over a period of 5–6 months.

C. Gluten-sensitive Enteropathy

Gluten-sensitive enteropathy (sprue) is characterized by an allergic reaction to gliadin, a substance contained in cereal proteins, in individuals with a genetic predisposition. The disease is associated with HLA-DR3 and -B8 antigens. Sprue is characterized by autoaggressive inflammation directed against the myoepithelial anchorage fibrils of the intestine. The immunological features include autoantibodies against endomysium and reticulin and antigliadin antibodies. The skin of the small intestine becomes atrophic (mucosal flattening) and lymphoepithelial infiltrates form. The clinical symptoms improve under a gluten-free diet. Along with malabsorption and steatorrhea, autoantibodies may cause dermatitis herpetiformis. These patients are also at increased risk of malignant lymphoma, which can develop from mucosa-associated lymphoid tissue.

Pathogenesis: Gliadin consumed in the diet penetrates through gaps in the epithelia and enters the lamina propria, where it is absorbed by (HLA-DQ- or HLA-DQ8-positive) APC and T cells. The tissue-bound transglutaminase forms cross-linkages in gliadin protein, leading to the formation of even more potent T-cell epitopes. A T_H1 response leads to an inflammatory reaction and structural changes, while cytokines of the T_H2 response activate B cells that form antibodies against gliadin and autoantibodies against transglutaminase and the gliadin–transglutaminase complex. The autoantibodies contribute to atrophy yet are directed against transglutaminase and therefore inhibit its potentiating effect.

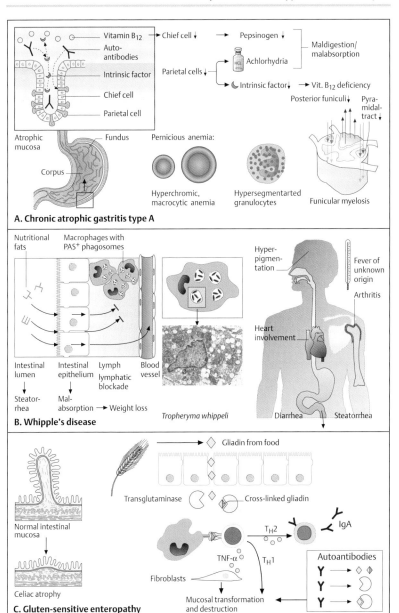

A. Chronic atrophic gastritis type A

B. Whipple's disease

C. Gluten-sensitive enteropathy

A. Crohn's Disease

Crohn's disease is a chronic granulomatous inflammation that can involve the entire digestive tract but, in most cases, initially presents as terminal ileitis or regional enterocolitis. The inflammation affects all layers of the intestinal wall, is restricted to disjointed segments of the bowel (skip lesions), and tends to produce fistulae, abscesses, and perforation. The radiological appearance of the disease is characterized by thickening, stenosis, and poor motility of the affected bowel segment (garden-hose appearance). Inflammatory conglomerate tumors develop due to abscess and fistula formation in adjacent structures (bladder or skin). The most common complications of Crohn's disease are therefore stenosis and bowel obstruction, malabsorption, and fistulization. An increased frequency of colorectal carcinoma and amyloidosis has also been observed. Crohn's disease is associated with HLA-DR1 and -DQw5 antigens. Many of the patients have a history of smoking, a reduced nursing period, and/or a high dietary intake of refined carbohydrates.

The mucosal lining of the intestine exhibits high levels of IL-12. When stimulated by bacteria, IL-12 allows naive T cells to differentiate into T_H1 cells. Accordingly, the T_H1 activity in the mucosa of these patients is high, as determined based on the concentration of IFN-γ, TNF-α, and IL-2. IgG subclass analyses reveal high levels of IgG2, an immunoglobulin that is particularly effective in recognizing bacterial carbohydrate antigens. The pathogenetic basis for Crohn's disease is therefore assumed to be a heightened immune response to exogenous antigens, such as fecal antigens (**D**).

Acute attacks are usually treated with sulfasalazine, 5-aminosalicylate drugs, and/or steroids. During remissions, patients may receive a triple drug combination consisting of azathioprine, methotrexate, and cyclosporin A. In refractory cases, TNF antagonists are used, such as infliximab. To prevent disease recurrence, the drugs should be continued in low-dose regimens. Surgical management is considered only if it is to be performed as minimally invasive surgery for treatment of complications or in cases refractory to drug therapy.

B. Ulcerative Colitis

Ulcerative colitis (UC) is a chronic, relapsing and remitting disease of the colon. It presents with diarrhea passed with blood or mucus and superficial mucosal ulcerations, and continuously spreads from the rectum to the more proximal regions of the bowel. Ulceration leads to flattening of the interstitial mucosae between the lesions and to depletion of goblet cells. Hyperregeneration leads to the formation of pseudopolyps. Double contrast enemas of the colon reveal a loss of haustra and an atypical, serrated pattern. The most dangerous complications are toxic megacolon and colorectal carcinoma. Ulcerative colitis can also manifest in extraintestinal sites; uveitis and arthritis are two of the main nonintestinal manifestations. Ulcerative colitis is also associated with IgA nephritis, autoimmune hepatitis, and primary biliary cirrhosis. The mucosa exhibits high levels of IL-5, which suggests increased T_H2 activity. IgG subclass analyses reveal high levels of IgG1 and IgG3. The additional presence of anti-neutrophil cytoplasmic antibodies (ANCA) and the association with certain autoimmune diseases suggests that ulcerative colitis is probably an autoimmune disease (**D**).

Acute attacks are treated with sulfasalazine and 5-aminosalicylate drugs. These drugs inhibit the synthesis of prostaglandin and leukotriene, but as in Crohn's disease, they intervene late in the inflammatory cascade. Surgical management can be achieved with proctocolectomy.

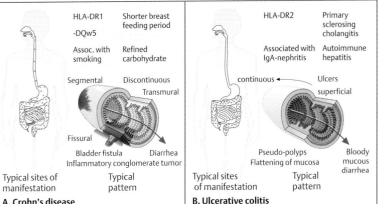

HLA-DR1   Shorter breast
-DQw5   feeding period

Assoc. with   Refined
smoking   carbohydrate

Segmental   Discontinuous
                 Transmural

Fissural

Bladder fistula   Diarrhea
Inflammatory conglomerate tumor

Typical sites of   Typical
manifestation   pattern

A. Crohn's disease

HLA-DR2   Primary
                 sclerosing
                 cholangitis

Associated with   Autoimmune
IgA-nephritis   hepatitis

continuous ←   Ulcers
                 superficial

Pseudo-polyps   Bloody
Flattening of mucosa   mucous
                           diarrhea

Typical sites   Typical
of manifestation   pattern

B. Ulcerative colitis

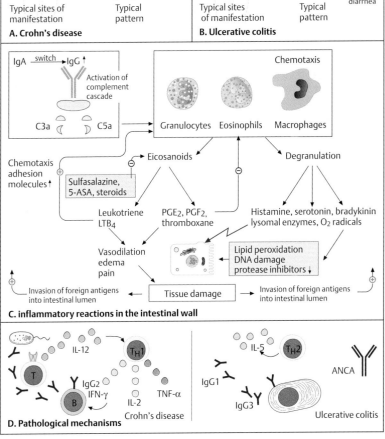

IgA $\xrightarrow{\text{switch}}$ IgG ↑

Activation of
complement
cascade

C3a   C5a

Chemotaxis

Granulocytes Eosinophils Macrophages

Chemotaxis
adhesion
molecules ↑

⊖ Eicosanoids   ⊖

Sulfasalazine,
5-ASA, steroids

Leukotriene   PGE₂, PGF₂,   Degranulation
LTB₄   thromboxane

Histamine, serotonin, bradykinin
lysomal enzymes, O₂ radicals

Vasodilation
edema
pain

Lipid peroxidation
DNA damage
protease inhibitors ↓

⊕
Invasion of foreign antigens   Tissue damage   Invasion of foreign antigens   ⊕
into intestinal lumen   into intestinal lumen

C. inflammatory reactions in the intestinal wall

IL-12   T_H1

T   IgG2
               IFN-γ   IL-2   TNF-α
B
                           Crohn's disease

IL-5   T_H2

                                    ANCA
IgG1

IgG3   Ulcerative colitis

D. Pathological mechanisms

A. Autoimmune Hepatitis

The etiology of autoimmune hepatitis is unknown. Hence, a number of criteria are required for the diagnosis. The disease occurs predominantly in women and is associated with HLA-DR3 and -DR4 antigens. The histological picture is that of chronic hepatitis, and serological tests reveal hypergammaglobulinemia. Immunosuppressive therapy leads to improvement of the symptoms. Autoimmune hepatitis is often associated with other autoimmune diseases, such as rheumatoid arthritis, glomerulonephritis, ulcerative colitis, Crohn's disease, and Hashimoto's disease. In 50% of cases, there are clinical signs of vasculitis, cryoglobulinemia, and Sjögren's syndrome. General signs of liver damage, such as jaundice, itching, nausea, diarrhea, fever, and hepatosplenomegaly, can also be observed. Transaminase levels (AST and ALT) are increased, and signs of cholestasis can be observed.

By immunological definition, this disease represents an autoimmune response to liver tissue structures. The pathogenetic role of the autoantibodies involved in the process is still unclear. The antibodies directed against structural proteins are called liver-kidney microsomal antibodies (LKM). LKM-1 targets cytochrome P450IID6, an enzyme that metabolizes certain drugs (e.g., beta-blockers, antiarrhythmic drugs, and antidepressants). LKM-1 often occurs in association with HCV antibodies. This suggests that autoimmune hepatitis is a disease originally induced by hepatotropic viruses.

The diagnosis can be established by demonstrating the presence of the autoantibodies. Viral hepatitis, liver damage due to other causes, such as drugs and alcohol, or genetic enzyme defects (e.g., α_1-antitrypsin deficiency, Wilson's disease) must always be considered in the differential diagnosis. HLA typing should always be performed. Immunosuppressive treatment consists of prednisolone alone or in combination with azathioprine.

B. Primary Biliary Cirrhosis (PBC)

Primary biliary cirrhosis, or nonpurulent, destructive cholangitis, is an inflammatory disease of the minor intrahepatic ducts that mainly afflicts women 40 years of age or older. In addition to signs of cholestasis, high levels of serum cholesterol can also be found. Elevated cholesterol levels can provoke the formation of cutaneous xanthoma. Other symptoms include jaundice, itching, skin pigmentation, and hepatobiliary indigestion. The presence of extrahepatic manifestations characterizes PBC as a multisystem disease. In some cases, the exocrine pancreas, lacrimal glands, and salivary glands are also affected (dry gland disease). Primary biliary cirrhosis is associated with Sjögren's syndrome in 50% of cases, and is also associated with other autoimmune diseases. Anti-mitochondrial antibodies (AMA) can be detected in the serum. AMA are primarily directed against the E2 subunit of pyruvate dehydrogenase complexes. Their role in the pathogenesis of PBC is unclear. One hypothesis suggests bacterial induction. Attempts at immunosuppressive therapy are usually without success.

C. Primary Sclerosing Cholangitis (PSC)

Primary sclerosing cholangitis is a chronic fibrotic inflammation of the intrahepatic and extrahepatic bile ducts. Wall thickening and stenosis ultimately lead to cholestasis. PSC is more common in men and is associated with HLA-B8 and -DR3 antigens. Concomitant ulcerative colitis is present in 50% of the patients. The diagnosis is established by demonstrating the presence of ANCA and bile duct changes. As in primary biliary cirrhosis, treatment is symptomatic.

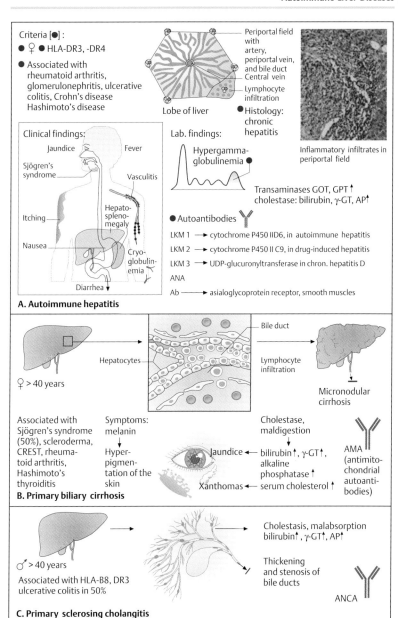

Criteria [●] :

● ♀ ● HLA-DR3, -DR4

● Associated with rheumatoid arthritis, glomerulonephritis, ulcerative colitis, Crohn's disease Hashimoto's disease

Lobe of liver

Periportal field with artery, periportal vein, and bile duct

Central vein

Lymphocyte infiltration

● Histology: chronic hepatitis

Inflammatory infiltrates in periportal field

Clinical findings:

Jaundice

Fever

Sjögren's syndrome

Vasculitis

Hepato-spleno-megaly

Itching

Nausea

Cryo-globulin-emia

Diarrhea

Lab. findings:

Hypergamma-globulinemia ●

Transaminases GOT, GPT ↑ cholestase: bilirubin, γ-GT, AP↑

● Autoantibodies

LKM 1 → cytochrome P450 IID6, in autoimmune hepatitis

LKM 2 → cytochrome P450 II C9, in drug-induced hepatitis

LKM 3 → UDP-glucuronyltransferase in chron. hepatitis D

ANA

Ab → asialoglycoprotein receptor, smooth muscles

A. Autoimmune hepatitis

Bile duct

Hepatocytes

Lymphocyte infiltration

♀ > 40 years

Micronodular cirrhosis

Associated with Sjögren's syndrome (50%), scleroderma, CREST, rheumatoid arthritis, Hashimoto's thyroiditis

Symptoms: melanin ↓ Hyper-pigmentation of the skin

Cholestase, maldigestion

Jaundice ← bilirubin ↑, γ-GT↑, alkaline phosphatase ↑

Xanthomas ← serum cholesterol ↑

AMA (antimito-chondrial autoanti-bodies)

B. Primary biliary cirrhosis

♂ > 40 years

Associated with HLA-B8, DR3 ulcerative colitis in 50%

Cholestasis, malabsorption bilirubin↑, γ-GT↑, AP↑

Thickening and stenosis of bile ducts

ANCA

C. Primary sclerosing cholangitis

Clinical Immunology

213

A. Genetic Predisposition

Bronchial asthma is a chronic disease characterized by intermittent, initially reversible obstruction of the airways, inflammatory changes, and bronchial hyperresponsiveness. As opposed to "intrinsic" or nonallergic asthma, "extrinsic" allergic (atopic) asthma is characterized by elevated serum IgE concentrations and association with other allergic manifestations in the patient and in the patient's family. However, the differentiation between the two is schematic, as some of the clinical and pathogenetic features of the entities overlap.

Bronchial hyperresponsiveness and the tendency to increased IL-4-dependent IgE production are commonly inherited through genes on chromosome 5q31-q33. The incidence is ca. 5% in adults and ca. 10% in children. Atopic asthma is by far the most common form.

B. Trigger Factors

Atopic (extrinsic) asthma can be induced by animal hair, dust mites, feathers, pollen, and mold. In intrinsic asthma, on the other hand, the bronchial hyperreactivity is caused by the inhalation of chemicals, such as sulfur dioxide (SO_2), ozone (O_3), and cigarette smoke as well as viral infections, cold air, exercise, and stress. Analgesics, including aspirin, can also cause an asthma attack.

C. Pathogenesis

Sensitization to the allergens may occur in early childhood (**1**). Antigen-presenting cells (APCs) in the bronchial mucosae capture the inhaled allergens and present them to CD4+ T cells, which then differentiate into T cells of the T_H2 phenotype. These cells secrete IL-4, IL-5, IL-9, IL-10, and IL-13, which promote a switch in B-lymphocyte immunoglobulin secretion, inducing them to produce IgE. In addition, IL-13 also induces activation of eosinophilic and basophilic granulocytes, as well as release of chemokines and proteolytic enzymes, such as metalloproteinases. The IgE molecules circulate, and then bind to high-affinity receptors (FcεRI) on mast cells and basophils and to low-affinity receptors (FcεRI, CD23) on eosinophils and macrophages. When reexposure occurs (**2**), the allergen can rapidly interact with the IgE molecules that are already bound to the cell surface. Histamine, proteases, leukotriene, prostaglandins, and platelet-activating

factor (PAF) are released. The bronchoconstrictive asthmatic response occurs in two phases. The lung function rapidly decreases within the first 10–20 minutes and gradually recovers during the next two hours. This "early response" involves histamine, prostaglandin-D_2 (PGD_2), cysteinyl-leucotrienes (LTC_4, LTD_4, LTE_4), and PAF. The cysteinyl-leucotrienes induce release of proteases: tryptase cleaves D3a and bradykinin from protein precursor molecules, which leads to bronchial muscle cell contraction and increased vascular permeability. Chymase, on the other hand, promotes mucus secretion. The induction of bronchoconstriction with mucosal edema and mucus secretion results in coughing, wheezing, and breathlessness. The "late reaction" (**3**) begins 4–6 hours later. LTB_4 and PAF attract eosinophils. They, in turn, attract major basic protein (MBP) and eosinophil cationic protein (ECP), which have a toxic effect on epithelial cells. Epithelial destruction occurs in the late stages. This ultimately leads to the accumulation of mucus in the bronchial lumen due to the increased number of goblet cells and hypertrophy of the submucosal mucous glands. Hypertrophy of smooth muscle in the basement membrane can also be observed. Since many of the effects described are induced by IL-13 via STAT 6 signaling, pharmacological blockade is being tested for therapeutic use.

D. Allergic Rhinitis

Allergic rhinitis is triggered by contact of allergens with the nasal mucosa. This reaction also implies prior sensitization because the allergens bind to sensitized IgE-bearing mast cells. Sneezing and mucus secretion (rhinorrhea) can occur within as little as 30–60 seconds after inhalation of the allergen. Due to a central reflex, the hypersecretion occurs not only on the exposed side, but also in the contralateral nostril. The allergens can be determined by prick testing, which involves intradermal injection of the dissolved antigens. In positive reactions, wheals form with reddening of the surrounding tissue within 15–30 minutes.

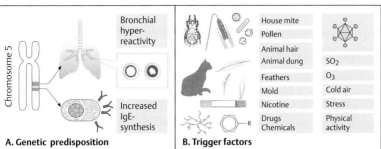

A. Genetic predisposition

Chromosome 5 — Bronchial hyper-reactivity — Increased IgE-synthesis

B. Trigger factors

House mite
Pollen
Animal hair
Animal dung
Feathers
Mold
Nicotine
Drugs
Chemicals

SO_2
O_3
Cold air
Stress
Physical activity

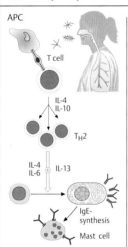

APC
T cell
IL-4
IL-10
T_H2
IL-4
IL-6 + IL-13
IgE-synthesis
Mast cell

1. Sensitization

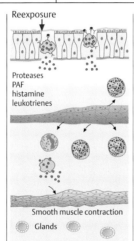

Reexposure
Proteases
PAF
histamine
leukotrienes
Smooth muscle contraction
Glands

2. Reexposure, early reaction

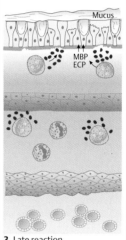

Mucus
MBP
ECP

3. Late reaction

C. Pathogenesis

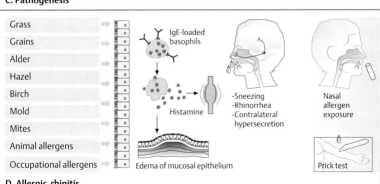

Grass
Grains
Alder
Hazel
Birch
Mold
Mites
Animal allergens
Occupational allergens

IgE-loaded basophils
Histamine
Edema of mucosal epithelium

-Sneezing
-Rhinorrhea
-Contralateral hypersecretion

Nasal allergen exposure

Prick test

D. Allergic rhinitis

Clinical Immunology

A. Sarcoidosis

Sarcoidosis is a multisystem disease characterized by the presence of noncaseating granulomas in multiple organs. The trigger factor is presumed to be the inhalation of a yet unidentified antigen (**1**). Antigen-presenting cells release IL-1, IL-15, IFN-γ, and TFN-α. They recruit activated T_H1 CD4 T cells, which leads to an oligoclonal T-cell alveolitis. Further release of monocyte chemoattractant protein-1 (MCP-1), monocyte inflammatory protein 1α (MIP-1α), CXCL10, and IL-16 induces migration of monocytes and T-cell proliferation. The monocytes produce fibrin, fibronectin, TGF-β, IL-3, IFN-γ, and TNF-α and then transform into epithelioid cells. Some of them coalesce to form multinucleate giant cells and form noncaseating (nonnecrotic) epithelioid cell granulomas. IL-4 and IL-6 lead to polyclonal B cell stimulation, which is reflected as hypergammaglobulinemia.

In many cases, the disease is incidentally discovered due to the presence of bilateral enlargement of the mediastinal lymph nodes (bilateral hilar lymphadenopathy) in chest radiograms (**4**). An acute form of the disease (Loefgren's syndrome) is characterized by bilateral hilar lymphadenopathy, fever, erythema nodosum, and acute arthritis, particularly of the knee and the ankle (**2**). Bronchoalveolar lavage (BAL) typically reveals the presence of CD4+ T-cell alveolitis (**3**). The BAL fluid often contains up to 10 times as many CD4+ T lymphocytes as the peripheral blood because lymphocytes are recruited from the peripheral blood and the skin (anergy to skin antigens) into the lung. In normal individuals, more than 90% of the cells in the BAL fluid are macrophages, and fewer than 1×10^6 lymphocytes are recovered; in sarcoidosis, ten or twenty times more lymphocytes are typically recovered. A decrease in the CD4/CD8 ratio in peripheral blood is also observed. Fever and malaise develop due to increased levels of TNF, IL-1, and IL-6 in serum.

Erythema nodosum, a nongranulomatous inflammation of the subcutaneous tissue, is the most common skin lesion. Eye involvement is common and may range from a harmless conjunctival nodule to blindness as a complication of intermediate and posterior uveitis (see pp. 244, 246). Granulomatous meningitis is a possible manifestation of neurosarcoidosis. Increased intestinal absorption of calcium occurs because the macrophages in the granulomas convert 25-hydroxyvitamin D to 1,25-hydroxyvitamin D. Osteolytic bone lesions ravely contribute to hypercalcemia and hypercalciuria. Ventricular tachycardia may occur due to the presence of granulomas in myocardial tissue. Small periportal granulomas or T cell infiltrates exhibiting various degrees of fibrosis are often found in the liver (**5**). The development of splenic granulomas can cause splenomegaly. The concentration of angiotensin-converting enzyme (ACE) in the serum increases due to the synthesis by granuloma tissue.

B. Idiopathic Pulmonary Fibrosis

Pulmonary fibrosis may occur in a number of diseases. Hence, idiopathic pulmonary fibrosis (IPF), or cryptogenic fibrosing alveolitis, is a diagnosis of exclusion. Activation of the alveolar macrophages presumably occurs in individuals with a genetic predisposition after contact with a yet unknown pathogen. Viruses or immune complexes are thought to be responsible. T-cell cytokines may also be involved in the activation process. Alveolar macrophages secrete IL-8 and leukotrienes, which recruit and activate neutrophil granulocytes. Granulocytic alveolitis is a typical feature of idiopathic pulmonary fibrosis, whereas lymphocytic alveolitis occurs in sarcoidosis. The alveolar macrophages also secrete fibroblast growth factors, such as TGF-β, insuline-like growth (IGF-1), and platelet-derived growth factor (PDGF). Oxidative processes enable the alveolar macrophages and neutrophils to destroy type I pneumocytes. This induces a compensatory increase in the number of type II pneumocytes, which produce chemotactic and fibrogenic factors. Extracellular matrix deposition occurs. This ultimately leads to the development of fibrotic cicatricial changes, which produce characteristic radiological and histological patterns (honeycomb lung). Corticosteroids have been used to treat this disease, although frequently with disappointing results. Interferon-γ together with corticosteroids may lead to clinical improvement.

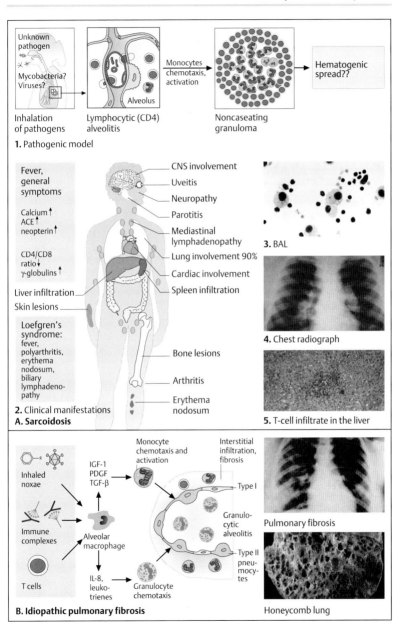

A. Sarcoidosis

Unknown pathogen

Mycobacteria?
Viruses?

Alveolus

Inhalation of pathogens

Lymphocytic (CD4) alveolitis

Monocytes chemotaxis, activation

Noncaseating granuloma

Hematogenic spread??

1. Pathogenic model

Fever, general symptoms

Calcium ↑
ACE ↑
neopterin ↑

CD4/CD8 ratio ↓
γ-globulins ↑

Liver infiltration

Skin lesions

Loefgren's syndrome:
fever, polyarthritis, erythema nodosum, biliary lymphadeno-pathy

CNS involvement
Uveitis
Neuropathy
Parotitis
Mediastinal lymphadenopathy
Lung involvement 90%
Cardiac involvement
Spleen infiltration

Bone lesions
Arthritis
Erythema nodosum

2. Clinical manifestations

3. BAL

4. Chest radiograph

5. T-cell infiltrate in the liver

B. Idiopathic pulmonary fibrosis

Inhaled noxae

Immune complexes

T cells

IGF-1
PDGF
TGF-β

Alveolar macrophage

IL-8, leuko-trienes

Monocyte chemotaxis and activation

Granulocyte chemotaxis

Interstitial infiltration, fibrosis

Type I

Granulo-cytic alveolitis

Type II pneumo-cytes

Pulmonary fibrosis

Honeycomb lung

Clinical Immunology

217

A. Extrinsic Allergic Alveolitis

1 Most common clinical syndromes. Extrinsic allergic alveolitis (EAA), or hypersensitivity pneumonitis, is caused by sensitization followed by secondary exposure to inhaled antigens. The causative antigens migrate together with dust particles into the alveoli, where they trigger a local immune response. The allergens may originate from bacteria, fungi, chemicals, animal products, or plant products. The resulting hypersensitivity reaction produces a uniform clinical picture, regardless of which type of antigen caused it. When bacteria and fungi are involved, they do not act invasively, but as antigens. More than 50 different occupational and environmental varieties have been described, and many of the names reflect the mode of exposure. Farmer's lung, for example, is caused by thermophilic actinomycetes found in moldy hay. Compost lung is caused by fungi (e.g., *Aspergillus*) that thrive in compost. Air conditioners, room humidifiers, whirlpools, and saunas provide ideal growth conditions for thermophilic actinomycetes, *Klebsiella*, amebae, *Candida*, and *Aureobasidium*. Bird breeder's lung is observed in individuals exposed to the excrement of pigeons and other birds. Isocyanates and anhydrides are the main chemicals involved in the development of chemical worker's lung. These chemicals are used to produce plastics, paints, and polyurethane foam. Despite the etiological variety, the underlying pathogenetic mechanism and clinical course of these different forms of the disease are uniform.

2 Immunological pathogenesis. The inhaled particles can induce the formation of precipitating IgG antibodies, which form complement-activating immune complexes. Complement activation can also occur in the absence of antibodies because the inhaled dust can directly activate the alternative complement pathway. The complement products have a chemotactic effect on neutrophil granulocytes, which are therefore recruited into the alveoli. Activated macrophages also release various monokines. Interleukin-8, for example, amplifies granulocytic chemotaxis. As a result, extensive granulocytic alveolitis occurs within 4–12 hours after exposure to the antigen. Other monokines recruit T cells into the alveolar septi and interstitial tissues or stimulate the release of autocrine factors. After 48–72 hours, additional T cells migrate into the alveoli and can be detected by bronchial lavage. As opposed to sarcoidosis, which causes CD4 alveolitis, these T cells are mainly CD8+. These cells display suppressor activity and can kill NK-sensitive targets; they express CD56 and CD57. Macrophages are also frequently found in the BAL. Histology reveals the presence of mononuclear cell infiltrates in the interstitial tissue and the early development of small granulomas. The pattern of alveolitis found in the BAL fluids can help in the differentiation of interstitial lung diseases of different etiology: while a prevalence of CD4+ T cells in the BAL is typical of sarcoidosis, tuberculosis, and berylliosis, a CD8+ T-cell alveolitis is found in hypersensitivity pneumonitis, silicosis, blastomycosis, and interstitial lung disease associated with HIV, collagen vascular disease and graft versus host disease.

3 Clinical course. Acute and chronic forms of the disease are distinguished. Acute EAA manifests soon after antigen exposure. Symptoms of fever, chills, cough, dyspnea, and myalgia usually develop after a latency of around 4–8 hours. The symptoms generally persist for 18–24 hours, then slowly reside if there is no further contact with the antigen. The symptoms then reoccur with each renewed contact. Radiographs may demonstrate nodular interstitial infiltrates in the lower pulmonary fields. In most cases, no special treatment is needed. In severe cases, steroids can be administered to alleviate symptoms. Chronic exposure to the allergens, i.e., at short intervals, produces symptoms that are much more severe. Weakness, anorexia, and weight loss may initially occur in absence of fever. Restrictive respiratory impairment with rest dyspnea ultimately develops. If there is long-term, chronic damage to the pulmonary tissue, the disease may ultimately progress to pulmonary fibrosis, which produces interstitial fibrotic changes on radiographs (**4**).

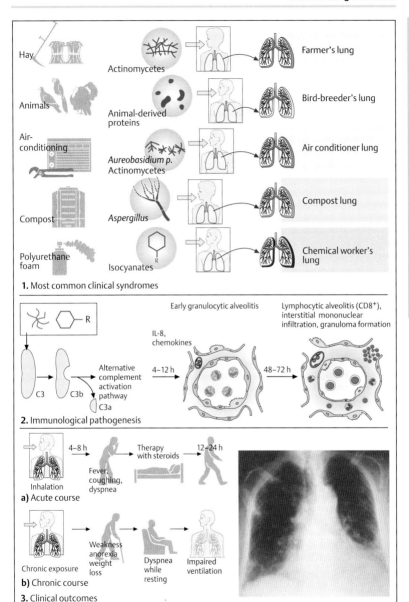

1. Most common clinical syndromes

2. Immunological pathogenesis

Early granulocytic alveolitis

Lymphocytic alveolitis (CD8+), interstitial mononuclear infiltration, granuloma formation

IL-8, chemokines

4–12 h

48–72 h

C3 → C3b → Alternative complement activation pathway → C3a

Inhalation
4–8 h
Fever, coughing, dyspnea
Therapy with steroids
12–24 h

a) Acute course

Chronic exposure → Weakness anorexia weight loss → Dyspnea while resting → Impaired ventilation

b) Chronic course

3. Clinical outcomes

A. Extrinsic allergic alveolitis

4. Chest radiograph

Hay — Actinomycetes → Farmer's lung

Animals — Animal-derived proteins → Bird-breeder's lung

Air-conditioning — *Aureobasidium p.* Actinomycetes → Air conditioner lung

Compost — *Aspergillus* → Compost lung

Polyurethane foam — Isocyanates → Chemical worker's lung

A. Tuberculosis

1 Air-borne infection. When they enter into the lungs, tuberculosis-inducing mycobacteria are phagocytosed by alveolar macrophages. The phagocytosis is mainly receptor mediated (**2**). Some receptors (e.g., Toll-like receptor, TLR) recognize certain surface antigen patterns common to all prokaryons, whereas others are specific for mycobacterial antigens (e.g., the CD14 molecule, which is specific for lipoarabinomannan (LAM) antibodies). Antibodies and complement factor C3 bind to molecules on the surface of the pathogen and are recognized by the corresponding receptors. Since the alveolar macrophages cannot effectively kill the phagocytosed mycobacteria, the bacteria can survive intracellularly. In fact, they can even replicate by blocking phagosome maturation. The migration of alveolar macrophages to the nearest lymph nodes activates a T-cell-mediated, specific immune response.

3 Induction of a specific immune response. *Mycobacterium tuberculosis* secretes proteins into the phagosome. Initially, these proteins are export proteins. They later form part of the cell wall and ultimately (after autolysis) represent intracellular proteins. Processed fragments consisting of 10–20 amino acids (AA) are presented on class II MHC molecules. Peptides consisting of 8–10 amino acids are presented on class I MHC molecules. CD1, a distant relative of class I MHC, presents bacterial lipoids that preferentially stimulate CD4 and CD8 double-negative T cells. In addition, γ/δ T cells are activated by mycobacterial antigens containing phosphate groups. No presenting molecule for this antigen group has yet been identified. It is assumed that the phospholigands are presented directly on the cell surface.

4 Granuloma. Activated CD4$^+$ T cells secrete chemokines that attract circulating monocytes to the site of inflammation. They also secrete TNF-α, which is responsible for granuloma formation. Complete intracellular killing of mycobacteria within the granuloma can occur due to the cytokine-mediated activation of macrophages. In most cases, however, the pathogen becomes concentrated within the granuloma, which becomes sealed off from the surroundings. The reason for this is TNF-α-mediated thickening and fibrosis of the granuloma wall and IL-4-induced coalescence of macrophages to form giant cells (Langhans' cells). In this case, the host is infected but does not develop tuberculosis (TBC) because the mycobacteria and the granuloma's defense system are at balance. IFN-γ activates tuberculostatic macrophages, for example, by promoting the synthesis of calcitriol, a substance that activates microbicidal effector function. The activated macrophages release O_2 metabolites and proteases and thus cause necrosis in the center of the granuloma. Activated CD8$^+$ cytotoxic T cells induce the lysis of macrophages, which release their contents into the necrotic granuloma center. The growth conditions there are less favorable for the mycobacteria because of the low O_2 tension within the center and because of the type of enzymes released.

Uncontrolled cell destruction, on the other hand, leads to caseation of the granuloma, which results in extensive tissue damage. The mycobacteria can now enter into the circulation and create new colonies in virtually any of the host's organs. If the ruptured granuloma gets access to a bronchus, the mycobacteria can be exhaled into the environment and can cause new infections (open TBC).

5 Complications. Disruption of the balance between the mycobacteria and the granuloma's defense system can lead to the further spread of the infection. Hilar lymph node tuberculosis, pleural effusion, and lesions in the apex of the lungs (Simon's apical foci) are typical complications. Generalization of the infection due to hematogenic spread leads to the formation of thousands of small nodules in the lung, liver, spleen, and meninges (miliary tuberculosis). Caseating pneumonia and acute tuberculous sepsis (Landouzy's sepsis) are usually lethal complications.

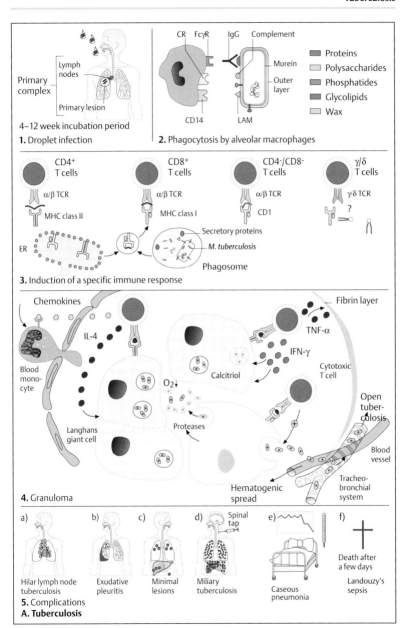

1. Droplet infection

Primary complex
- Lymph nodes
- Primary lesion

4–12 week incubation period

2. Phagocytosis by alveolar macrophages

CR   FcγR   IgG   Complement
Murein
Outer layer
CD14   LAM

- Proteins
- Polysaccharides
- Phosphatides
- Glycolipids
- Wax

3. Induction of a specific immune response

CD4+ T cells — α/β TCR — MHC class II
CD8+ T cells — α/β TCR — MHC class I
CD4-/CD8- T cells — α/β TCR — CD1
γ/δ T cells — γ/δ TCR — ?

ER   Secretory proteins   M. tuberculosis   Phagosome

4. Granuloma

Chemokines
IL-4
Blood monocyte
Langhans giant cell
O_2↓
Proteases
Calcitriol
TNF-α
IFN-γ
Cytotoxic T cell
Fibrin layer
Open tuberculosis
Blood vessel
Tracheo-bronchial system
Hematogenic spread

5. Complications

a) Hilar lymph node tuberculosis
b) Exudative pleuritis
c) Minimal lesions
d) Miliary tuberculosis — Spinal tap
e) Caseous pneumonia
f) Death after a few days — Landouzy's sepsis

A. Tuberculosis

Clinical Immunology

221

Many renal diseases have underlying immunological mechanisms. Antibody-mediated effects are primarily involved, whereas cellular mechanisms are less important. Immunological diseases of the kidney mainly affect the glomerulus, which is most likely due to its filter function. Immunological processes related to vasculitic processes have not been taken into account in this chapter, but they are outlined in the Appendix (see Tab. 6).

A. Immunological Mechanisms

A schematic illustration of the most important glomerular structures is presented in (**1**). In order to leave the circulation and enter into the urinary space of the glomerulus, a solute must first migrate through the fenestrated endothelium of the capillaries and then penetrate the glomerular basement membrane (GBM). The GBM consists of collagen, laminin, polyanionic proteoglycans, fibronectin, and other glycoproteins. The next layer is made up of visceral epithelial cells (podocytes) and their foot processes. The urinary space is located between the visceral and parietal epithelia of Bowman's capsule. The entire glomerulus is supported by the mesangium, a matrix that forms a meshwork in which mesangial cells are scattered. These mobile phagocytic cells secrete matrix, collagen, and a number of biological mediators.

Antibody-mediated renal diseases are induced by three mechanisms (**2**). Circulating, preformed immune complexes accumulate subendothelially, on the capillary aspect of the basement membrane (**2a**). Alternatively, the antibodies may react in situ with the GBM (**2b**) or with antigens of the visceral cells (so-called Heymann's nephritis) (**2c**). The immunoglobulins and complement can be made visible using fluorescent antisera. Preformed immune complexes and antibodies to epithelial antigens appear as granular, discontinuous fluorescent structures, whereas antibodies against the basement membrane produce a linear, continuous pattern.

Antibody deposits can cause direct damage to epithelial or endothelial cells due to complement activation and pore formation (**3**). On the other hand, the antibodies can also bind to the Fc receptors of monocytes, macrophages, granulocytes, and platelets. This leads to the activation or, in the case of platelets, aggregation of the cells. Complement cleavage products, especially C5a, enhance the activation

process. Proteases, cytokines, eicosanoids, oxidants, and nitric oxides are ultimately released. The cytokines can attract and activate T cells.

The glomerular damage can cause two distinct symptom complexes: the nephrotic syndrome (**B**) and the nephritic syndrome (**C**). In nephrotic syndrome, damage to the endothelial cells, basement membrane, and/or visceral epithelium leads to an increased filtration of proteins in the urinary space. This causes extensive proteinuria and an associated loss of low-molecular-weight substances, such as albumin and immunoglobulins. As a result, there is a relative increase in α_2- and β-globulins in serum. Due to the hypoalbuminemia, the osmotic pressure of the blood decreases, resulting in generalized edema with pleural effusions and ascites. A reactive increase in lipoprotein synthesis occurs in the liver, thereby inducing hyperlipidemia. The compensatory secretion of aldosterone leads to sodium retention and hypertension. Hyaline and granular casts can be detected in the urinary sediment. The causes of nephrotic syndrome differ in children and adults. The childhood form is usually characterized by minimal change glomerulonephritis with a benign course, whereas the adulthood form is usually associated with a systemic disease and has a more severe prognosis.

Nephritic syndrome occurs more frequently in childhood. The onset of the disease is usually characterized by the sudden appearance of blood in the urine and reduced urinary secretion in association with acute renal failure (oliguria) and hypertension. The disease is usually precipitated by postinfectious or rapidly progressive glomerulonephritis.

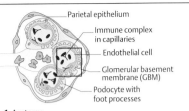

- Parietal epithelium
- Immune complex in capillaries
- Endothelial cell
- Glomerular basement membrane (GBM)
- Podocyte with foot processes

1. Anatomy

2a. Immune complex deposition

2b. Anti-GBM Ab

2c. Anti-epithelial cell Ab

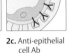

Direct damage (C5b–C9)

Secondary T cell migration

Cytotoxicity

C5a

Platelet aggregation

Neutrophil activation

Monocyte activation

Mesangial cell activation

Proteases, eicosanoids, NO, cytokines, growth factors

3. Mediators of glomerular damage

A. Mechanisms

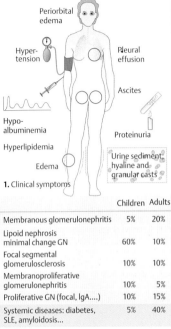

- Periorbital edema
- Hyper-tension
- Pleural effusion
- Ascites
- Hypo-albuminemia
- Proteinuria
- Hyperlipidemia
- Edema

Urine sediment: hyaline and granular casts

1. Clinical symptoms

	Children	Adults
Membranous glomerulonephritis	5%	20%
Lipoid nephrosis minimal change GN	60%	10%
Focal segmental glomerulosclerosis	10%	10%
Membranoproliferative glomerulonephritis	10%	5%
Proliferative GN (focal, IgA....)	10%	15%
Systemic diseases: diabetes, SLE, amyloidosis...	5%	40%

2. Causes of nephrotic syndrome

B. Nephrotic syndrome

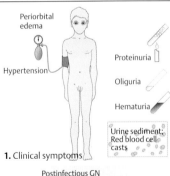

- Periorbital edema
- Hypertension
- Proteinuria
- Oliguria
- Hematuria

Urine sediment: Red blood cell casts

1. Clinical symptoms

Postinfectious GN
Rapidly progressive GN
IgA nephropathy

2. Causes of the nephritic syndrome

C. Nephritic syndrome

A. Minimal Change Nephropathy

Minimal change nephropathy, or "lipoid nephrosis," is a benign disease. It is the most common cause of childhood nephrotic syndrome. The glomeruli appear normal upon light microscopy, and electron microscopy reveals the loss or fusion of foot processes of the visceral epithelial cells. Deposits (see arrow on photograph) can be detected in the podocytes directly opposite to the basement membrane. The formation of so-called microvilli (M) is another typical feature. The cause of minimal change nephropathy is unknown. T-cell cytokines are presumed to destroy the podocyte architecture. The loss of podocyte function leads to an increase in protein filtration. The changes caused by minimal change nephropathy are completely reversible. Ninety percent of all cases respond to corticosteroids, although some patients require long-term therapy. In adults, larger doses of steroids must be used, and the rate of recurrence is much higher compared with children.

B. Focal Segmental Glomerulosclerosis

Focal segmental glomerulosclerosis (FSGS) is characterized by the occurrence of sclerosis in only a few glomeruli; moreover, only some parts (segments) of the involved glomeruli are affected (see photograph). These changes occur in association with HIV infection, drug abuse, and IgA nephropathy, or as a secondary complication of compensatory hypertrophy. The cause is often unknown. Around 10% of all nephrotic syndromes are attributable to focal segmental glomerulosclerosis. These changes presumably represent a more severe variant of "minimal change disease." The accumulation of lipids, fibrin, C3 complement, and IgM immunoglobulins leads to a mesangial reaction associated with hyalinosis and sclerosis. Histological sections (see photograph) clearly reveal the segmental nature of sclerotic involvement. FSGS responds poorly to corticosteroids. Approximately 50% of the patients develop renal failure within 10 years.

C. Membranous Glomerulonephritis

Membranous glomerulonephritis is characterized by the formation of immune complexes on the subepithelial surface of the basement membrane. The antibodies react in situ with endogenous podocyte antigens or with antigens that were filtered and have gormed deposits. The disease is idiopathic in 80% of cases; it is sometimes associated with systemic diseases or with the use of certain medications. Exposure to toxic agents can also induce membranous glomerulonephritis. Typical features include diffuse thickening of the basement membrane with fusion of the foot processes. The inhomogeneous distribution of the IgG and C3 deposits results in a granular pattern upon immunofluorescence (see photograph). Glomerular sclerosis may occur in the later stage of the disease. Clinically, membranous glomerulonephritis appears as a relatively mild nephrotic syndrome. Around 40% of the patients gradually develop progressive renal failure. The response to corticosteroids is poor.

D. Membranoproliferative Glomerulonephritis

Membranoproliferative glomerulonephritis (MPGN) is characterized by changes in the basement membrane and proliferation of mesangial cells and glomerular cells. There are two subtypes, which are classified according to their different pathomechanisms. *Type I* (approximately two-thirds of all cases) is associated with SLE, hepatitis B, and hepatitis C. The subendothelial tissue contains complement and immunoglobulins, which presumably represent preformed immune complexes. *Type II* (around one-third of cases) is associated with an antibody against C3 convertase, called *C3 nephritic factor*. The antibodies stabilize convertase, leading to a constant activation of C3. Deposits containing C3 and other substances are located within the glomerular basement membrane. Electron microscopy reveals the presence of characteristic, *heavy electron-dense deposits* in the basement membrane (see photograph). In both types of MPGN, the capillary wall appears as a double-lined structure (tramtrack appearance) due to the accumulation of mesangial matrix between the basement membrane and the endothelial cells. The disease, especially the type II form, has a poor prognosis. Only around 30% of patients do not develop renal failure. There is no effective treatment. The value of corticosteroids is controversial.

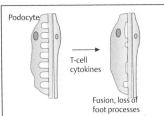

Loss of digital extensions
↓
Albuminuria
↓
Lipid aggregation
in tubular cells
↓
Nephrotic
syndrome

Good response
to corticosteroids,
good prognosis

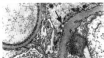

Electron microscopy

A. Minimal change glomerulonephritis (GN)

HIV-infection,
heroin
abuse

Secondary to
other GN

Secondary to
compensatory
hypertrophy

Idiopathic

Deposition
of IgM, fibrin

Loss of
foot processes

Damage to
epithelial cell
↓
Deposition of
proteins,
lipids, fibrin
↓
Mesangial
proliferation

Poor response
to corticosteroids

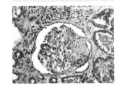

Segmental sclerosis

B. Focal segmental glomerulosclerosis

Idiopathic >80%
(genetic predisposition)
  Infections
  Carcinomas
  SLE
  Drugs
  Gold, mercury

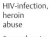

Loss of
foot processess

Thickening of
basement membrane
↓
Nonselective
proteinuria
↓
40% - Progressive
course with
renal failure

Poor response
to corticosteroids

Granular IgG deposits

C. Membranous glomerulonephritis

Type I

Hepatitis B, C
SLE
Infections?

Subendothelial
IgG, complement
deposition

Nephrotic
syndrome
acute nephritis

↓

40% - Progressive
renal failure

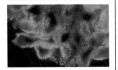

Tramtrack effect

Type II
Ab against
C3-convertase
↓
Complement
activation,
consumption

Intramembranous
C3 deposition

30% - Partial
renal failure

30% - Persistent
nephrotic
syndrome

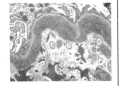

EM: Dense deposits

D. Membranoproliferative GN (MPGN)

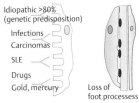

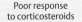
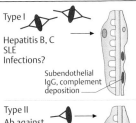
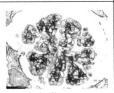

Clinical Immunology

A. Postinfectious (Diffuse Proliferative) Glomerulonephritis

Acute poststreptococcal glomerulonephritis (APSGN) is the prototype postinfectious glomerulonephritic disease, but GN may also be caused by pneumococci, staphylococci, and viruses. In most cases, fever and hematuria develop within a few weeks after *Streptococcus*-induced pharyngitis or skin infection. IgG-bearing immune complexes and complement accumulate in the subepithelial portion of the basement membrane. Histological sections present a cell-rich picture with diffuse proliferation of endothelial and mesangial cells and an increased number of leukocytes in the capillary lumina. The prognosis is good, particularly in children: chronic renal failure rarely occurs. However, chronic progression develops in around 50% of adult patients.

B. Rapidly Progressive Glomerulonephritis

Rapidly progressive glomerulonephritis (RPGN) should be considered a syndrome rather than a specific disease. Regardless of the etiology, the disease is characterized by the formation of "crescents" within the glomeruli. The crescents occur because of leakage of fibrin into the urinary space due to the proliferation of the parietal epithelial cells of Bowmann's capsule and infiltration with monocytes and macrophages. There are three subtypes of RPGN, which are classified according to immunohistological features.

Type I is characterized by the formation of autoantibodies directed against the (glomerular) basement membrane (anti-GBM antibodies). These antibodies sometimes cross-react with the basement membrane of alveoli in the lung and cause "Goodpasture's syndrome," a disease associated with renal failure and pulmonary hemorrhage. Immunohistological specimens (see photograph) exhibit diffuse, linear deposition of IgG and, in many cases, C3 along the glomerular basement membrane.

Type II is characterized by the deposition of immune complexes. This subtype of RPGN is observed in severe streptococcal nephritis, IgA nephropathy, SLE, and Schönlein–Henoch purpura or may occur as an idiopathic disease.

In *Type III*, neither anti-GBM antibodies nor immune complexes are detected. Hence, the disease is described as "pauci-immune." This subtype often occurs in conjunction with vasculitis associated with anti-granulocyte antibodies (ANCA, see p. 184).

The clinical picture of RPGN is that of a nephritic syndrome with oliguria and acute renal failure. The prognosis depends on the number of glomeruli involved. Aggressive immunosuppressive therapy is sometimes successful. Phasmapheresis is indicated in the presence of anti-GBM antibodies.

C. IgA Nephropathy

IgA nephropathy is the most common glomerular disease worldwide. In children and teenagers, the disease typically appears after a preceding bout of a flu-like illness. Genetic predisposition is assumed. The hallmark of the disease is the deposition of IgA in the mesangium (see photograph). Schönlein–Henoch purpura also leads to mesangial IgA deposition, but the deposits are also present in the gastrointestinal tract, joints, and skin. The mesangial IgA immune complexes trigger activation of the alternative complement pathway and cell proliferation. Depending on the severity of the disease, the features may include focal segmental changes (see p. 210) or crescents similar to those of RPGN. Children have a good prognosis. In adults, the disease has a chronic progressive course. More than 50% of the patients develop terminal renal failure.

D. Tubulointerstitial Nephritis

Inflammatory changes in the interstitial tissues may occur due to infections or medications or may occur without any identifiable cause. A clinical investigation reveals generalized symptoms, oliguria, and acute renal impairment; dehydration can further worsen the clinical picture. The morphological findings reveal infiltration of the interstitial tissues by mononuclear cells, granulocytes, and eosinophils (see photograph); granulomas may also occur due to protracted drug exposure. A delayed-type hypersensitivity reaction is assumed. The fact that some patients exhibit increased levels of IgE suggests that a type I hypersensitivity reaction may play a role in some cases. Complete normalization occurs after discontinuation of the offending medication.

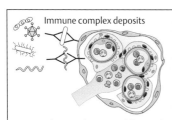

Immune complex deposits

Common symptoms, hematuria

↓

Hypercellularity in all glomeruli

↓

Children → >80% Healing

Adults → ~50% Healing

No specific therapy

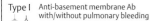

Hypercellularity

A. Postinfectious (acute proliferative) GN

Type I Anti-basement membrane Ab with/without pulmonary bleeding

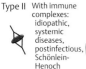

Type II With immune complexes: idiopathic, systemic diseases, postinfectious, Schönlein-Henoch

Type III Pauci-immune: idiopathic, Wegener's, PAN

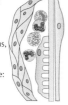

Renal insufficiency in 90%

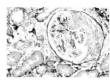

Aggressive immunosuppression: high-dose steroids cyclophosphamide

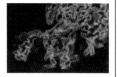

B. Rapidly progressive GN

Crescent

Linear IgG deposition

Genetic predisposition, infections

↓

Increased IgA synthesis

IgA immune complexes

Mesangial IgA deposition, mesangial proliferation

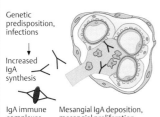

Infection of airways

↓

Hematuria, kidney pain

↓   ↓

Children   Adults

↓   ↓

High healing rate   Slowly progressive

No specific therapy

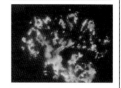

IgA deposits

C. IgA immune complexes

Idiopathic

?

Infections   Drugs

↓

Interstitial deposition

↓

Granuloma formation

Interstitial edema, kidney enlargement

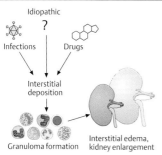

Medications

↓

Fever, eosinophilia, exanthema (25%)

↓

Renal damage (hematuria, proteinuria, leukocyturia)

↓

Renal insufficiency (avoid dehydration)

Rehydration Steroids??

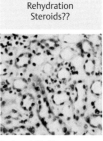

Eosinophil infiltrates

D. Tubulointerstitial nephritis

Clinical Immunology

A. Autoantigens of the Thyroid Gland

The anterior pituitary produces thyroid-stimulating hormone (TSH), which binds to TSH receptors (TSHR) on thyroid cells. Iodide is subsequently oxidized to iodine (I_2) and incorporated into tyrosine. Monoiodotyrosine (MIT) and diiodotyrosine (DIT) bind to thyroglobulin (Tg) and are transformed to triiodothyronine (T_3) and tetraiodothyronine (T_4) by thyroid peroxidase (TPO). After cleavage of thyroglobulin, T_3 and T_4 are released into the circulation. The aforementioned proteins can be immunogenic targets, and antibodies can be found in the blood of patients with thyroid diseases.

B. Most Important Autoantibodies

The pathogenetically relevant autoantibodies are mainly those directed against the receptor for TSH. They can imitate the normal action of TSH (thyroid-stimulating immunoglobulin, TSI), leading to thyroid hyperactivity (hyperthyroidism), or may completely block TSH stimulation (thyroid stimulation-blocking immunoglobulin, TSBI), thereby inhibiting thyroid gland function (hypothyroidism). A third group of antibodies (TSH binding-inhibiting immunoglobulins, TBII) is capable of stimulating TSH receptors while simultaneously blocking the binding of natural TSH. This can result in either hyperthyroidism or hypothyroidism.

C. Graves' Disease

Graves' disease is the prototype immunogenic hyperthyroid disease. It occurs mainly in women and is associated with the haplotypes HLA-DR3 and HLA-B8. The main feature is diffuse enlargement of the thyroid (goiter); other typical features include protrusion of the eyeballs (exophthalmos) and pretibial myxedema, a skin thickening due to the accumulation of mucopolysaccharides. The increased production of thyroid hormones T_3 and T_4 increases the patient's sensitivity to catecholamines, resulting in nervousness, sweating, heat intolerance, weight loss, diarrhea, tremor, and tachycardia.

Autoimmunity to the TSH receptor is presumably caused by viral antigens with a high degree of homology with the receptor (**2**). T cells of the T_H2 type induce plasma cell differentiation and antibody formation via IL-4 and IL-6. Autoantibodies acting as agonists (TSI) bind to the TSH receptor, thereby stimulating hormone production more persistently than naturally occurring TSH. TBII are also present in patients with Graves' disease (**B**). These immunoglobulins block the binding of TSH throughout the entire extracellular domain of the TSH receptor. Depending on the extent to which this occurs, the affected patient will have either hyperthyroidism, euthyroidism, or hypothyroidism.

Endocrine orbitopathy (**3**) mainly occurs in association with Graves' disease, but may also occur independently. Exophthalmos (see photograph) is caused by edema of ocular muscles (see CT image), proliferation of retro-orbital connective tissue, and infiltration with leukocytes. The ocular muscles possibly share cross-reactive epitopes with TSH. Retro-orbital fibroblasts appear to secrete TSHR-like molecules and adhesion molecules that make them receptive to TSHR autoantibodies.

D. Hashimoto's Thyroiditis

Destruction of the thyroid gland due to Hashimoto's thyroiditis (HT) is a common cause of hypothyroidism. Fatigue, cold intolerance, bradycardia, and weight gain are typical symptoms (**E**). Myxedema, a generalized cutaneous edema most commonly detected on the face (see photograph), is caused by the swelling of mucopolysaccharides in the skin. The underlying cause of HT appears to be T_H1 type T cells that release TNF, IL-2, and IFN-γ, thereby stimulating the CD8+ T cells responsible for the destruction of thyroid tissue. The T-cell-mediated damage to thyroid cells presumably leads to the release of antigens and to secondary production of TPO-specific or thyroglobulin-specific autoantigens. Infiltration with lymphocytes and, in some cases, formation of complete lymph follicles can be detected in thyroid tissue (see photograph). Hashimoto's thyroiditis is closely associated with HLA-DR3 and HLA-DR5 and mainly occurs in females. The patients often remain asymptomatic for many years and develop clinical symptoms of hypothyroidism only after advanced destruction of the thyroid follicles has occurred.

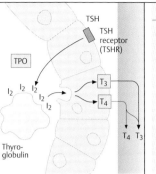

A. Autoantigens of thyroid

Target	Ab	Effect of antibody
Thyroglobulin (Tg)	Tg-Ab	
Microsomal antigen, thyroid-peroxidase TPO	TPO-Ab	Decreased iodination of Tg
TSH-Receptor	TSI	**T**hyroid **s**timulating **i**mmunoglobulin: hyperthyroidism (Graves' disease)
	TBII	**T**SH-**b**inding **i**nhibitory **i**mmunoglobulin: hyper- or hypothyroidism
	TSBI	**T**hyroid-**st**imulation **b**locking **i**mmunoglobulin: hypothyroidism

B. Most important autoantibodies

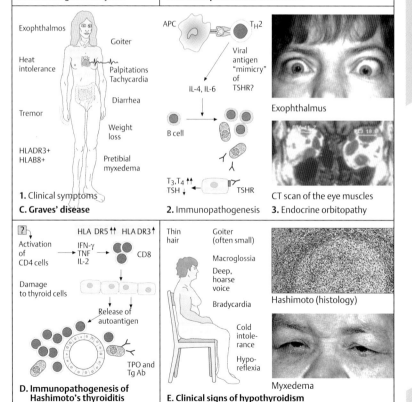

Exophthalmos

Goiter

Heat intolerance

Palpitations Tachycardia

Diarrhea

Tremor

Weight loss

HLADR3+ HLAB8+

Pretibial myxedema

1. Clinical symptoms
C. Graves' disease

APC T_H2

Viral antigen "mimicry" of TSHR?

IL-4, IL-6

B cell

T_3, T_4 ↑↑
TSH ↓ TSHR

2. Immunopathogenesis

Exophthalmus

CT scan of the eye muscles

3. Endocrine orbitopathy

?

Activation of CD4 cells

HLA DR5 ↑↑ HLA DR3 ↑

IFN-γ
TNF
IL-2 CD8

Damage to thyroid cells

Release of autoantigen

TPO and Tg Ab

D. Immunopathogenesis of Hashimoto's thyroiditis

Thin hair

Goiter (often small)

Macroglossia

Deep, hoarse voice

Bradycardia

Cold intolerance

Hyporeflexia

Hashimoto (histology)

Myxedema

E. Clinical signs of hypothyroidism

Clinical Immunology

Insulin, a metabolic hormone, regulates the entry of glucose from the blood into the cells. Diabetes mellitus can develop due to insulin deficiency (type I diabetes; insulin-dependent diabetes mellitus, IDDM) or due to target tissue resistance to insulin (type II diabetes). Type I diabetes is most commonly attributable to a pathological autoimmune reaction.

A. Clinical Manifestations

Type I diabetes occurs mainly in younger patients. The inability to incorporate glucose into the cells results in increased blood glucose levels and increased plasma osmolarity. This, in turn, leads to osmotic diuresis with increased urinary frequency (polyuria), thirst, and increased fluid intake (polydipsia). The patients have an increased appetite (polyphagia), but lose weight because the body is unable to use the glucose. Fatty acids are released from fatty tissues and are metabolized by the liver into ketone bodies, leading to metabolic acidosis. Vessel damage (diabetic microangiopathy) is due to accumulation of glycosylated proteins and polypeptides in the vessel wall. Glycosylation end-products cause cross-links between polypeptides, trapping of lipoproteins, and cell activation, leading to atherosclerosis. This is a major late complication of diabetes, which can lead to stroke, kidney failure, blindness, and heart failure.

B. Genetic Predisposition in IDDM

The presence of HLA-DQ and -DR alleles, which contain a serine, alanine, or valine group at position 57 of the β chain, increases the risk of IDDM (see also p. 54). The presence of aspartate in this position is associated with a decreased incidence of IDDM. So-called "diabetogenic" alleles apparently bind peptides with a negative charge at position 9, whereas diabetes-resistant alleles with an aspartate molecule at position 57 bind peptides with a positively charged serine, glycine, or alanine molecule at peptide position 9. Such peptides appear to turn the immune response towards a T_H2-type response, whereas negatively charged peptides tend to induce a cytotoxic immune response of the T_H1 type.

C. Pathogenetic Concepts

The serum of IDDM patients contains autoantibodies to various islet cell autoantigens, such as insulin, heat shock protein 60 (hsp60) and, most importantly, glutamate decarboxylase 65 (GAD65). Since Coxsackievirus proteins have a great degree of homology with the GAD65 antigen, the production of cross-reacting antibodies is assumed to occur. The antibodies cause inflammation outside the pancreatic beta islet cells (peri-insulitis), which results in the recruitment of antigen-presenting cells. These can capture antigens from the damaged islet cells and induce a T-cell response within the beta islet cells (intra-insulitis). A cytotoxic T_H1 response predominates in individuals with the predisposing HLA alleles. Once the primary infection has occurred, several years may pass before the full-blown disease manifests because small quantities of insulin are sufficient to prevent symptoms.

D. Autoimmune Polyglandular Syndrome (APS)

APS develops as a result of multiple genetic defects which occur simultaneously or due to an immune response against antigens expressed by different endocrine organs. Three subtypes can be distinguished. *Type I* is most common in teenagers and manifests as adrenocortical insufficiency (immune response to 21-hydroxylase, 21-OH), hypoparathyroidism (autoantibodies to parathyroid calcium sensor), and recurrent mucocutaneous candidal infections. Hypogonadism sometimes occurs due to autoantibodies to p450 side chain cleavage enzyme (p450scc) and 17α-OH enzyme. APS is sometimes associated with chronic active hepatitis (autoantibodies to microsomal antigens of the liver and kidney). Pernicious anemia may also occur if autoantibodies to intrinsic factor are present (see p. 208).

Age-independent *type II* APS is characterized by the co-occurrence of adrenocortical insufficiency and autoimmune thyroid disease (see p. 214). This subtype is associated with IDDM in 50% of cases. *Type III* is characterized by the joint occurrence of thyroid disease and other autoimmune diseases in the absence of adrenocortical insufficiency.

Clinical Immunology

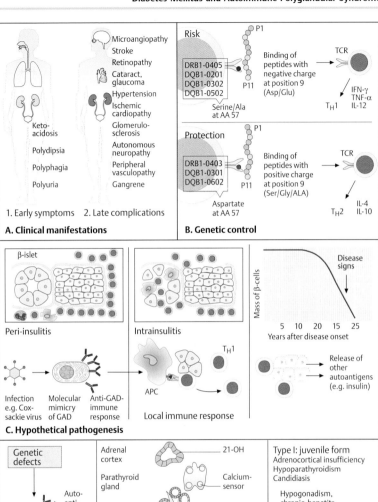

Risk

DRB1-0405
DQB1-0201
DQB1-0302
DQB1-0502

Serine/Ala at AA 57

P1 · P11

Binding of peptides with negative charge at position 9 (Asp/Glu)

TCR

T_H1 — IFN-γ, TNF-α, IL-12

Protection

DRB1-0403
DQB1-0301
DQB1-0602

Aspartate at AA 57

P1 · P11

Binding of peptides with positive charge at position 9 (Ser/Gly/ALA)

TCR

T_H2 — IL-4, IL-10

Microangiopathy
Stroke
Retinopathy
Cataract, glaucoma
Hypertension
Ischemic cardiopathy
Glomerulo-sclerosis
Autonomous neuropathy
Peripheral vasculopathy
Gangrene

Keto-acidosis
Polydipsia
Polyphagia
Polyuria

1. Early symptoms   2. Late complications

A. Clinical manifestations

B. Genetic control

β-islet

Peri-insulitis

Intrainsulitis

T_H1

Mass of β-cells

Disease signs

5 10 20 15 25
Years after disease onset

Infection e.g. Coxsackie virus → Molecular mimicry of GAD → Anti-GAD-immune response

APC

Local immune response

Release of other autoantigens (e.g. insulin)

C. Hypothetical pathogenesis

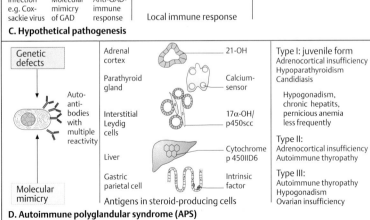

Genetic defects

Auto-anti-bodies with multiple reactivity

Molecular mimicry

Adrenal cortex — 21-OH

Parathyroid gland — Calcium-sensor

Interstitial Leydig cells — 17α-OH/p450scc

Liver — Cytochrome p 450IID6

Gastric parietal cell — Intrinsic factor

Antigens in steroid-producing cells

Type I: juvenile form
Adrenocortical insufficiency
Hypoparathyroidism
Candidiasis

Hypogonadism,
chronic hepatits,
pernicious anemia
less frequently

Type II:
Adrenocortical insufficiency
Autoimmune thyropathy

Type III:
Autoimmune thyropathy
Hypogonadism
Ovarian insufficiency

D. Autoimmune polyglandular syndrome (APS)

Clinical Immunology

231

A. Rheumatic Fever

Rheumatic fever (RF) is an inflammatory process involving the heart, joints, skin, and central nervous system (**1**), which usually begins around 1–3 weeks after a tonsillar infection with group A streptococci. The acute symptoms, which may persist for a few weeks up to several months, sometimes cause irreversible damage. Valvular fibrosis, for example, is one of the most common causes of acquired heart disease in children and teenagers. Carditis and polyarthritis are the most common clinical manifestations. The carditis may involve the endocardium (valves), myocardium, and pericardium; mitral valve involvement is typical. The articular involvement manifests as migratory polyarthritis mainly involving the large joints. Twenty percent of patients have involuntary muscle coordination disorders (Sydenham's chorea). Other less common manifestations include erythema marginatum, a nonpruritic, evanescent rash producing reddish spots with rounded borders and a pale center, and subcutaneous nodules on the extensor surface of the joints. The aforementioned manifestations represent the major diagnostic criteria (Jones criteria) for rheumatic fever. The minor criteria are fever, elevated ESR and CRP, and a prolonged PR interval (EKG).

Pharyngotonsillitis due to infection with group A β-hemolytic *Streptococcus* always precedes rheumatic fever (**4**). However, only around 3 % of all untreated cases of streptococcal pharyngitis lead to RF; streptococcal infections of the skin never do. Only virulent, encapsulated strains that induce a strong immune response to streptococcal antigens (**2**) are capable of inducing RF. These *Streptococcus* strains are mainly M types 1, 3, 5, 6, and 18. The streptococcal antigens cross-react with human cardiac tissue, especially sarcolemmic proteins and cardiac myosin, but also with antigen structures in the joints or brain. Epidemiological studies have demonstrated a familial disposition associated with the HLA haplotypes DR1, DR2, DR3, and DR4.

The granulomas associated with RF are referred to as *Aschoff's bodies*. These typically develop near the smaller vessels of the heart (**3**). They are characterized by central areas of fibrinoid necrosis (degeneration of collagen) with bundled muscle fibers that are surrounded by mononuclear cells and fibrohistiocytic Aschoff's cells and, in some cases, multinucleate Aschoff's giant cells. Aschoff's bodies develop as a result of direct cell damage and immune complex precipitation after the rapid formation of antibodies to various cross-reacting streptococcal antigens. Induction of this immune response takes place in local lymph tissue during pharingitis/tonsillitis (**4**).

B. Myocarditis

Myocarditis is caused by a number of pathogens. In the Western world, Coxsackieviruses are the most common cause. In South America, on the other hand, it is most often caused by parasites (Chagas' disease, caused by *Trypanosoma cruzi*). In the initial phase, replication of the pathogen in the myocytes leads to cell lysis and myonecrosis. MHC molecules and cell adhesion molecules, especially ICAM-1, are expressed on the myocytes. Local presentation of viral antigens then occurs, leading to the induction of humoral and cellular immune responses. TNF promotes the generation of cytotoxic T cells, and cross-reacting antibodies lead to increased cell damage. The destruction of myocardial tissues leads to the release of intracellular proteins, such as myosin, which were previously ignored by the immune system.

C. Dressler's Syndrome and Postpericardiotomy Syndrome

Post-myocardial infarction syndrome (*Dressler's syndrome*) is an acute disease associated with fever, pericarditis, and pleuritis which, in most cases, starts within 1–2 weeks to a few months after acute myocardial infarction. *Post-pericardiotomy syndrome* manifests with similar symptoms and develops within 2 weeks of heart surgery. Both diseases are associated with the formation of antimyocardial antibodies that induce fever and pericardial inflammation. Since it occurs in the absence of a strong inflammatory stimulus, the autoimmune process is self-limited. Treatment consists mainly of bed rest and nonsteroidal anti-inflammatory drugs.

Clinical Immunology

A. Rheumatic fever

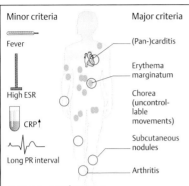

Minor criteria

Fever

High ESR

CRP↑

Long PR interval

Major criteria

(Pan-)carditis

Erythema marginatum

Chorea (uncontrollable movements)

Subcutaneous nodules

Arthritis

1. Primary manifestations

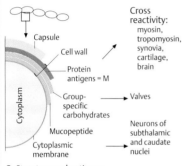

Capsule

Cell wall

Protein antigens = M

Group-specific carbohydrates

Mucopeptide

Cytoplasmic membrane

Cytoplasm

Cross reactivity: myosin, tropomyosin, synovia, cartilage, brain

Valves

Neurons of subthalamic and caudate nuclei

2. Streptococcal antigens

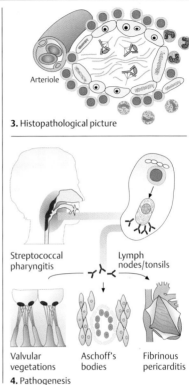

Arteriole

3. Histopathological picture

Streptococcal pharyngitis

Lymph nodes/tonsils

Valvular vegetations

Aschoff's bodies

Fibrinous pericarditis

4. Pathogenesis

B. Myocarditis

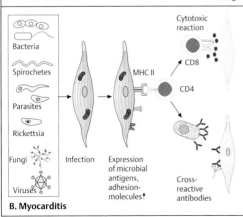

Bacteria

Spirochetes

Parasites

Rickettsia

Fungi

Viruses

Infection

Expression of microbial antigens, adhesion-molecules↑

MHC II

CD8

CD4

Cytotoxic reaction

Cross-reactive antibodies

C. Dressler's syndrome

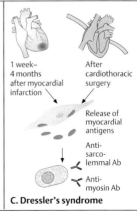

1 week–4 months after myocardial infarction

After cardiothoracic surgery

Release of myocardial antigens

Anti-sarcolemmal Ab

Anti-myosin Ab

Multiple sclerosis (MS) is a disease of the central nervous system of unknown etiology. It is characterized by the presence of multiple foci of de-myelinization (plaques) that later become sclerotic.

A. Morphological and Histopathological Findings

Degradation of the lipid-rich isolating layer of nerve processes (axons), which is formed by oligodendrocytes, occurs in the demyelinization zones. Early lesions (**1**) appear as perivenular zones of lymphoplasmacytic infiltration with demyelinization of individual axons. Late lesions are characterized by the involvement of multiple axons (**2**). Glial fibrils and foamy cells are present. These include macrophages or microglial cells (the CNS-resident macrophages) that have phagocytosed myelin. The foci of demyelinization can be visualized on magnetic resonance imaging (MRI); their location constantly changes over the course of time (**3**).

B. Experimental Autoimmune Encephalomyelitis (EAE)

An animal model for MS can be induced by immunizing animals (mice, rats) with purified myelin proteins, such as myelin basic protein (MBP), proteolipid protein (PLP), myelin-oligo-dendrocyte glycoprotein (MOG), and myelin-associated glycoprotein (MAG). Activated T cells from the immunized animals can transmit the disease to healthy animals.

C. Immunopathogenetic Mechanisms

A genetic predisposition (HLA association: DR15/DQ6) together with external factors (presumably viral infection, e.g., with human herpesvirus 6) can lead to the migration of auto-reactive T cells through the blood–brain barrier into the CNS. This is mediated by the expression of adhesion molecules on lymphocytes and endothelial cells. Microglia present myelin peptides to the activated T cells, which differentiate locally into T_H1 and T_H2 cells. The T_H2 cells induce B-cell activation and the production of myelin-reactive autoantibodies, which can increase myelin degeneration and induce the additional release of antigens. This is reflected by findings of an oligoclonal γ-globulin fraction in cerebrospinal fluid (CSF). T_H1 cells activate astrocytes, microglia, and macrophages which, in turn, release IL-1, TNF-α, nitric oxide (NO), H_2O_2, and free radicals. These induce apoptosis of oligodendrocytes and promote their phagocytosis by microglia and macrophages.

D. Clinical Features

The demyelinization of axons can impair or enhance neuronal signal transmission, depending on whether stimulatory or inhibitory neurons are affected. If stimulatory neurons are damaged, limb weakness, impaired vision, and ataxia can occur. Enhancement of signal transmission due to the damage of inhibitory neurons leads to tonic contractions, paresthesia, and Lhermitte's sign (the occurrence of electric-like shocks that spread from the neck down to the legs upon flexion of the head). The disease presents in most cases with acute episodes followed by partial remissions (relapsing-remitting MS), but has a chronic progressive course in about 10–15%. The symptoms are mild in ca. 25% of the patients.

E. Approaches to Treatment

Corticosteroids are the most important drugs for treatment of relapsing-remitting MS (**1**). Around one-third to one-half of the patients respond to IFN-β, but the drug's exact mechanism of action is unknown. Synthetic polypeptide combinations (glutiramer acetate) imitate the structure of MBP antigens and are reported to restore tolerance. Azathioprine, a purine analogue, inhibits both antibody production and the cellular immune response. Intravenous high-dose immunoglobulins can be beneficial. A monoclonal antibody to $\alpha4$ integrin has recently shown clinical activity.

Treatment of chronic progressive MS requires stronger immunosuppressants, such as methotrexate, cyclophosphamide, and cyclosporine; IFN-β also appears to be effective in some of these patients (**2**). Experimental treatment strategies, including the use of anticytokine antibodies or myelin peptides to anergize myelin-reactive T cells, had disappointing results or induced worsening of the disease. In particular, trials with TNF-blocking antibodies were stopped because of worsening of symptoms.

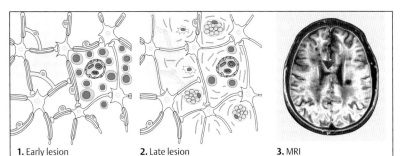

1. Early lesion   **2.** Late lesion   **3.** MRI

A. Morphological and histopathological findings

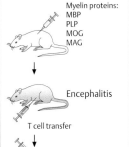

Myelin proteins:
MBP
PLP
MOG
MAG

Encephalitis

T cell transfer

Disease
transfer

**B. Experimental autoimmune
encephalitis (EAE)**

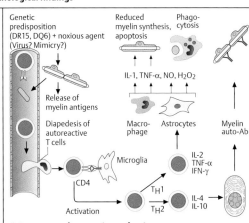

Genetic
predisposition
(DR15, DQ6) + noxious agent
(Virus? Mimicry?)

Release of
myelin antigens

Diapedesis of
autoreactive
T cells

Activation

CD4

Microglia

T_H1

T_H2

Reduced
myelin synthesis,
apoptosis

Phago-
cytosis

IL-1, TNF-α, NO, H_2O_2

Macro-
phage

Astrocytes

Myelin
auto-Ab

IL-2
TNF-α
IFN-γ

IL-4
IL-10

C. Immunopathogenetic mechanisms

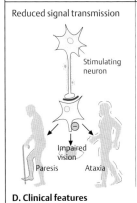

Reduced signal transmission

Stimulating
neuron

Impaired
vision

Paresis   Ataxia

D. Clinical features

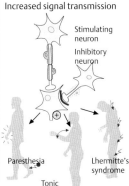

Increased signal transmission

Stimulating
neuron

Inhibitory
neuron

Paresthesia

Tonic
contractions

Lhermitte's
syndrome

1. Treatment of
relapsing-remitting MS

Corticosteroids, IFN-β,
polypeptides (glutiramer),
azathioprine,
intravenous immunoglobulins

2. Treatment of primary
progressive MS

Methotrexate,
cyclophosphamide, (IFN-β),
cyclosporine

E. Treatment approaches

Clinical Immunology

A. Guillain–Barré Syndrome

Guillain–Barré syndrome (GBS), or "*acute poly-neuroradiculitis*," is an acute demyelinizing inflammation of the peripheral nerves characterized by ascending, symmetrical motor paralysis of the muscles of the limbs, eyes, face, and respiratory tract (**1**). The prognosis is good. Unless severe respiratory failure develops, most patients recover completely. The mortality rate is around 5%. More than two-thirds of the patients report a preceding infection, usually with *Campylobacter jejuni*, but also with cytomegalovirus (CMV) or Epstein–Barr virus (EBV). This suggests that molecular mimicry with peripheral myelin is involved in the development of GBS (**2**). Surgical interventions that cause the release of neuron antigens can also precipitate the disease, as can lymphomas that induce autoreactive T-cell proliferation. The autoantigens involved are thought to be myelin antigens (P0, P1, P2) and gangliosides. Activated antigen-presenting cells (APCs) present the autoantigens and induce T_H1 and T_H2 responses. Activated macrophages phagocytose myelin and produce proinflammatory cytokines, reactive oxygen radicals, nitric oxide, and proteases. Plasma cells stimulated by T_H2 cells produce autoantibodies to myelin. Since the autoantibodies play an important role in the pathogenesis of GBS, it is not surprising that plasmapheresis has a beneficial effect on the clinical course of the disease (**3**). High-dose intravenous immunoglobulins (IVIGs) seem to be even more effective. IVIGs contain naturally occurring anti-idiotypic antibodies that probably inhibit the binding of myelin-specific autoantibodies. The immunoglobulins also saturate the Fc receptors on macrophages, thereby inhibiting the phagocytosis of autoantibody-coated peripheral nerve cells.

B. Rasmussen's Encephalitis

Rasmussen's encephalitis is a disease of childhood, which is characterized by severe, untreatable epileptic attacks with dementia and focal cerebral inflammation. Autoantibodies to the third subunit of the glutamate receptor (GluR3) can be detected in some of the patients. Glutamate is an excitatory neurotransmitter that leads to the depolarization of central neurons. Anti-GluR3 autoantibodies act as receptor agonists that bind to the receptor much longer than glutamate. Hence, receptor stimulation by the agonist is much more long-acting than under physiological conditions and therefore leads to massive epileptic neural excitation, as shown by the depolarization curve in the presence of autoantibodies.

C. Paraneoplastic Neurological Syndromes

Paraneoplastic neurological syndromes (PNS) usually develop as an immune response to antigens that are expressed by tumor cells but which also occur in the normal nervous system. Neurological symptoms often precede the tumor diagnosis. The most widely recognized among these antigens is the Hu antigen, a nuclear protein that is present in all central and peripheral neurons. Hu proteins are expressed in small-cell lung cancer and neuroblastoma. Anti-Hu antibodies are associated with sensory neuropathy and encephalomyelitis. Patients with small-cell lung carcinoma and low titers of anti-Hu antibodies without signs of PNS tend to have smaller tumors, respond better to treatment, and survive longer—which suggests that these antibodies may mediate an effective antitumoral response.

Unlike the Hu protein, the neuronal nuclear protein Ri is restricted to the central nervous system. Ri protein has been identified as a target of autoantibodies in patients with gynecological tumors and breast cancer with concomitant eye movement disorders (opsoclonus).

Yo proteins are expressed in the cytoplasm of Purkinje cells (neurons of the cortex cerebelli) and are also expressed in some gynecological tumors and breast cancers. As a result of an antibody reactivity against Yo antigens, many of these patients suffer from paraneoplastic degeneration of the cerebellum. Most patients with central paraneoplastic syndromes do not benefit from plasmapheresis or immunosuppressants. Tumor removal or remission induction by medical or radiotherapy treatment can lead to an improvement of symptoms.

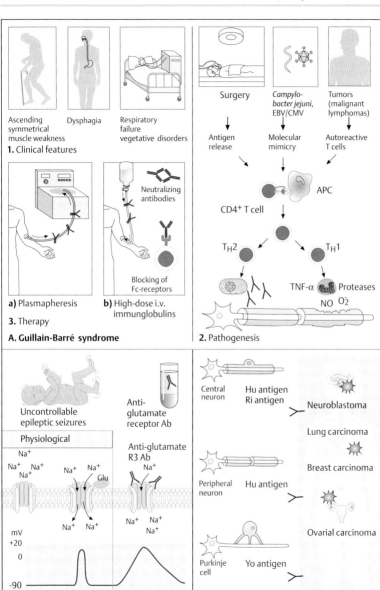

1. Clinical features

Ascending symmetrical muscle weakness

Dysphagia

Respiratory failure vegetative disorders

3. Therapy

a) Plasmapheresis

b) High-dose i.v. immunglobulins

Neutralizing antibodies

Blocking of Fc-receptors

A. Guillain-Barré syndrome

2. Pathogenesis

Surgery

Campylo-bacter jejuni, EBV/CMV

Tumors (malignant lymphomas)

Antigen release

Molecular mimicry

Autoreactive T cells

APC

$CD4^+$ T cell

T_H2

T_H1

TNF-α Proteases

NO O_2^-

B. Rasmussen's encephalitis

Uncontrollable epileptic seizures

Anti-glutamate receptor Ab

Physiological

Na^+

Na^+ Na^+
Na^+

Na^+ Na^+
Glu

Anti-glutamate R3 Ab

Na^+

Na^+ Na^+

Na^+ Na^+

Na^+ Na^+

mV
+20
0
-90

C. Paraneoplastic neurological syndromes

Central neuron

Hu antigen
Ri antigen

Neuroblastoma

Lung carcinoma

Breast carcinoma

Peripheral neuron

Hu antigen

Ovarial carcinoma

Purkinje cell

Yo antigen

Clinical Immunology

A. Myasthenia Gravis

1 Clinical features. Myasthenia gravis (MG) is an autoantibody-mediated, progressive, exercise-dependent disease characterized by weakness and premature fatigue of the voluntary muscles. Initial involvement of the eye muscles is common. The typical feature is drooping of the eyelids (ptosis) and double vision (diplopia). When the patient looks up for a while, the fatigued eyelids begin to droop (see photographs). The disease remains limited to the ocular muscles in 20% of patients, but becomes generalized in most cases (**1b**). The ability to chew, swallow, and speak may be impaired. MG may spread to the extremities and even to the respiratory tract. Electrophysiological studies (**1c**) show a typical decremental decrease in muscle potential after repeated stimulation. The potential amplitude drops by more than 10% from the 1st to 5th stimulus. After administration of an acetylcholine esterase inhibitor, the muscle potential remains at a constant level and an improvement of ptosis can be observed.

2 Pathogenesis. The arrival of an action potential at the terminal axon induces the release of acetylcholine (ACh) to the synaptic cleft, where it binds to the acetylcholine receptor (AChR). Activation of the AChR leads to subsequent depolarization of the muscle cell (**2a**).

Depolarization is then terminated by acetylcholinesterase-mediated hydrolysis of acetylcholine. Patients with myasthenia gravis have a decreased neuromuscular transmission capacity due to the presence of AChR antibodies. These antibodies inhibit AChR activity by inducing complement-mediated lysis at the postsynaptic membrane (**2b**). AChR autoantibodies can also block ACh binding sites. Furthermore, the rate of AChR degradation increases once it has been internalized upon formation of the autoantibody–receptor complex. The ACh concentration in the synaptic cleft can be maintained at higher levels by acetylcholinesterase inhibitors, leading to a temporary improvement of symptoms. Apart from AChR, proteins of the striated muscles (e.g., actin, myosin, and titin) may also act as autoantigens.

Myasthenia gravis is associated with small, usually benign epithelial thymomas in around 30% of cases (**2c**). The tumors generally exhibit abnormal expression of neurofilaments, which share epitopes with AChR and titin. As a result of molecular mimicry, AChR-specific and titin-specific T cells are positively selected in the thymus and activated outside the thymus, allowing the production of autoantibodies.

Approximately 70% of patients with MG have a lymphofollicular thymitis (**2d**). The infiltrating B cells form complete germinal centers (see photograph). MG is frequently associated with the HLA-B8 and HLA-DR3 alleles. AChR-bearing cells that resemble muscle cells (myoid cells) are present in the thymus. The myoid cells form thymic aggregates with dendritic APCs, which are thought to be capable of presenting AChR antigens to CD4+ T cells, resulting in the production of AChR-specific antibodies directly in the thymus. This is supported by the fact that the autoantibodies found in thymitis-associated MG specifically recognize the embryonal form of AChR, which is found postpartum only in the thymus and the eye muscles.

B. Lambert–Eaton Syndrome

Lambert–Eaton myasthenic syndrome (LES) is similar to myasthenia gravis but is characterized by primary involvement of the pelvic muscles as opposed to the facial muscles. Unlike MG, LES produces autonomic symptoms, such as mouth dryness and micturition disturbances. Anticalcium channel antibodies that inhibit the release of ACh are present in the presynaptic membrane of patients with LES. This blocks the transmission of stimuli to the postsynaptic membrane. After serial stimulation, the presynaptic block is temporarily overcome and acetylcholine can be released in higher concentrations, leading to an increase of the potential amplitude over the baseline level. LES was first described as a paraneoplastic syndrome associated with certain types of cancer, especially small-cell lung carcinoma. It sometimes precedes cancer detection. There is evidence suggesting that certain antibodies may cross-react with the tumor cells.

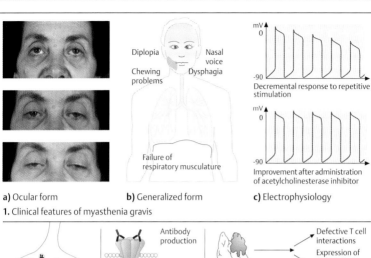

a) Ocular form   **b)** Generalized form   **c)** Electrophysiology

Decremental response to repetitive stimulation

Improvement after administration of acetylcholinesterase inhibitor

Diplopia   Nasal voice

Chewing problems   Dysphagia

Failure of respiratory musculature

1. Clinical features of myasthenia gravis

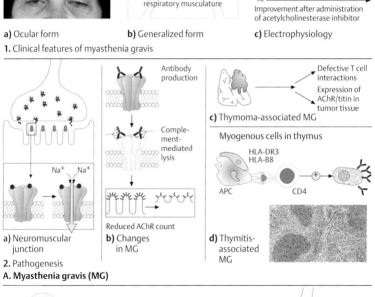

a) Neuromuscular junction   **b)** Changes in MG

Antibody production

Complement-mediated lysis

Reduced AChR count

c) Thymoma-associated MG

Defective T cell interactions

Expression of AChR/titin in tumor tissue

Myogenous cells in thymus

HLA-DR3
HLA-B8

APC   CD4

d) Thymitis-associated MG

2. Pathogenesis

A. Myasthenia gravis (MG)

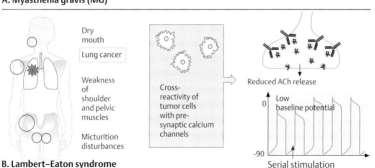

Dry mouth

Lung cancer

Weakness of shoulder and pelvic muscles

Micturition disturbances

Cross-reactivity of tumor cells with pre-synaptic calcium channels

Reduced ACh release

Low baseline potential

Serial stimulation

B. Lambert–Eaton syndrome

Clinical Immunology

239

Like the skin and the mucous membranes, the eye is constantly exposed to environmental factors, such as bacteria, viruses, dust, and ultraviolet light. The eye has a limited reaction potential, and its anatomic structures are complex and fragile. Moreover, the eye contains an extensive network of blood vessels, where immune complexes can easily accumulate and where immune cells can rapidly migrate from the circulation. Even slight pathological changes in the ocular vessels can have a dramatic impact on visual power and acuity. Hence, such changes become clinically manifest much more quickly than similar changes in the vessels of the internal organs. Furthermore, pathological processes in the blood vessels of the eye can be directly observed because the retinal vessels of the fundus are visible.

A. Anatomy of the Eye

A distinction is made between extraocular and intraocular inflammation. The conjunctiva, cornea, and sclera are extraocular structures, whereas the iris, lens, ciliary body, vitreous body, retina, and choroid are intraocular structures. The cornea, lens, and vitreous body do not contain blood vessels. The sclera is sparsely vascularized, whereas the iris, ciliary body, and choroid are densely vascularized with a spongelike network of vessels. This vessel-rich part of the eye is called the *uvea*. The retina also has an extensive network of capillaries. The endothelial cells of the ciliary body and choroid are fenestrated and thus pervious to large protein molecules.

B. Immunological Pathomechanisms

The eyelids, conjunctiva, and a thin layer of tear fluid protect the eye from environmental irritants. If any of these structures is damaged, bacteria, viruses, dust particles, and other exogenous noxae can exert their effects on the internal structures of the eye. The eye does not have a great deal of resistance to mechanical damage. In perforating wounds, the otherwise well-isolated structures of the eye are directly exposed to pathogens and foreign antigens. Therefore, even a relatively mild inflammatory response can have a dramatically harmful effect.

Since the uvea has a particularly rich blood supply, secondary colonization of bacteria or viruses can occur due to hematogenic spread. Antibodies and preformed immune complexes can also accumulate in the eye. Cross-reactivity between bacterial, viral, parasitic, or fungal antigens and endogenous antigens of the eye may occur due to molecular mimicry. The modification of autoantigens by interaction with the microorganisms can also induce a reaction against normal structures.

Another unique feature of the eye is the "sequestration" of antigens in the lens, cornea, and vitreous body due to the lack of blood vessels; atigens within these structures are inaccessible to the immune system. However, if the protective barrier is damaged, these antigens are set free and can be recognized by cells of the immune system. This mechanism plays an important role in the development of phacogenic uveitis (see p. 246).

C. Experimental Autoimmune Uveoretinitis

Destruction of the retinal photoreceptors can be induced experimentally by immunizing certain animals (guinea pigs, mice, rats, and primates) with retinal antigens (e.g., retina-S antigen or interphotoreceptor retinoid-binding protein, IRBP). This animal model is called experimental autoimmune uveoretinitis (EAU) and is assumed to reflect the pathogenesis of some autoimmune diseases of the human eye. Transfusion of T lymphocytes from the immunized animals can induce the disease in healthy animals. However, only a portion of the animals will develop EAU after the transfusion. Only animals with a T_H1-type immune response instead of a T_H2-type response are susceptible. This response may be due to APCs, such as dendritic cells, which release IL-12 when activated, thereby inducing a T_H1 response. Exogenous IL-12 can indeed render resistant animals susceptible to EAU. Experimental autoimmune uveoretinitis is used as an animal model to study the development of sympathetic ophthalmia (see p. 246).

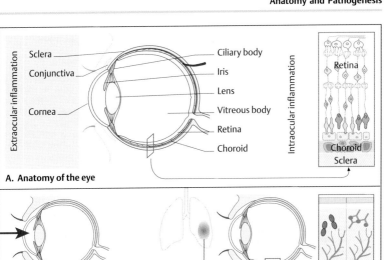

Extraocular inflammation

- Sclera
- Conjunctiva
- Cornea

- Ciliary body
- Iris
- Lens
- Vitreous body
- Retina
- Choroid

Intraocular inflammation

Retina

Choroid

Sclera

A. Anatomy of the eye

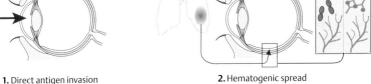

1. Direct antigen invasion

a) Loss of protection

b) Perforating wound

2. Hematogenic spread of germs or deposition of preformed immune complexes

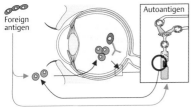

Foreign antigen

Autoantigen

3. Modification of autoantigens, molecular mimicry

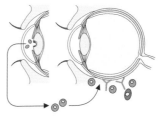

4. Release of lens antigens induces autoimmune reaction against different eye antigens

B. Immunological pathomechanisms

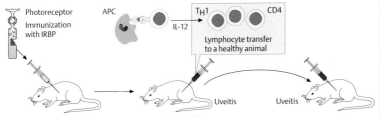

Photoreceptor

Immunization with IRBP

APC

IL-12

T_H1

CD4

Lymphocyte transfer to a healthy animal

Uveitis

Uveitis

C. Experimental autoimmune uveoretinitis (EAU)

A. Protective Mechanisms

The eyelids form a mechanical barrier that protects the eyeball. They contain sebaceous glands, sweat glands, and lacrimal glands. The regular blink reflex ensures that the conjunctiva stays moist. The tear fluid constantly rinses germs and dust particles out of the eye. Tears also have an antimicrobial effect because they contain IgA antibodies, lysozyme, lactoferrin, and complement along with monocytes and granulocytes. Hence, tear fluid serves as a primary, nonspecific barrier that wards off infections and antigens. APCs are also present in the conjunctiva.

B. Conjunctivitis

Bacteria, viruses, fungi, parasites, and chemical and physical irritants (e.g., acids, UV light) can induce conjunctivitis. The initial phase is characterized by increased blood supply (hyperemia), itching, and light intolerance (photophobia). The inflammation is more severe in patients with reduced tear production. In Sjögren's syndrome, for example, the production of tear fluid is severely reduced and the composition of the fluid is altered (see photograph and p. 190).

C. Allergic Conjunctivitis

Pollen and grass are the most common causes of seasonal allergic conjunctivitis, whereas dust, feathers, house dust mites, and animal hair cause chronic, seasonally independent conjunctivitis. Both forms of the disease represent anaphylactic type I hypersensitivity reactions (see p. 67) in which degranulation of mast cells and basophils occurs. The IgE levels in serum and tear fluid are elevated. Many patients also have watery nasal discharge (rhinorrhea). The co-occurrence of allergic conjunctivitis and atopic dermatitis is referred to as *atopic keratoconjunctivitis*.

Vernal conjunctivitis is a bilateral, recurrent, conjunctival inflammation characterized by the occurrence of cobblestone-like giant papillae of the upper conjunctiva (see photograph). The condition occurs mainly in children with eczema or asthma. The presence of mast cells, eosinophils, and CD4+ T cells in the giant papillae suggests that a delayed type cellular hypersensitivity reaction (type IV) must occur after the type I hypersensitivity reaction. *Giant papillary conjunctivitis* produces manifestations similar to those of vernal conjunctivitis but is caused by hypersensitivity to contact lenses.

D. Pathology of the Cornea

The cornea is a crystal clear, transparent structure, which forms together with the sclera the most important protective wall for the eye. Inflammation of the cornea is called *keratitis* and can lead to scarring and blindness. The most common cause of keratitis is infection with herpes simplex virus (HSV). Type 1 HSV contains proteins that are structurally related to those of the normal cornea. A keratogenic peptide has recently been isolated. Local infection with HSV induces neovascularization and increases the chance of a cross-reactive immune response to this peptide. The penetration of vessels in the normally avascular cornea leads to the migration of lymphoid and inflammatory cells to the cornea. The release of cytokines leads to epithelial damage; *corneal ulcers* may also develop (see photograph).

E. Pathology of the Sclera

The sclera is the white part of the eye. It makes up the outer layer of the eyeball and gives it strength and support. Several blood vessels pass through it, but its own blood supply is meager. *Episcleritis* is an inflammation of the superficial layers of the sclera, whereas *scleritis* involves the deep layers. The inflammation is often due to infection, but in many cases it is difficult to distinguish between the direct effects of a pathogen and a pathological immune response. Scleral inflammations often occur in conjunction with a systemic disease, such as rheumatoid arthritis, connective tissue disorders, or vasculitis. Immune complexes may accumulate in and around blood vessels, leading to complement activation, chemotaxis of granulocytes and, ultimately, necrosis (see photograph). The most serious complication is perforation of the eyeball.

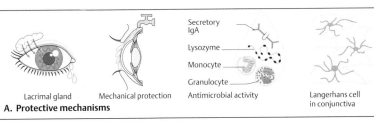

Secretory IgA
Lysozyme
Monocyte
Granulocyte

Lacrimal gland   Mechanical protection   Antimicrobial activity   Langerhans cell in conjunctiva

A. Protective mechanisms

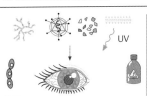
UV

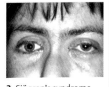

1. Causes   **2.** Dry eye   **3.** Sjögren's syndrome

B. Conjunctivitis

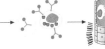
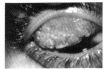

Pollen, grass, blossoms   IgE-bound antigens   Binding to mast cells   Histamine release   Vernal conjunctivitis

C. Allergic conjunctivitis

Tear film

Viruses (HSV), bacteria, parasites

Idiopathic form, GVHD

Cornea

Rheumatoid arthritis, Sjögren's syndrome, panarteritis, SLE, Wegener's granulomatosis

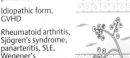

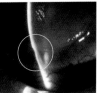

1. Normal cornea   **2.** Etiology   **3.** Neovascularization   **4.** Epithelial lesion   Corneal ulcer

D. Pathology of the cornea

Retina

Viruses (HSV, HZV), fungus, parasites

Choroid

Idiopathic form 50%

Sclera

Rheumatoid arthritis, Sjögren's syndrome, panarteritis, SLE, Wegener's granulomatosis

Episclera

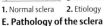

1. Normal sclera   **2.** Etiology   **3.** Episcleritis   **4.** Scleritis   Necrotizing scleritis

E. Pathology of the sclera

Uveitis is an inflammation of the uveal tract, the vessel-rich part of the eye consisting of the iris, the ciliary body, and the choroids. Inflammatory processes of the retina (retinitis) and vitreous body (vitritis) may also be referred to by this name. For didactic reasons, we will use an anatomical classification of uveitis.

A. Anterior Uveitis

Anterior uveitis (AU) is an inflammation of the iris (iritis), ciliary body (cyclitis), or both (iridocyclitis). AU may occur in conjunction with HLA-B27-associated spondylarthropathy (see p. 176), infectious diseases, or systemic diseases. The common "idiopathic" forms of anterior uveitis are closely associated with HLA-B27. *Heterochromic uveitis* (Fuchs' disease) is a subtype characterized by depigmentation and fading of the affected iris and a minimal inflammatory response. Molecular mimicry apparently leads to the production of cross-reacting antibodies that subsequently accumulate as immune complexes and induce further damage. The main clinical features (see photograph) are edematous swelling, depigmentation and fading of the iris, and contraction of the pupil (irritative miosis). In iridocyclitis, opacity of the vitreous body is also observed. Adhesion of the iris to the anterior capsule of the lens can occur due to the exudation of secretions into the anterior chamber. These secretions are usually gelatinous but sometimes hemorrhagic.

B. Intermediate Uveitis

Inflammations of the vitreous body (vitritis), pars plana of the ciliary body (pars planitis), or anterior segments of the retina (peripheral retinitis) are usually idiopathic (70–80%). Sarcoidosis, multiple sclerosis, and Lyme disease are rare causes. The disease is caused by migration of leukocytes into the vitreous body, where they aggregate, forming "snowballs." This leads to progressive opacity of the vitreous body. The glia over the pars plana proliferate, causing so-called "snowdrifts." In the late stages, the vitreous body may shrink and detach from the retina, and edemas may form in the macula. It is assumed that activated T cells that secrete IFN-γ induce the formation of so-called high-endothelial venules (HEV, see p. 64). These activated endothelial cells exhibit increased expression of adhesion molecules and MHC class II molecules. This enables the HEV to present autoantigens to the T lymphocytes, thereby triggering an autoimmune response. Moreover, HEV can contribute to the local recruitment of T cells.

C–G. Posterior Uveitis: Causes, Associations, and Clinical Features

The most common form of posterior uveitis is chorioretinitis; isolated choroiditis is rare. These inflammations are caused by bacterial, viral, parasitic or mycotic infections, systemic diseases (e.g., vasculitis), and granulomatous diseases, especially sarcoidosis. The causes of some subtypes are unknown, e.g., birdshot retinopathy, acute posterior multifocal placoid pigment epitheliopathy (APMPPE), and serpiginous choroiditis. A few important entities will be presented below.

Toxoplasmosis (**D**) is one of the most common causes of uveitis in immunocompetent patients. The condition may occur as a multisystem disease acquired via the placenta or as isolated retinochoroiditis in adulthood. Vitritis is usually present, and retinitis with macular edema and segmental vasculitis may also be found. Treatment with antibiotics is required particularly if posterior lesions are present and for immunocompromised patients.

In *sarcoidosis* (**E**), granulomas may be present in all parts of the eye, causing conjunctivitis, keratitis, iridocyclitis, retinal vasculitis, and granulomatous papillitis, which can destroy the nerve fibers of the papilla. Retinal involvement occurs in conjunction with CNS involvement.

In *histoplasmosis* (**F**), hypersensitivity to antigens of *Histoplasma capsulatum* results in a chronic immune response with subretinal proliferation. Scars may form in the macula and in peripapillary and peripheral regions of the choroid.

There is an extremely strong association between HLA-A29 and *birdshot chorioretinopathy*, a rare disease of middle-aged, otherwise healthy individuals (**G**). The relative risk (RR) for HLA-A29 individuals is 224 times increased. An immune response to retinal peptides appears to be responsible for the granulomatous changes within and below the retina, which appear as "cream-colored spots" in the fundus. Focal depigmentation of choroidal melanocytes in analogy to vitiligo of the skin is presumed.

Clinical Immunology

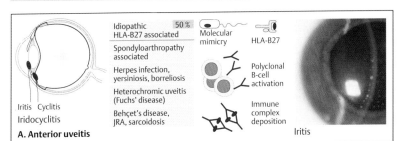

Iritis Cyclitis
Iridocyclitis

Idiopathic 50 %
HLA-B27 associated

Spondyloarthropathy associated

Herpes infection, yersiniosis, borreliosis

Heterochromic uveitis (Fuchs' disease)

Behçet's disease, JRA, sarcoidosis

Molecular mimicry   HLA-B27

Polyclonal B-cell activation

Immune complex deposition

Iritis

A. Anterior uveitis

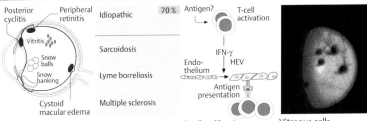

Posterior cyclitis   Peripheral retinitis

Vitritis

Snow balls

Snow banking

Cystoid macular edema

Idiopathic 70 %

Sarcoidosis

Lyme borreliosis

Multiple sclerosis

Antigen?   T-cell activation

IFN-γ

Endo-thelium   HEV

Antigen presentation

T-cell proliferation

Vitreous cells

B. Intermediate uveitis

Syphilis
Tuberculosis
Borreliosis
Leprosy
Whipple's disease
Brucellosis

CMV
EBV
HSV
VZV
HIV

Histoplasmosis

Toxoplasmosis

PAN
Behçet's disease

Sarcoidosis

Birdshot retinopathy

ApMPPE

Sepiginous choroiditis

C. Posterior uveitis: Causes/associations

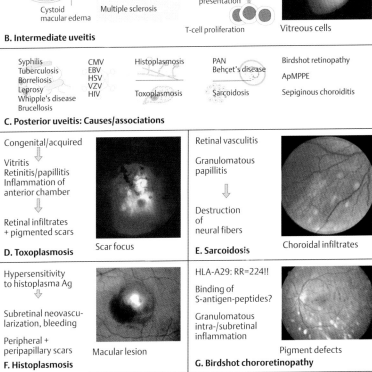

Congenital/acquired

Vitritis
Retinitis/papillitis
Inflammation of anterior chamber

Retinal infiltrates + pigmented scars

Scar focus

D. Toxoplasmosis

Retinal vasculitis

Granulomatous papillitis

Destruction of neural fibers

Choroidal infiltrates

E. Sarcoidosis

Hypersensitivity to histoplasma Ag

Subretinal neovascularization, bleeding

Peripheral + peripapillary scars

Macular lesion

F. Histoplasmosis

HLA-A29: RR=224!!

Binding of S-antigen-peptides?

Granulomatous intra-/subretinal inflammation

Pigment defects

G. Birdshot chororetinopathy

Clinical Immunology

245

A. Panuveitis: Causes and Associations

Panuveitis is an inflammation of the entire uveal tract. It is commonly caused by bacterial infections, especially with spirochetes (e.g., Lyme borreliosis and syphilis), viral infections (especially CMV and HIV), autoimmune reactions triggered by autoantigens of the eye, chronic granulomatous diseases, and vasculitis.

B. Uveitis in Behçet's Disease

Behçet's disease (see p. 180) is one of the most common causes of acquired blindness in the Middle East and Japan. Haplotype HLA-B5 is associated with the disease; the relative risk is 7. Eye involvement occurs in 80–90% of all patients with Behçet's disease. The recurrence of sterile *hypopyons*, which are aseptic pus deposits in the anterior chamber of the eye (see photograph), is a typical feature of the disease. Examination of the ocular fundus reveals vasculitis with perivascular exudation involving both arteries and veins, which become dilated and tortuous. Necrotizing leukocytoclastic vasculitis ultimately occurs due to the local accumulation of immune complexes and complement and the local recruitment of neutrophil granulocytes by IL-8.

C. Vogt–Koyanagi–Harada Syndrome

Vogt–Koyanagi–Harada (VKH) syndrome is characterized by the expression of class II MHC molecules on melanocytes due, perhaps, to a viral infection. Class II MHC expression permits the presentation of autoantigens to T cells. HLA-DR4+ and HLAw53+ individuals, respectively, have an increased relative risk of 16 and 34 to acquire the disease. Uveitis starts with symptoms of bilateral hyperemia and edema formation in the posterior choroid. Subretinal fluid accumulation then occurs. Iritis and edema formation in the ciliary body may also occur in the later course of the disease. Meningism and headache are typical CNS symptoms, which may be associated with hearing loss, tinnitus, and vertigo. Patchy depigmentation of the skin (vitiligo) and eyebrows (poliosis) and hair loss (alopecia) may also occur.

D. Multifocal Choroiditis and Panuveitis

The cause of this disease is unknown. The condition is a form of chorioretinitis characterized by the presence of multiple fresh lesions and fibrotic changes. It often occurs in association with vitritis. Infection with Epstein–Barr virus has been proposed as a possible cause.

E. Sympathetic Ophthalmia

Sympathetic ophthalmia (SO) is a bilateral, granulomatous inflammation of the uvea that may result in blindness. Genetic factors have a predisposing effect. The condition is usually triggered by a penetrating wound to the eye and, rarely, due to eye surgery. Inflammatory changes occur in the injured eye around two weeks to three months after the injury. Autoantigens are presumably presented to CD4+ T cells by retinal epithelial cells and Müller's cells. Multiple granulomas later develop in the entire uveal tract of the affected eye and in the healthy "sympathizing" eye. Cytotoxic T cells are the predominant cell type at this point. A typical feature of the disease is the presence of *Dalen–Fuchs nodules*, which consist of histiocytes and depigmented cells of the pigmented layer of the retinal epithelium. Although immunosuppression can slow down the progression of the disease, early enucleation of the injured eye is the only way to totally avoid sympathetic ophthalmia.

Phacogenic uveitis is an autoimmune reaction induced by the presence of lens antigens in the vitreous body following cataract surgery. The disease has become increasingly rare due to improvements in surgical technique.

F. Ocular Manifestations of Systemic Disease

Ocular manifestations are associated with a number of systemic diseases, such as rheumatoid arthritis (RA), spondyloarthropathies (SPA), systemic lupus erythematosus (SLE), Sjögren's syndrome (SJS), juvenile rheumatoid arthritis (JRA), Wegener's granulomatosis (WG), panarteritis nodosa (PAN), Behçet's disease (Behçet), and sarcoidosis. The most common associations are presented in the table.

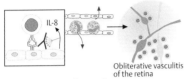

Syphilis
Borreliosis
Yersiniosis

CMV
EBV
HIV

Sympathetic
ophthalmia

Phacogenic
uveitis

Behçet's disease

Sarcoidosis

Vogt-Koyanagi-Harada
syndrome

Multifocal chorioiditis and
panuveitis

A. Panuveitis: Causes and associations

IL-8

Obliterative vasculitis
of the retina

Hypopyon

Neuritis, accompanying
vasculitis

B. Uveitis with Behçet's disease

Bilateral panuveitis

CNS symptoms
 Meningism
 Headache
 Pleocytosis

Hearing loss, tinnitus

Vitiligo, alopecia

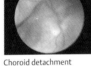

Choroid detachment

C. Vogt-Koyanagi-Harada Syndrome

EBV??

Vitritis

Chorioretinal
lesions (fundus)

Scar formation
in macula

Chronic outcome
with recurrent disease

Choroid lesions

D. Multifocal choroiditis and panuveitis

HLA-A11

Per-
forating
wound

CD8

Anti-S-100
Anti-IRBP

Injured
eye

CD8

Attack
on
healthy
eye

CD4

TNF

Müller cells

CD8

Granuloma
formation

E. Sympathetic ophthalmia

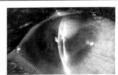

Right eye: scar

Left eye: beginning iritis

	RA	SPA	SLE	SJS	JRA	Wegener	PAN	Behçet	Sarcoidosis
Conjunctivitis sicca	+		+	++	+				
Keratitis, corneal ulcer	++		+	++	+	+		+	
Episcleritis, scleritis	++		+			++	+		
Anterior uveitis	+	++	+		++		+	++	++
Vasculitis	+		++			+	++	++	++
Choroiditis, panuveitis					+		+	++	

F. Ocular manifestations of systemic diseases

Clinical Immunology

A. Immune-Mediated Infertility

Male infertility can occur due to the development of autoantibodies to spermatoza-specific acrosomal antigens or membrane peptide antigens that immobilize the sperm (**1**). *Female infertility* may be caused by isoantibodies to sperm or autoantibodies to zona pellucida antigens that inhibit the accumulation and penetration of sperm in the egg cell (**2**). Attempting to lower the antibody concentration by preventing antigen exposure or by immunosuppression is a possible approach to treatment (**3**). Intrauterine insemination is another alternative. The best results are achieved by in vitro fertilization. Intracytoplasmic sperm injection (ICSI) makes it possible to completely evade the immunological barriers.

B. Maternofetal Tolerance

For the mother, the fetus represents a kind of allogeneic transplant against which an immune response must be suppressed. In a normal pregnancy, humoral immunity prevails due to an increased release of T_H2 cytokines. The humoral immune response changes from a cytotoxic IgG2 (T_H1-induced) response to noncytotoxic IgG1 (T_H2-induced) antibody production. A predominating T_H1-type response is associated with a tendency to spontaneous abortion. Secondly, progesterone induces the production of progesterone-induced blocking factor (PIBF) in lymphocytes. PIBF suppresses the proliferation of lymphocytes, the activation of NK cells, and the production of TNF. In women with multiple miscarriages, only a very small number of lymphocytes secrete PIBF. Moreover, progesterone and PIBF promote T_H2-type immune responses.

The trophoblast also produces an immunosuppressive factor. The antiabortive effects of IL-10 observed in animal studies suggest that it is an important cytokine in pregnancy. Furthermore, the human placenta lacks the classic class I HLA antigens A, B, and C. This prevents recognition of the paternal antigens present in the placenta by maternal T cells but makes placental tissues a target for natural killer cells, which can recognize cells without class I HLA molecules. However, the nonclassic class Ib HLA molecule, HLA-G, is expressed on the maternal side of the placenta, and this interacts with inhibitory receptors on NK cells, protecting the placenta from NK-mediated cytotoxicity. An additional protective mechanism is the expression of Fas ligands on trophoblastic tissue. This ensures the elimination of Fas-expressing activated maternal T lymphocytes by apoptosis.

C. Neonatal Autoimmune Syndromes

Maternal autoantibodies can cross the placenta and thereby be transmitted to the fetus. In immune thrombocytopenic purpura (ITP, see p. 126), autoantibodies against platelet glycoproteins enter into the fetus, where they may produce hemorrhagic symptoms ranging from mild bleeding to intracranial hemorrhage. Frequently, this occurs shortly after birth. TSH binding-inhibiting immunoglobulins (TBII) can induce transient congenital hypothyroidism in infants born to mothers with autoimmune thyroiditis (see p. 228). The thyroid-stimulating immunoglobulins (TSI) that occur in Graves' disease can cause neonatal hyperthyroidism. Neonatal transitory myasthenia (see p. 238) may develop due to the transmission of anti-AChR autoantibodies.

Anticardiolipin autoantibodies increase the risk of thrombosis, which may result in transitory ischemic attacks or apoplexy. Another potential complication is placental infarction, which is responsible for the increased rate of miscarriages in lupus patients. The presence of anticardiolipin antibodies in the pregnant woman is frequently associated with thrombocytopenia. Neonatal lupus (see pp. 188, 190) can occur in infants born to mothers with SLE or Sjögren's syndrome due to the transplacental transfer of SS-A (anti-Ro) and SS-B (anti-La) autoantibodies. Neonatal lupus is characterized by a transient rash similar to that seen in discoid lupus, cytopenia, and congenital atrioventricular heart block with bradycardia.

Clinical Immunology

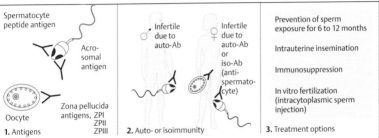

1. Antigens   **2.** Auto- or isoimmunity   **3.** Treatment options

A. Immune-mediated infertility

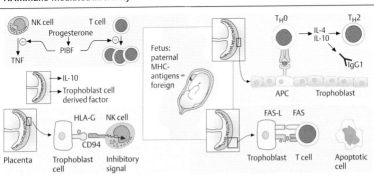

B. Maternofetal tolerance

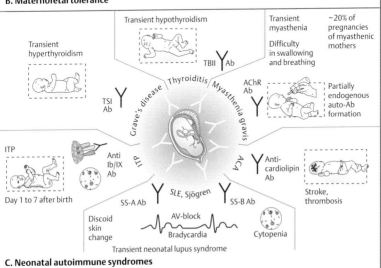

C. Neonatal autoimmune syndromes

A good vaccine must fulfill many requirements. The goal of the immunization is to protect the recipient from the disease in question while causing as few side effects and risks as possible. The protective action of the vaccine should ideally be complete and long-lasting (for several years or a lifetime). The costs of manufacturing the vaccine should be low enough to make it affordable to a large portion of the population. Moreover, the vaccine should be widely available and have a long shelf-life. The need for a vaccine depends on the current epidemiological situation and the goal of immunization, e.g., individual protection, herd immunity (certain pathogens do not become endemic when only a proportion of the population is immunized), or total eradication of the pathogen, as was possible with the smallpox virus vaccination. The vaccines for active immunization can be divided into four groups: toxoids, split virus vaccines, inactivated vaccines, and live vaccines.

Toxoids: When the immune response is directed against certain products produced by a pathogen, e.g., against the toxins of *Corynebacterium diphtheriae* or *Clostridium tetani*, it is possible to create a vaccine using only that portion of the toxin responsible for the neutralizing immunity. The toxoid is usually administered together with a carrier substance (adjuvant) that further enhances the immune response.

Split-virus vaccines are vaccines made of purified subunits of a virus, usually the coat. However, if carbohydrate capsule-forming bacteria are used, the immunization usually will not be sufficient, especially in small children.

Inactivated vaccines are prepared using inactivated bacteria and are effective against extracellular organisms. They induce an adequate humoral immune response, for example, to cholera. The antibody protection provided by these vaccines is of only limited duration. Hence, frequent booster shots are required.

Live vaccines have the highest rate of side effects and the highest risk of inducing illness. However, they are most effective in inducing adequate vaccine protection, especially when the immune response to the target organism is mediated by T cells.

A. Vaccination Calendar in Childhood

In Germany, the publicly recommended vaccinations start in early childhood and follow a regular immunization schedule established using continuously updated information. The schedule includes vaccinations for tetanus, diphtheria, poliomyelitis, *Haemophilus influenzae*, measles, mumps, rubella, and hepatitis B. The fact that these vaccinations are recommended by the public health services ensures that the costs will be covered by insurance companies and that compensation will be paid in recognized cases of vaccination-related damage. In Germany, BCG and pertussis vaccinations are recommended only in high-risk situations. Hence, they are considered to be optional or need-only vaccinations (**B**).

The following factors are considered to be general contraindications for immunization: acute infectious diseases, hematological diseases, congenital and acquired immune defects, hypersensitivity to any ingredients in the vaccination. All live vaccines except the live oral poliovirus vaccine are strictly contraindicated during pregnancy. Inactivated vaccines, such as the cholera vaccine, can also induce violent immune responses. Live vaccines should not be administered within less than approximately four weeks of each other.

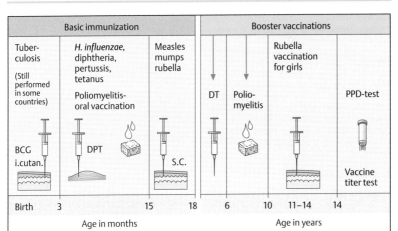

A. Vaccination calendar in childhood

Pathogen	Indications	Side effects	Contraindications
HBV recombinant HBsAg-vaccine	– Hospital staff, – Dialysis patients, – Family members of HBV-carriers – prostitutes – Homosexuals – Drug users – Travel in endemic regions	Short fever reaction	– Pregnancy – Known allergy
Influenza killed vaccine	Very ill patients > 60 y	Allergic reactions (rare)	– Acute diseases – Egg albumin allergy
Rabies killed vaccine	– After exposure (animal bite) – Before exposure in veterinarians, forest-workers, hunters, etc.	Fever, lymph node swelling	Before exposure: allergy to neomycin and tetracycline in vaccine
Pneumococci dead vaccine capsular polysaccharides in 14 serotypes	– Splenectomy – Sickle cell anemia	Mild local reaction	Ongoing pneumococcal infection, chronic purulent diseases
For journeys in endemic regions			
Cholera killed vaccine		Low grade fever	Allergies
Yellow fever live vaccine attenuated D17-strain		Low grade fever	– Pregnancy – Egg albumin allergy
Typhoid fever live vaccine		No problems	Use killed vaccine in high-risk patients

B. Optional vaccinations

Clinical Immunology

Thanks to the vaccines available today, many infectious diseases can now be largely prevented or almost completely eradicated in many areas of the world. However, there is still a lack of vaccines for long-term control of many pathogens with different mechanisms for evading the host's immune defense system. Some prominent examples are mycobacterial infections (e.g., tuberculosis) and parasitic diseases (e.g., malaria and leishmaniasis). Researchers are currently focusing on the development of new vaccines by techniques of genetic engineering.

A. Synthetic Peptides

Synthetic peptides contain only the epitope of a protective antigen. Other parts of the protein that exert negative (suppressive) effects on the immune response, have toxic effects, or cross-react with endogenous proteins are therefore absent. Most peptides induce a humoral immune response, the potency of which varies depending on the respective HLA type. Optimal vaccine protection can therefore be achieved in only a proportion of the population.

B. Recombinant Proteins

Recombinant proteins can be manufactured in large quantities. The main advantage is that, unlike conventional vaccines, they are free from the harmful fragments of the pathogen responsible for side effects. Engineered vaccines can also be used in cases where the pathogen cannot be cultured or is very difficult to cultivate (e.g., viruses). However, their use requires a suitable expression system (e.g., in *E. coli*) and easy removal of the vaccine from the cells in which it was produced.

C. Recombinant Vaccine Strains

If a recombinant protein is unable to induce an adequate immune response, especially of T cells, it is possible to clone its gene in a suitable carrier medium (e.g., in vaccinia or BCG). Together with antigens in the carrier medium, the recombinant protein can then exert protective immunity.

D. Deletion Mutants

The deletion of genes essential for the virulence or viability of a pathogen within a host organism can make the pathogen incapable of producing a disease in the host. However, the reduced survival time of the pathogen must be long enough to induce a protective immune response.

Purified DNA

Purified DNA preparations used as vaccines contain the gene for the pathogenic antigen and a suitable "promoter." Once integrated into the host cells, enough of the DNA vaccine is transcribed to ensure that the antigen is released. This enables the antigen to produce a B-cell response, provided that the antigenic gene contains the sequence required by the signal peptide. A fraction of the processed antigens can be processed intracellularly and presented on the cell surface together with class I MHC molecules, leading to the stimulation of a T-cell response. The use of purified DNA vaccines in experimental animals produced promising results. These substances were recently proposed as a vaccine for AIDS (see p. 113**B**). However, a number of questions must be answered before they can be used in humans. The main questions involve their fate in the host, i.e., their potential for transforming into virulent DNA, how long they persist in the host genome, and whether they replicate there.

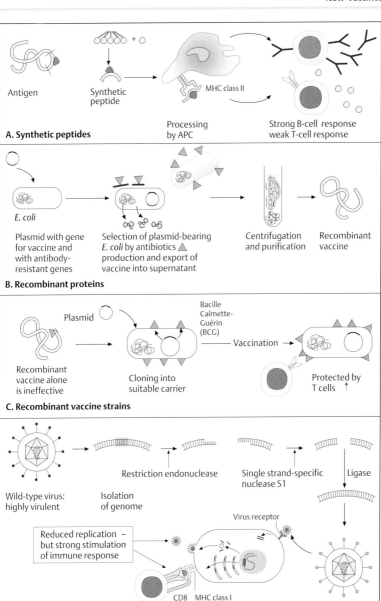

A. Synthetic peptides

Antigen

Synthetic peptide

MHC class II

Processing by APC

Strong B-cell response weak T-cell response

B. Recombinant proteins

E. coli

Plasmid with gene for vaccine and with antibody-resistant genes

Selection of plasmid-bearing E. coli by antibiotics △ production and export of vaccine into supernatant

Centrifugation and purification

Recombinant vaccine

C. Recombinant vaccine strains

Plasmid

Bacille Calmette-Guérin (BCG)

Recombinant vaccine alone is ineffective

Cloning into suitable carrier

Vaccination

Protected by T cells ↑

D. Deletion mutants

Restriction endonuclease

Single strand-specific nuclease S1

Ligase

Wild-type virus: highly virulent

Isolation of genome

Virus receptor

Reduced replication – but strong stimulation of immune response

CD8   MHC class I

Low virulence

A. Nonsteroidal Anti-Inflammatory Drugs (NSAIDs)

NSAIDs interfere with the prostaglandin metabolism by inhibiting cyclooxygenase. Phospholipase A_2 triggers the release of arachidonic acid from phospholipids in the cell membrane. Arachidonic acid serves as a substrate for the production of eicosanoids, leukotrienes, thromboxane, prostacyclin, and prostaglandins. The most important step in the synthesis of prostaglandins is the production of prostaglandin H_2 through cyclooxygenase. Two of their isoenzymes, COX1 and COX2, have been identified.

COX1 is responsible for the production of prostaglandins with physiological functions, e.g.:
- Regulation of peripheral resistance, renal blood flow, and sodium elimination,
- Cytoprotection of the gastric mucosa by increasing the flow of mucus and inhibiting acid secretion,
- Enhancement of pain receptor sensitivity,
- Bronchodilation.

COX2 is induced in monocytes, macrophages, endothelial cells, and synoviocytes by inflammatory stimuli exerted, for example, by endotoxins or IL-1. It enhances prostaglandin synthesis during an inflammatory response.

Cyclooxygenase inhibition by NSAIDs therefore has an anti-inflammatory effect and blocks the COX1-mediated physiological effects of prostaglandins. The anti-inflammatory effect is therapeutically useful in acute and chronic joint inflammations. Inhibition of COX1-mediated effects is the cause of most side effects associated with these drugs, including gastric wall damage and ulcer formation. Inhibition of the enzyme can also cause renal failure and blood pressure disorders in certain patients.

B. Glucocorticoids

The anti-inflammatory effect of glucocorticoids plays a key role in the treatment of rheumatic diseases. The action of these drugs is dose-dependent and occurs at different sites in the cell. Most of their activities are induced by altered transcription. After binding to a glucocorticoid receptor in the cytosol, the receptor dissociates from heat shock protein (hsp) complexes and becomes capable of binding to certain sites of genomic DNA in the cell nucleus (the so-called *hormone response elements*). This leads to the activation of certain genes, the products of which inhibit the spread of inflammation. Moreover, the production of inflammation-enhancing proteins (e.g., enzymes involved in prostaglandin metabolism) are also inhibited by interactions with NFκB and other transcription factors on the gene level.

In higher concentrations, effects that cannot be attributed to genomic activities occur in certain types of cells after a short period of time. It has therefore been postulated that a membrane-bound, rapidly activating glucocorticoid receptor must be present.

When the glucocorticoid concentration is very high, increasing numbers of glucocorticoid molecules are integrated into the cell membrane, causing nonspecific changes in the physical properties of the membrane (fluidity, permeability). Transmembranous cation transport then decreases and the overall activation capacity of the cell is reduced.

Glucocorticoids have many ways of interfering in inflammatory processes and cellular immune responses. For example, they inhibit the migration of leukocytes to the site of inflammation, modulate the various function of effector cells, and decrease the production of inflammation mediators.

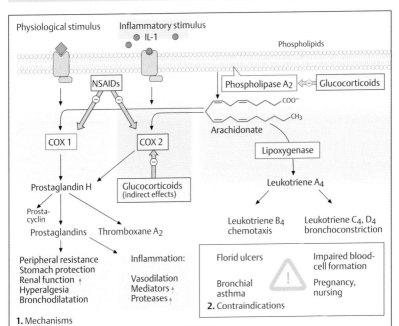

Physiological stimulus   **Inflammatory stimulus**
● IL-1 ●

Phospholipids

NSAIDs

Phospholipase A₂ ⇐ Glucocorticoids

COO⁻

CH₃

Arachidonate

COX 1   COX 2

Lipoxygenase

Prostaglandin H

Glucocorticoids (indirect effects)

Prosta-cyclin

Prostaglandins   Thromboxane A₂

Leukotriene A₄

Leukotriene B₄ chemotaxis   Leukotriene C₄, D₄ bronchoconstriction

Peripheral resistance
Stomach protection
Renal function ↑
Hyperalgesia
Bronchodilatation

Inflammation:

Vasodilation
Mediators ↑
Proteases ↑

Florid ulcers   Impaired blood-cell formation

⚠

Bronchial asthma   Pregnancy, nursing

1. Mechanisms

2. Contraindications

A. Nonsteroidal anti-inflammatory drugs (NSAIDs)

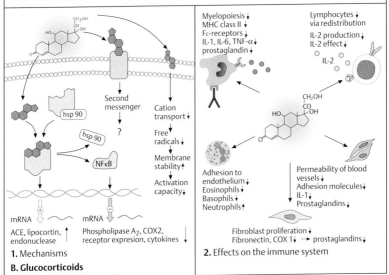

Myelopoiesis ↓
MHC class II ↓
Fc-receptors ↓
IL-1, IL-6, TNF-α ↓
prostaglandin ↓

Lymphocytes ↓
via redistribution
IL-2 production ↓
IL-2 effect ↓

○ IL-2
○

hsp 90

Second messenger
?

Cation transport ↓

Free radicals ↓

Membrane stability ↑

Activation capacity ↓

hsp 90

NFκB

Adhesion to endothelium ↓
Eosinophils ↓
Basophils ↓
Neutrophils ↑

Permeability of blood vessels ↓
Adhesion molecules ↓
IL-1 ↓
Prostaglandins ↓

mRNA ⊕
ACE, lipocortin, ↑
endonuclease

mRNA ⊖
Phospholipase A₂, COX2,
receptor expresion, cytokines ↓

Fibroblast proliferation ↓
Fibronectin, COX 1 ↓ → prostaglandins ↓

1. Mechanisms

2. Effects on the immune system

B. Glucocorticoids

255

A. Antimetabolites

Methotrexate (MTX) acts as an antimetabolite that interferes with folic acid metabolism. By binding to the enzyme dihydrofolate reductase, it inhibits the intracellular reduction of folate to tetrahydrofolate, thereby blocking C1 metabolism, which is required for thymidine and purine biosynthesis. The decreased DNA and RNA synthesis leads to functional deficits and cell death (mainly in B cells). MTX also inhibits cell growth in other rapidly proliferating tissues, e.g., hematopoietic bone marrow, gonads, mucosal linings, tumors, and psoriatic skin. High doses of MTX have a primarily cytostatic effect, whereas low doses (one-fifth to one-tenth of the immunosuppressive dose) have an antiphlogistic effect due to the inhibition of adhesion molecules and cytokines. Apart from the side effects in the rapidly proliferating tissues, hepatotoxicity and pulmonary toxicity may also occur.

Azathioprine is a particularly effective inhibitor of T-cell growth. After enteral absorption, the drug is converted to 6-mercaptopurine, a sulfurous adenine that inhibits purine biosynthesis by acting as a "wrong end product" that transmits negative feedback. Moreover, it is incorporated as a false component into DNA and RNA, thereby damaging the molecules. The antigout agent allopurinol is an inhibitor of xanthine oxidase. The drug therefore inhibits the metabolism and efficacy of 6-mercaptopurinol, but increases its toxicity. Gastrointestinal disorders and reversible pancytopenia may occur as side effects.

B. Cyclophosphamide

Cyclophosphamide, a cytostatic drug, is one of the most potent immunosuppressive agents. Once it has been converted in the liver to the active form, 4-hydroxycyclophosphamide, it can alkylate and thus inactivate various structures within the cells. The alkylation of bases in DNA and RNA molecules leads to the cross-linkage of opposing base pairs and, ultimately, to cell death. The inhibition of functional activity and the numeric reduction in cells affects B and T cells equally. The most significant side effect of cyclophosphamide is hemorrhagic cystitis, the risk of which can be reduced by coadministration of 2-mercapto-ethanesulfonic acid (MESNA).

C. Sulfasalazine

Sulfasalazine is one of the most sparingly absorbed sulfonamide derivatives. It is used in the treatment of ulcerative colitis and Crohn's disease. The drug binds to collagen and elastin fibers of the subepithelial tissue in mucosal lesions in the deep layers of the small intestine. A fraction of the drug is converted to the active components sulfapyridine and 5-aminosalicylate (5-ASA) by cleavage of azo bonds by intestinal bacteria. The active components inhibit inflammatory responses in the intestinal wall. The later absorption of sulfapyridine is responsible for some of the drug's side effects (dizziness, nausea, sulfonamide fever, arthralgia). The constituents are acetylated and excreted in the urine. The side effects are most severe in so-called "slow-acetylating" patients.

D. Gold

Gold preparations are part of the disease-modifying therapy regimen for rheumatoid arthritis. The mechanism of action is still unexplained. One hypothesis is that immunomodulation occurs due to chemical modification of peptides presented by MHC molecules. Another theory is that macrophages have a stabilizing function due, presumably, to inhibition of mediator and enzyme release. The side effects of gold (dermatitis, stomatitis, thrombocytopenia, and agranulocytosis) make it necessary to monitor the blood and urine status at regular intervals.

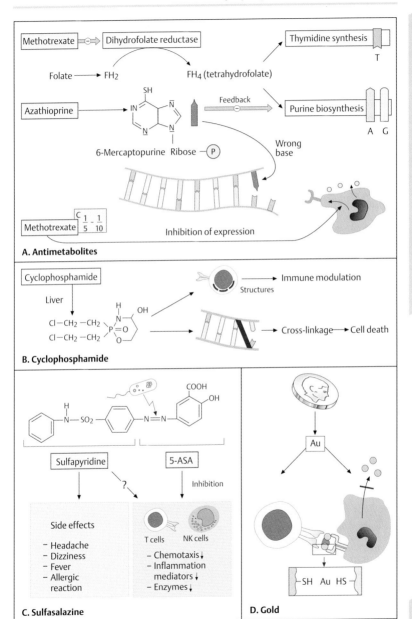

A. Antimetabolites

B. Cyclophosphamide

C. Sulfasalazine

D. Gold

Clinical Immunology

257

A. Cyclosporin A

Cyclosporin A is a cyclic peptide produced by the soil fungus *Tolypocladium inflatum*. There are 11 amino acids in the molecule. The immunosuppressive effect of cyclosporin A is due to the inhibition of cytokine production, especially that of IL-2, at an early phase of T-cell activation. The molecular mechanism of the drug was recently explained as follows. Cyclosporin A binds to the cytoplasmic receptor cyclophilin, a proline isomerase. The cyclosporin A and cyclophilin complex inhibits calcineurin, which acts as the protein-phosphate phosphatase responsible for the activation of transcription factor NFAT (nuclear factor of activated T cells). The absence of dephosphorylation inhibits the migration of active NFAT into the cell nucleus and, thus, inhibits transcription of the IL-2 gene. Cyclosporin A also interferes with the signal transduction of pathway of TCR. It inhibits protein kinase Cβ (PKCβ), thereby blocking the induction of nuclear components of NFAT.

Cyclosporin A inhibits the production of other cytokines to a small degree (e.g., IL-1 in macrophages and IL-3, IL-4, IL-8, and IFN-γ). Hence, it has a primary impact on cellular immunity.

Tacrolimus (FK506), a macrolide antibiotic, is also used to suppress cellular immunity. Its mechanism of action is very similar to that of cyclosporin A. After binding to a cytoplasmic receptor, *FK-binding protein* (FK-bp), the tacrolimus–FK-bp complex inhibits the phosphatase calcineurin and, thus, indirectly inhibits cytokine production.

Rapamycin, another macrolide antibiotic, inhibits IL-2-dependent processes in the target cell after binding to a cytoplasmic receptor. The drug therefore interferes with the T-cell activation sequence somewhat later than cyclosporin A and tacrolimus and, thus, acts synergistically with them.

B. Mycophenolate

Mycophenolate is a new immunosuppressive drug that has achieved good results in the treatment of transplant rejection. It was clinically tested in patients with rheumatoid arthritis and psoriasis. The prodrug mycophenolate-mofetil is quickly converted to mycophenolate after intravenous administration. Mycophenolate causes reversible inhibition of inosine monophosphate dehydrogenase (IMP-DH) and, thus, of the de novo biosynthesis of purines. Since lymphocytes are especially dependent on de novo synthesis, a sharp drop in the concentration of guanine nucleotides occurs. The damage to lymphocytes occurs by different routes. The dGTP deficiency leads to a reduction of DNA and RNA synthesis. There is an additional lack of guanosine 5'-diphosphate-fucose, which is required for *N*-glycosylation of glycoproteins, such as adhesion molecules. The deficiency of GTP-cyclohydrolase-1 causes a lack of tetrahydrobiopterin. This reduces the number of redox reactions in the cell, especially the formation of NO.

C. Leflunomide

Leflunomide is another new immunosuppressant that especially targets lymphocytes. Its mechanism of action is similar to that of mycophenolate. By inhibiting the enzyme dihydroorotate dehydrogenase (DHO-DH), it interferes in the early phase of de novo pyrimidine biosynthesis. The drug equally inhibits B and T cells. Resting lymphocytes have only a small pool of pyrimidines. If only a few pyrimidines can be synthesized due to the inhibition of DHO-DH during activation, a reduction of DNA and RNA synthesis will occur. The synthesis of adhesion molecules will also be reduced.

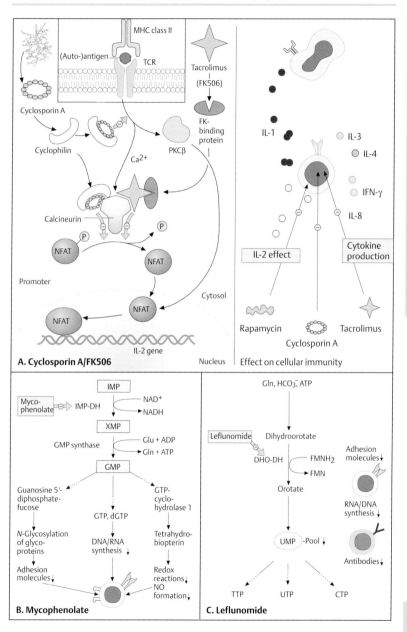

A. Cyclosporin A/FK506

Effect on cellular immunity

B. Mycophenolate

C. Leflunomide

A. Monoclonal Antibodies

The manufacture of large quantities of antibodies of a given specificity by fusion of a B cell with a myeloma cell has gained great significance, especially in diagnostic applications. However, monoclonal antibodies (MAbs) are derived from mice (murine), and they represent a foreign antigen when introduced into the human body. In response, the body produces antibodies to neutralize the MAb. This antibody response limits the use of monoclonal antibodies in therapeutic applications. Since human monoclonal antibodies are much more difficult to produce, researchers are attempting to reduce the antigenicity of murine monoclonal antibodies. One approach is to *humanize* the monoclonal antibodies by linking the antigen-specific murine Fab segment with a human Fc segment. Another way to engineer monoclonal antibodies is to incorporate only those parts of the murine Fab fragment important for antigen recognition (complementarity-determining regions, CDR) into the human antibody (CDR grafting).

One example of a chimeric antibody design with murine and human elements is the anti-TNF antibody, which consists of a murine Fab fragment with high affinity for human TNF and a human Fc fragment. In TNF-R–Fc fusion protein, the Fab fragment is replaced with recombinant human soluble TNF receptor. The receptor is normally present in serum and binds TNF-α. Both types of engineered TNF blockers were investigated in clinical studies and found to be effective for treatment of rheumatoid arthritis, psoriatic arthritis, and ankylosing spondylitis. Anti-TNF antibodies inhibit the induction of an inflammatory reaction by TNF-α, which can affect the blood vessels, the migration of immune cells, inflammations of the synovia and cartilage, and the bone metabolism. One side effect of anti-TNF-α therapy is the possible activation of latent tuberculoosis (see p. 221).

Another important clinical application for monoclonal antibodies is the inhibition of CD4+ cells to reduce the immune response in autoimmune diseases. Anti-CD4 MAb are directed against the extracellular domain of the CD4 molecule. Once bound, they can modulate the activation capacity of T cells or induce apoptosis. Complement activation with subsequent lysis, phagocytosis of the target cells by macrophages, and antibody-dependent cell-mediated cytotoxicity (ADCC) by CD8+ killer cells are other potential cytotoxic effects of monoclonal antibodies. The target cell can, to a certain degree, cleave or *shed* the CD4 molecule and attached antibody or internalize them, thereby avoiding damage. Several monoclonal antibodies have entered the clinic in the last 2–3 years: B-cell-specific CD20 antibody rituximab has become an important tool for the treatment of B-cell Hodgkin's lymphomas, and the anti-HER-2/neu antibody trastuzumab is successfully used in breast cancer treatment.

Adhesion molecule blockade is another way to inhibit the inflammatory process and the activation of immune cells. Monoclonal antibodies directed against ICAM-1 (CD54) prevent adhesion molecules from binding to LFA-1 (CD11a/CD18) and, thus, from adhering to endothelial cells and activating T cells. Clinical trials are currently being carried out to evaluate the efficacy of these monoclonal antibodies in the treatment of autoimmune diseases.

B. Polyclonal Antibodies

Polyclonal antibodies can interfere in immune responses in several ways. They can reduce the immune response in patients with autoimmune diseases by preventing APCs from capturing and presenting antigens to T cells. They can also impede the phagocytosis of antigens by macrophages and inhibit B-cell activation. The interception of pathogenic autoantibodies is a very important point of attack of polyclonal antibodies.

Peptide Vaccination

The latest attempts to inhibit the cellular immune response in autoimmune diseases have to do with the interactions of MHC molecules and TCR. Anti-MHC antibodies have been successfully used in vitro and in animals to inhibit T-cell activation by inhibiting MHC recognition and/or anti-TCR and anti-CD4 antibodies.

Peptide vaccination involves the use of peptides specific for the T-cell clones active in a disease process. These peptides competitively displace the pathogenic peptides from the MHC molecules. They have been shown to reduce the level of disease activity in experimental animals.

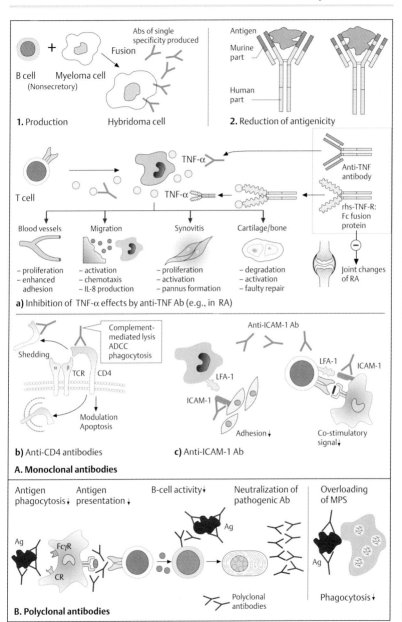

1. Production

Abs of single specificity produced

B cell   Myeloma cell
(Nonsecretory)

Fusion

Hybridoma cell

2. Reduction of antigenicity

Antigen
Murine part
Human part

T cell

TNF-α

TNF-α

Anti-TNF antibody

rhs-TNF-R: Fc fusion protein

Blood vessels
– proliferation
– enhanced adhesion

Migration
– activation
– chemotaxis
– IL-8 production

Synovitis
– proliferation
– activation
– pannus formation

Cartilage/bone
– degradation
– activation
– faulty repair

Joint changes of RA

a) Inhibition of TNF-α effects by anti-TNF Ab (e.g., in RA)

Complement-mediated lysis
ADCC
phagocytosis

Shedding

α β
TCR CD4

Modulation
Apoptosis

b) Anti-CD4 antibodies

Anti-ICAM-1 Ab

LFA-1

ICAM-1

Adhesion↓

LFA-1   ICAM-1

Co-stimulatory signal↓

c) Anti-ICAM-1 Ab

A. Monoclonal antibodies

Antigen phagocytosis↓

Antigen presentation↓

B-cell activity↓

Neutralization of pathogenic Ab

Overloading of MPS

Ag

FcγR

CR

Polyclonal antibodies

Ag

Phagocytosis↓

B. Polyclonal antibodies

Clinical Immunology

261

Table 1: ACR Criteria for Classification of Rheumatoid Arthritis (RA) (shortened)

Criterion	Short definition
1. Morning stiffness	Morning stiffness in or around the joints (for at least 1 hour)
2. Arthritis in three or more joint regions	Concurrent involvement of at least three joint regions with soft tissue swelling or effusion
3. Arthritis in the joints of the hand: wrist, MCPs, or PIPs	Soft tissue swelling or effusion in at least one of these regions
4. Symmetrical swelling (arthritis)	Concurrent involvement of the same joint regions on both sides of the body
5. Rheumatoid nodules	Subcutaneous nodules over bony excrescences, extensor surfaces, or in other areas proximal to the joints
6. Rheumatoid factor in serum	Detection of abnormally high quantities of serum rheumatoid factors
7. Radiological changes of rheumatoid arthritis	Detection of typical changes, such as erosions and decalcification proximal to the joints

Table 2: ESSG Classification of Spondylarthropathy

Inflammatory spinal pain
   or
Synovitis
   asymmetric or
   predominantly in the lower limbs
and one or more of the following:
Positive family history
Psoriasis
Inflammatory bowel diseases
Urethritis, cervicitis, or acute diarrhea within 1 month before arthritis
Buttock pain alternating between right and left gluteal areas
Enthesopathy
Sacroiliitis

Table 3: Antinuclear Antibodies in Rheumatic Diseases

Specificity	Staining pattern (HEP-2 cells)	Incidence of disease
Nucleic acids		
• Double-stranded DNA (dsDNA), identical antigenic determinants in dsDNA and ssDNA	Homogeneous, circular	Detectable in 60–70% of patients with SLE (diagnostic marker of SLE)
• Single-stranded DNA (ssDNA), antigenic determinants related to purines and pyrimidines	Homogeneous, circular	Detectable in over 95% of patients with SLE; also observed in other diseases, even nonrheumatoid conditions
Histones		
• Antigenic determinants on H1, H2a, H2b, H3, H4 or conglomerated with H2a-H2b, H3-H4	Homogeneous, circular	Detectable in 30–70% of patients with SLE, in 15–20% of patients with RA, and in up to 95% of patients with drug-induced SLE
Nuclear proteins		
• SM antigen Antigenic determinant complexes with small nuclear RNA (snRNA)	Coarsely granular	Detectable in 25–35% of patients with SLE; disease-specific marker
• U1-RNP Antigenic determinant complexes with U1-RNA	Coarsely granular	High titers detectable in 95% of patients with MCTD and in 35–45% of patients with SLE; low titers are detected in patients with progressive systemic sclerosis, discoid SLE, and Sjögren's syndrome
• SS-A(Ro) Antigenic determinants 2 proteins: 61 kDa, 52 kDa	Finely granular + cytoplasm	Detectable in 30–40% of patients with SLE and in 60–70% of patients with Sjögren's syndrome; significant in neonatal SLE associated with congenital heart block
• SS-B/La Antigenic determinant related to a 43 kDa protein, complexes with RNA	Finely granular + cytoplasm	Detectable in 15% of patients with SLE and in 40–60% of patients with Sjögren's syndrome; significant in neonatal SLE in association with congenital heart block
• PCNA (proliferating cell nuclear antigen) Antigenic determinant related to a 33 kDa protein	Nuclear fluorescence of variable intensity	Detectable in 3% of patients with SLE
• Scl 70 (topoisomerase I)	Nucleolar and homogeneous	Detectable in 30% of patients with progressive systemic sclerosis
• Jo-1 (histidyl-synthetase)	Granular in cytoplasm	Detectable in 5% of patients with dermatomyositis and in 30% of those with polymyositis
• Centromere (kinetochore antigen)	Spotted	Detectable in 70% of patients with the limited form of scleroderma

Appendix

Table 4: Significance of Autoantibodies in the Diagnosis of Autoimmune Diseases

Auto-antibody	Associated disease							
	SLE	MCTD	Sclero-derma	Myo-sitis	Sjögren's syndrom	Rheuma-toid arthritis	Primary vasculitis	Anti-phospho-lipid syndrome
ANA	+++	+++	+++	+	+++	+	+	+
dsDNA	+++	-	-	-	-	-	-	-
SM	++	-	-	-	-	-	-	-
U1-RNP	+	+++	+	+	-	-	-	-
Ribosomal P	++	-	-	-	-	-	-	-
PCNA	+	-	-	-	-	-	-	-
Ro	++	+	+	-	+++	+	-	-
La	++	+	+	-	+++	+	-	-
RA33	++	++	-	-	+	++	-	-
Scl70	-	-	+++	-	-	-	-	-
Centromere	-	-	+++	-	-	-	-	-
Jo-1	-		-	++	-	-	-	-
PM-Scl	-	-	+	+	-	-	-	-
Cardiolipin	+++	+	+	-	+	+	-	+++
ANCA	-	-	-	-	-	-	+++	-
Rheumatoid factor	++	+	+	+	+++	+++	+	-

Table 5: ACR Criteria for Classification of SLE (shortened)

Criterion	Definition
Malar rash	Flat or raised rash on both cheeks that skips the bridge of the nose
Discoid rash	Erythematous raised spots with keratotic scales and atrophic scars, primarily at sites exposed to light
Photosensitivity	Rash that rapidly develops after exposure to sunlight (or corresponding family history)
Oral ulcers	Painless oral or nasopharyngeal ulcers observed by the attending physician
Arthritis	Nonerosive arthritis in more than two peripheral joints (tenderness, swelling, effusion)
Serositis	Documented occurrence of pleuritis or pericarditis
Renal disorder	Persistent proteinuria of >0.5 g/day or cylindruria (hyalinic, erythrocytic, granulated)
Neurological disorder	Convulsions or psychoses in the absence of metabolic or drug-related causes
Hematological disorder	Immunohemolytic anemia (reticulocytosis, positive Coombs' test or leukopenia of $<4000/m^3$ or lymphopenia of $<1500/mm^3$ or thrombocytopenia of $<100\,000/mm^3$
Immunological disorder	Positive LE cell test or detection of dsDNA antibodies or detection of Sm antibodies or false–positive syphilis reaction
Antinuclear antibodies	Abnormally high ANA titer in patient not taking any drugs that could lead to "drug-induced SLE"

The simultaneous or serial detection of four or more of these 11 criteria in a patient during a given observation period is classified as diagnostic of SLE.

Appendix

Table 6: Chapel Hill Definition of Systemic Vasculitis

Vasculitis involving large vessels	
Giant cell (temporal) arteritis	Granulomatous arteritis of the aorta and its major branches; predilection for the extracranial branches of the carotid artery. Temporal artery is commonly affected (age: >40 years). Commonly associated with polymyalgia rheumatica.
Takayasu's arteritis	Granulomatous inflammation of the aorta and its major branches (age: >40 years).

Vasculitis involving medium-sized vessels	
Polyarteritis nodosa	Necrotizing inflammation of the medium-sized or small arteries without glomerulonephritis and without vasculitis of the arterioles, capillaries, and venules.
Kawasaki's disease	Arteritis of the large, medium-sized, and small arteries; commonly associated with mucocutaneous lymph node syndrome. The coronary arteries are often affected. Involvement of the aorta and veins may also be observed (usually in children).

Vasculitis involving small vessels	
Wegener's granulomatosis	Granulomatous inflammation of the respiratory tract and necrotizing vasculitis of the small to medium-sized blood vessels. Necrotizing glomerulonephritis.
Churg–Strauss syndrome	Eosinophilia and granulomatous inflammation of the respiratory tract with necrotizing inflammation of the small to medium-sized blood vessels; associated with asthma and eosinophilia.
Microscopic polyangiitis	Necrotizing inflammation of the small vessels without or with only minimal immune depots. Necrotizing arteriitis of the small and medium-sized arteries may be present. Necrotizing glomerulonephritis, pulmonary capillaritis.
Schönlein–Henoch purpura	Small vessel vasculitis with in situ immune deposits containing mainly IgA. Characterized by involvement of the skin, gastrointestinal tract, and glomeruli in conjunction with arthralgia and/or arthritis.
Essential cryoglobulinemic vasculitis	Small vessel vasculitis associated with cryoglobulin immune deposits in situ and with cryoglobulins in serum. Glomerular involvement is common.
Cutaneous leukocytoclastic angiitis	Isolated leukocytoclastic angiitis of the skin without systemic vasculitis or glomerulonephritis.

Table 7: Reference Laboratory Values

	Conventional units	SI units
Erythrocyte sedimentation rate (ESR)	Males: 3–8 mm (1 h), 5–18 mm (2 h) Females: 6–11 mm (1 h), 6–20 mm (2 h)	

Reference values for blood

Leukocytes	$4.3–10.0 \times 10^3/\mu l$	4.3–10.0 G/l
Thrombocytes	$150–350 \times 10^3/l$	150–350 G/l
Hemoglobin (Hb)	Males: 13–18 g/dl	8.1–11.2 mmol/l
	Females: 12–16 g/dl	7.4–9.9 mmol/l
Erythrocytes	Males: $4.5–6.9 \times 10^6/\mu l$	
	Females: $4.0–5.2 \times 10^6/\mu l$	

Differential cell count

Granulocytes	
• Segmented neutrophils	$57 \pm 10\%$
• Stab neutrophils	$5 \pm 3\%$
• Eosinophils	$3 \pm 2\%$
• Basophils	<1%
Lymphocytes	$30 \pm 10\%$
Monocytes	$6 \pm 4\%$
Plasma cells	<0.1%

Distribution of lymphocyte subpopulations

T cells: $CD4^+ CD8^-$	ca. 47%	$610–1400/\mu l$
$CD8^+ CD4^-$	ca. 31%	$400–930/\mu l$
$\gamma\delta$	ca. 1–5%	$26–60/\mu l$
$CD4^- CD8^-$	<1%	
B cells	<20%	$260–600/\mu l$

Electrophoresis

Albumin	54–65%	0.54–0.65
α_1-globulins	2–5%	0.02–0.05
α_2-globulins	7–10%	0.07–0.10
β-globulins	9–12%	0.09–0.12

Plasma proteins	6.6–8.5 g/dl	66–85 g/l
Protein, total	20–30 mg/dl	200–300 mg/l
Albumin	3.6–5.0 g/dl	36–50 g/l
α_1-Antitrypsin	90–200 mg/dl	0.9–2.0 g/l
α_2-Macroglobulin	130–300 mg/dl	1.3–3.0 g/l
β_2-Microglobulin (β_2m)	8–24 mg/dl	0.8–2.4 mg/l
Myoglobulin	<70 µg/l	<70 µg/l
Ferritin	30–300 µd/dl	30–300 µd/dl
Transferrin	200–360 md/dl	2.0–3.6 g/l
Haptoglobin	70–380 mg/dl	0.7–3.8 g/l
Ceruloplasmin	15–60 mg/dl	0.15–0.6 g/l
C-reactive protein (CRP)	<0.8 mg/dl	<0.008 g/l

(**Table 7:** Reference Laboratory Values, continued)

	Conventional units	SI units
Immunoglobulins		
IgA	70–400 mg/dl	0.9–4.5 g/l
IgA subclasses		
IgA$_1$	57–321 mg/dl	0.57–3.21 g/l
IgA$_2$	4.7–82 mg/dl	0.047–0.82 g/l
IgG	700–1600 mg/dl	7–16 g/l
IgG subclasses		
IgG$_1$	422–1292 mg/dl	4.22–12.92 g/l
IgG$_2$	117–747 mg/dl	1.17–7.47 g/l
IgG$_3$	41–129 mg/dl	0.41–1.29 g/l
IgG$_4$	<291 mg/dl	<2.91 g/l
IgG in urine	10 mg/l	10 mg/l
IgM	40–230 mg/dl	0.4–2.3 g/l
IgE	<24 mg/dl *or*	<0.24 g/l *or*
	10–120 units/ml	10–120 units/ml
C1q	180 μg/ml	
C1 inhibitor	60–140 %	60–140 %
C3 complement	55–120 mg/dl	0.55–1.2 g/l
C4 complement	20–50 mg/dl	0.2–0.5 g/l
IL-2 receptor	200–1000 units/ml	
IL-8	<70 ng/l	
Enzymes		
ACE	15–80 units/l	
Alkaline phosphatase	60–180 units/l	
Creatine kinase (CK)	<80 units/l	
Coagulation		
Thromboplastin time (quick)	70–130 %	0.9–1.15 INR*
Partial thromboplastin time (PTT)	23–35 s	
Fibrinogen	200–400 mg/dl	5.88–11.76 μmol/l
Tumor markers		
α$_1$-Fetoprotein (AFP)	<10 μg/l	<10 μg/l
CEA	<5 μg/l	<5 μg/l
CA 125	<35 U/ml	
CA 15-3	<28 U/ml	
CA 19-9	<37 U/ml	
CA 72-4	<6.0 U/ml	
CA 19-9	<37 U/ml	
CA 72-4	<6.0 U/ml	

*INR = international normalized ratio = patient plasma (Quick)/pool plasma (Quick)

Appendix

(Table 7: Reference Laboratory Values, continued)

	Conventional units	SI units
Cerebrospinal fluid (CSF)		
Cell count	<15/3 μ/l	
Albumin	11–35 mg/dl	110–350 mg/dl
IgA	<0.6 mg/dl	<6 mg/l
IgG	0.9–2.6 mg/dl	9–26 mg/l
IgM	0.09–0.25 mg/dl	0.9–2.5 mg/l
Cortisol		
Morning	171–800 nmol/l	171–800 nmol/l
Evening	82.8–477 nmol/l	82.8–477 nmol/l
Antibodies		

Antibodies, such as antinuclear antibodies and anti-DNA antibodies, are not listed here because of the great degree of measurement variations from one test system to another. The reference values must be provided by the responsible laboratory.

Appendix

Table 8: CD Nomenclature

Monoclonal antibodies (MAb) make it possible to obtain a quantitative assessment of cell populations in the blood, to sort them, and to classify them according to their surface antigens. The various names for the monoclonal antibodies and their antigens were processed by the WHO-IUIS Standardization Committee on Leukocyte Differentiation Antigens and compiled to form the simplified international terminology. Monoclonal antibodies with virtually identical specificity for a given membrane antigen were grouped together and defined using cluster of differentiation (CD) numbers. The following table provides an overview of the monoclonal antibodies and their antigens. The new CD clusters and subclusters presented at the 7th International Workshop in Harrogate, United Kingdom, in 2000 ("HLDA7"), which have recently been published (Leukocyte Typing VII), are also included.

CD number	Other designation/Molecule/Antigen	Cellular reactivity
CD1a,	Presentation molecule for mycobacterial lipids	Thymocytes, LHC, DC
CD1b,		Thymocytes, DC
CD1c;		Thymocytes, LHC, DC, B
CD1d	Constitutively expressed, interaction with NKT cells	M, T cells
CD2	T11, Tp50, sheep erythrocyte receptor, receptor for CD48, CD58, CD59	T cells, NK cells
CD2R	CD2 epitope on activated T cells	T cells, NK cells
CD3	CD3 complex	T cells
CD4	T4, MHC class II, HIV receptor	T cells, monocytes
CD5	Tp67, CD72 receptor	T cells, B cells
CD6	T12	T cells, B cells
CD7	IgM Fc receptor	T cells, NK cells
CD8	T8, MHC class I-specific receptor	T cells, NK cells
CD8b	T8, MHC class I-specific receptor	T cells
CD9	p24	pre-B, M, Plt, Eo
CD10	Neutral endopeptidase, gp100, common ALL antigen (CALLA)	cALL, germinal center B cells, granulocytes
CD11a	Leukocyte function antigen 1 (LFA-1)	Leukocytes
CD11b	C3bi receptor (CR3), Mac-1, Mo-1	M, G, NK
CD11c	C3bi receptor (CR3), C3dgR, CR4	M, G, NK, B
CDw12	Unknown function	M, G, Plt
CD13	Aminopeptidase N, gp150, coronavirus-R	Monocytes, granulocytes
CD14	LPS/LBP receptor, gp55	M, G, DC, B
CD15	Lewis (Le-x), 3-FAL, x-hapten, lacto-N-fucopentatose III, SSEA	G, M, Reed–Sternberg cells
CD15s	Sialyl-Lewis (sLe-x), CD62e ligand	Leukocytes, EC
CD15u	Sulfated CD15	
CD16	FcRIIIa for IgG, gp 50–65	NK, G, macrophages
CD16b	FcRIIIb for IgG (with GPI anchor)	Granulocytes
CDw17	Lactosylceramide	G, M, platelets
CD18	β_2-Integrin chain with CD11a, b, c	Leukocytes
CD19	Bgp95, SIg family	B cells
CD20	B1, Bp35, Ca²⁺ channels	B cells
CD21	C3d-R (CD2), gp140, EBV-R, CD23R	Mature B cells, FDC
CD22	Bgp135, CD45R0 receptor	B cells
CD23	Low-affinity Fc-IgE receptor, FcεRII, Gp50–45, CD21 receptor	Mature B, M, FDC, Eo

(**Table 8:** CD Nomenclature, continued)

CD number	Other designation/Molecule/Antigen	Cellular reactivity
CD24	Heat-stable antigen (HSA) homologue	B cells, granulocytes
CD25	IL-2 receptor α chain, Tac antigen	Activ. T, B, M
CD26	Dipeptidylpeptidase IV, gp120, Ta1	Activ. T, B, MP
CD27	CD70 receptor, TNFR-like protein	T cells, thymocytes, NK, B
CD28	Tp44, CD80 receptor, CD86 receptor	T cells, activ. B
CD29	β_1-Integrin chain, platelet gpIIa	Leukocytes
CD30	Ki-1 antigen, TNFR-like protein	Activ. B cells, T cells; Reed–Sternberg cells
CD31	PECAM-1, platelet gpIIa, endocam	Platelets, M, G, B, T
CD32	FcRII for IgG, gp40	M, G, B, Eo
CD33	My9, unknown function	M, myeloid precursors
CD34	My10	Hematopoietic precursors, Eo
CD35	C3b/C4b receptor (CR1)	Ery., G, M, B (T, NK, FDC)
CD36	Platelet gpIV (gpIIIb), thrombospondin receptor, collagen type I/III receptor	M, Plt, EC
CD37	gp40–45	B cells, (T), myeloid cells
CD38	T10, gp45 (NAD glycohydrolase and ADP ribosylcyclase activity)	Plasma cells, early B and T, activated T cells
CD39	gp80	B cells, NK, EC, M, DC
CD40	gp50, CD40L-R, from TNFR family	B, M, DC, basal EC
CD40L	gp39, TRAP-1, CD40 ligand	T cells
CD41	Receptor for fibrinogen and vWF	Plt, megakaryocytes
CD42a	Platelet gpIX	Plt, megakaryocytes
CD42b	Platelet gpIb-α	Plt, megakaryocytes
CD42c	Platelet gpIb-β	Plt, megakaryocytes
CD42d	Platelet GPV	Platelets
CD43	Leukosialin, gp95, sialophorin, gp115, leukocyte sialoglycoprotein	Leukocytes, except resting B
CD44	Pgp-1, gp80–95, hyaluronic acid-R, HCAM	T, B, G, M, erythrocytes
CD44R	Restricted CD44	Erythrocytes
CD45	T200, leukocyte common antigen (LCA), tyrosine phosphatase	All hematopoietic cells
CD45RO	Restricted T200, gp180, CD22-R	T subsets, B-subsets, M
CD45RA	Restricted T200, gp220, LCA isoform	T subsets, B, M
CD45RB	Restricted T200, LCA isoform	T subsets, B, G, M
CD46	Membrane cofactor protein (MCP), gp45–70, measles virus receptor	Leukocytes
CD47	Integrin-associated protein, OA3, 1D8	All cells
CD48	gp41, putative CD244 receptor	Leukocytes
CD49a	VLA α_1 chain (VLA-1); laminin and collagen receptor	Activated T, B; M
CD49b	VLA α_2 chain (VLA-2); platelet GPIa; laminin and collagen receptor	Platelets, cultured T cells
CD49c	VLA α_3 chain (VLA-3); laminin, collagen, and fibronectin receptor	B cells
CD49d	VLA α_4 chain (VLA-4); fibronectin and VCAM receptor	M, T, B, thrombocytes
CD49e	VLA α_5 chain (VLA-5), fibronectin R	Memory T, M, Plt
CD49f	VLA α_6 chain (VLA-6), laminin R	Plt, T

(**Table 8:** CD Nomenclature, continued)

CD number	Other designation/Molecule/Antigen	Cellular reactivity
CD50	Intercellular adhesion molecule 3 (ICAM-3), CD11a/CD18 (LFA-1) receptor	Numerous, but not on EC
CD51	α Chain of vitronectin receptor (VNR)	(Plt), EC, fibroblasts
CD52	Campath-1, gp21–28	Leukocytes
CD53	MEM-53	Only on leukocytes, but not on platelets
CD54	Intercellular adhesion molecule 1 (ICAM-1), CD11a/CD18 (LFA-1) receptor, MAC-1 ligand	Numerous
CD55	Decay-accelerating factor (DAF)	Numerous
CD56	NKH1, isoform of neural cellular adhesion molecule (NCAM)	NK
CD57	HNK1, gp110, unknown function	NK, B, T subsets, brain
CD58	Lymphocyte function-associated antigen 3 (LFA-3), CD2 receptor	Leukocytes, epithelium
CD59	gp18–20, Ly-6 similarity, homologous restriction factor 20 (HRF-20), CD2 receptor, protectin	Numerous
CD60a	Ganglioside GD3	T cells, platelets
CD60b	9-O-acetyl-GD3	T cells, platelets
CD60c	7-O-acetyl-GD3	T cells, platelets
CD61	β_2-Integrin chain (gpIIIa)	Platelets, megakaryocytes
CD62E	E-selectin, ELAM-1	Activ. EC
CD62L	L-selectin, LAM-1, Leu-8, TQ1, MEL14	Numerous
CD62P	P-selectin, gmp140, PADGEM	Activ. EC, Plt
CD63	Plt 53 kDa activation antigen, LIMP	Activ. Plt; M, (G, T, B)
CD64	FcRI for IgG, high-affinity FcR for IgG	Monocytes
CD65	VIM2 antigen, ceramide dodecasaccharide 4c	Granulocytes, (monocytes)
CD66a	Biliary glycoprotein (BGP)	Granulocytes
CD66abce	Ab to BGP, NCA95, NCA90	Granulocytes
CD66acd	Ab to BGP, NCA90, CGM1	Granulocytes
CD66acde	Ab to BGP, NCA90, CGM1, CEA	Granulocytes
CD66ace	Ab to BGP, NCA90, CEA	Granulocytes
CD66ade	Ab to BGP, CGM1, CEA	Granulocytes
CD66ae	Ab to BGP, CEA	Granulocytes
CD66b	CD67, p100, CGM6, nonspecific cross-reacting antigen (NCA) 95	Granulocytes
CD66be	Ab to NCA95, CEA	Granulocytes
CD66c	NCA90	Granulocytes
CD66ce	Ab to NCA90, CEA	Granulocytes
CD66d	CGM1	Granulocytes
CD66de	Ab to CGM1, CEA	Granulocytes
CD66e	Carcinoembryonic antigen (CEA)	Colon epithelial cells
CD67	Now CD66b	—
CD68	gp110, macrosialin	M, Mμ, neutrophils, basophils
CD69	Activation inducer molecule (AIM), EA1, MLR, Leu23	Early activ. T cells, B cells, macrophages, NK
CD70	CD27 receptor, Ki-24	T, B-EBV, pre-BLL, Reed–Sternberg cells
CD71	Transferrin receptor, T9 antigen	Activ. T, B, proliferating cells

(**Table 8:** CD Nomenclature, continued)

CD number	Other designation/Molecule/Antigen	Cellular reactivity
CD72	Lyb-2, CD5 receptor	B cells, not plasma cells
CD73	Ecto-5′-nucleotidase (ecto-5′-NT)	B cells, T cells
CD74	MHC class II-specific chaperone invariant chain	B cells, monocytes
CD75	Lactosamines, perhaps a CD22 ligand	Mature B cells, T subsets
CD76	α-2,6-sialated lactosamines	B cells, T cells, EC
CD77	Globotriaosylceramide (Gb3), Burkitt's lymphoma antigen (BLA)	Germinal B cells, Burkitt's lymphoma cells
CD79α	mb-1, Ig-α	B cells
CD79β	B29, Ig-β	B cells
CD80	B7/BB1; CD28 and CTLA-4 receptor	B subset
CD81	Target of antiproliferative antibody (TAPA-1), M38	Lymphocytes
CD82	R2, 4F9, C33, IA4	M, Activ. B, T, LGL
CD83	HB15	LHC, DC, erythrocytes
CDw84	p75, 2G7, unknown function	B, T, M, platelets
CD85	ILT/LIR family	Dendritic cells
CD86	FUN-1, BU-63, B7-2; CD28 and CTLA-4 ligand	B cells, monocytes, DC
CD87	Urokinase plasminogen activator receptor (uPAR)	Monocytes, granulocytes, endothelial cells
CD88	C5a receptor (C5aR), GR10	Granulocytes, monocytes, smooth muscle cells
CD89	IgA Fc receptor	G, M, B, T
CD90	Thy-1	Precursor cells, brain
CD91	α₂-Macroglobulin receptor (α₂MR)	Monocytes
CD92	p70, VIM15, unknown function	Granulocytes, monocytes, EC
CD93	p120, GR11, unknown function	M, G, EC
CD94	KP43	NK cells, T cells
CD95	APO-1, Fas	Activ. T cells, MP
CD96	TACTILE (T-cell activation increased late expression)	T cells, NK cells
CD97	p74/80/89, TNFR family, GR1, binds CD55	G, M, T, B
CD98	4F2	T, B, NK, platelets
CD99	E2, MIC2	Numerous
CD99R	Restricted CD99	Numerous
CD100	p150	Numerous
CD101	p140	G, M, T, DC
CD102	Intercellular adhesion molecule-2 (ICAM-2)	Numerous, including ECs and monocytes
CD103	HML1, αEβ₇ integrin	Intraepithelial lymphocytes of the intestines, hairy cells
CD104	β₄-Integrin chain	Thy.
CD105	Endoglin; TGF-β₁ and -β₃ receptor	EC, activ. M
CD106	VCAM-1, INCAM110, VLA-4 receptor	Activ. endothelial cells
CD107a	LAMP1	Activ. EC, platelets, T
CD107b	LAMP2	Activ. EC, platelets, T
CD108	GPI-gp80 (with GPI anchor)	Ery., circulating lymphocytes
CD109	(Has GPI anchor)	EC, T cells, platelets
CD110	MPL, TPO R	Platelets
CD111	PRR1/Nectin1	Myeloid cells

(Table 8: CD Nomenclature, continued)

CD number	Other designation/Molecule/Antigen	Cellular reactivity
CD112	PRR2	Myeloid cells
CD114	G-CFR receptor	Granulocytes, monocytes
CD115	Colony-stimulating factor-1 receptor (CSF-1R), M-CSFR	Monocytes, macrophages
CD116	GM-CSF receptor (GM-CSFR)	Monocytes, granulocytes
CD117	Stern cell factor receptor, c-kit	Mast cells, myeloid precursors
CD118	for IFN-α, β receptor	Numerous
CD119	Interferon-γ receptor (IFN-γ-R)	M, G, B, NK
CD120a	55 kDa TNF type I receptor (TNFRI)	Numerous
CD120b	75 kDa TNF type II receptor (TNFRII)	Numerous
CD121a	Interleukin-1 type I receptor (IL1RI)	T, thymocytes
CDw121b	Interleukin-1 type II receptor (IL1RII)	G, M, B, macrophages
CD122	IL-2R β chain	Activ. T cells, cultured NK cells, monocytes
CD123	gp70, IL-3R α chain	Myeloid precursors
CD124	IL-4R α chain, IL-13R α chain	Mature B/T cells, M, hematopoietic precursors
CD125	gp60, IL-5 receptor	Myeloid precursors
CD126	IL-6R α chain	Activ. B, plasmacytes, endothelial cells
CD127	IL-7R α chain	Lymphoid precursors, pro-B cells
CDw128	gp58–67, IL-8 receptor	G, T, M, keratinocytes
CD129	Not assigned; reserved for IL-9 receptor	—
CD130	gp130, IL-6R β chain	Numerous
CDw131	gp95–120, transducing β chain of IL-3R, IL-5R, and GM-CSFR	M, G, Eo
CD132	γ Chain of IL-2R, IL-4R, IL-7R, IL-9R, and IL-15R	T cells, B cells, lymphoid precursor cells
CD133	AC133	Stem/progenitor cells
CD134	OX40, TNFR family	Activ. T cells
CD135	Flt3/Flk2, tyrosine kinase Ig subfamily	Early lymphoid precursors
CDw136	gp180, proto-oncogene c-ron, macrophage-stimulating protein receptor	Numerous
CDw137	gp30, 4–1BB, TNFR family	T cells
CD138	Syndecan-1, heparan sulfate proteoglycan, extracellular matrix receptor	B cells
CD139	gp209–228, unknown function	B cells, follicular DCs
CD140a	PDGFR α chain	Numerous
Cd140b	PDGFR β chain	EC, stroma, mesangium
CD141	Thrombomodulin	EC, smooth muscle cells
CD142	Tissue factor, initiates clotting, binds factor VIIa	EC, epithelium, monocytes, keratinocytes
CD143	Angiotensin-converting enzyme (ACE), peptidyl dipeptidase	Endothelial cells, epithelium, macrophages
Cd144	VE-cadherin	Endothelial cells
CDw145	pg25–90–110, panendothelial marker, also on basement membrane	—
CD146	MUC18, S-endo	EC

(**Table 8:** CD Nomenclature, continued)

CD number	Other designation/Molecule/Antigen	Cellular reactivity
CD147	Neurothelin, basigin, TCSF, EMMPRIN, M6	ECs, myeloid and lymphoid precursor cells
CD148	HPTP-η, DEP-1, phosphotyrosine phosphatase	Numerous; lost in breast, bladder, and hepatocellular carcinoma cells
CD150	Ig subfamily, surface lymphocyte activation molecule (SLAM)	B cells, T cells, thymocytes
CD151	PETA-3, tetraspan	Plt, ECs, epithelium, granulocytes
CD152	CTLA-4, Ig subfamily; CD80 and CD86 ligand	Activ. T cells
CD153	CD30 ligand, TNF family	T cells
CD154	CD40 ligand, gp39, TNF family	Activ. CD4⁺ T cells
CD155	Polio virus receptor (PVR), Ig subfamily	Numerous, e.g., M, Mµ, Thy., neurons in CSF
CD156a	EGF subfamily, ADAM8 (a disintegrin and metalloprotease)	M, G, Mµ
CD156b	TACE/ADAM17	Adhesion structures
CD157	Bone marrow stromal antigen (BST-1)	Bone marrow stromal cells, G, M, EC, FDC
CD158	KIR family	NK cells
CD159a	NKG2A	NK cells
CD160	BY55	T cells
CD161	NKRP1A, C-lectin subfamily	NK cells, T cells
CD162	P-selectin glycoprotein ligand-1 (PSGL-1), GD62P ligand	M, G, T, (B)
CD162R	PEN5	NK cells
CD163	M130, scavenger RI/II, unknown function	(Monocytes, macrophages)
CD164	MGC-24, mucin-like homodimer	M, G, T (B)
CD165	AD2	Plt, T, NK, Thy.
CD166	ALCAM, CD6 ligand, Ig subfamily	EC, M
CD167a	Discoidin domain R (DDR1)	Adhesion structures, EC
CD168	RHAMM	Adhesion structures, breast cancer cells
CD169	Sialoadhesin	Adhesion structures, subset of macrophages
CD170	Siglec-5	Adhesion structures, neutrophils
CD171	L1	Adhesion structures, numerous
CD172a	SIRPα	Adhesion structures, numerous
CD173	Blood group H type 2	Carbohydrate structures
CD174	Lewis y	Carbohydrate structures
CD175	Tn	Carbohydrate structures
CD175s	Sialyl-Tn	Carbohydrate structures
CD176	TF	Carbohydrate structures
CD177	NB1	Myeloid cells
CD178	Fas ligand	Activ. T
CD179a	Vpre-B	Early B

(Table 8: CD Nomenclature, continued)

CD number	Other designation/Molecule/Antigen	Cellular reactivity
CD179b	Lambda 5	B
CD180	RP105	B
CD183	CXCR-3	Numerous
CD184	CXCR-4	Numerous
CD195	CCR5	Numerous
CDw197	CCR7	Numerous
CD200	OX2	Nonlineage molecules
CD201	EPC R	EC
CD202b	Tie2 (Tec)	EC
CD203c	NPP3/PDNP3	Myeloid cells
CD204	Macrophage scavenger R	Myeloid cells
CD205	DEC205	DC
CD206	Macrophage mannose R	Macrophages, EC
CD207	Langerin	DC
CD208	DC-LAMP	DC
CD209	DC-SIGN	DC
CDw210	IL-10R	Numerous
CD212	IL-12R	Activ. CD4$^+$, CD8$^+$ T
CD213a1	IL-13-Rα1	B, M, EC, fibroblasts
CD213a2	IL-13-Rα2	B, M, EC, fibroblasts
CDw217	IL-17R	Activ. memory T cells
CD220	InsulinR	Numerous
CD221	IGF-1R	Numerous
CD222	Mannose 6-phosphate/IGF-2 R	Numerous
CD223	LAG-3	Activ. T, NK
CD224	γ-Glutamyltransferase	Numerous
CD225	Leu13	Numerous
CD226	DNAM-1 (PTA1)	T subset, NK, platelets, M
CD227	MUC.1	Numerous
CD228	Melanotransferrin	Numerous, human melanomas
CD229	Ly9	Lymphocytes
CD230	Prion protein	Numerous
CD231	TALLA-1/A15	Numerous
CD232	VESP R	Numerous
CD233	Band 3	Erythroid cells
CD234	Fy-glycoprotein (DARC)	Erythroid cells
CD235a	Glycophorin A	Erythroid cells
CD235b	Glycophorin B	Erythroid cells
CD235ab	Glycophorin AB	Erythroid cells
CD236	Glycophorin C/D	Erythroid cells
CD236R	Glycophorin C	Erythroid cells
CD238	Kell	Erythroid cells
CD239	B-CAM	Erythroid cells
CD240CE	Rh30CE	Erythroid cells
CD240D	Rh30D	Erythroid cells
CD240DCE	Rh30D/CE cross-reactive	Erythroid cells
CD241	RhAg	Erythroid cells
CD242	ICAM-4	Erythroid cells
CD243	MDR-1	Stem/progenitor cells

(**Table 8:** CD Nomenclature, continued)

CD number	Other designation/Molecule/Antigen	Cellular reactivity
CD244	2B4	NK cells
CD245	P220/240, NPAT	T cells
CD246	Anaplastic lymphoma kinase	Numerous
CD247	Zeta chain	T, NK

Key to abbreviations: Activ. = activated, ALL = acute lymphoid leukemia, B = B cells, EC = endothelial cells, Eo = eosinophil granulocytes, Ery. = erythrocytes, FDC = follicular dendritic cells, DC = dendritic cells, G = granulocytes, L = ligand, LGL = large granular lymphocytes, LHC = Langerhans cells, M = monocytes, MP = macrophages, NK = NK cells, Plt = platelets, R = receptor, T = T cells, Thy. = thymocytes. If not specified, the function of the antigen is unknown.

Table 9: Most Important Cytokines and Chemokines in Immunology

Key to abbreviations: AA = amino acids, activ. = activated, DC = dendritic cells

Cytokine	Other designations	Gene locus	Structure
IL-1	Lymphocyte activating factor, endogenous pyrogen, leukocyte endogenous mediator, mononuclear cell factor, catabolin	2q12-q21, 2q13-q21	Two molecules with slight homology: IL-1α (271 AA) and in IL-1β (269 AA). Both bind to the same receptor. IL-1 receptor antagonist (IL-1Ra) also binds to it and cancels the effect of IL-1.
IL-2	T-cell growth factor (TcGF)	4q26-q27	133 AA, 15 kDA
IL-3	Multi-colony stimulating factor (M-CSF), mast cell growth factor (MCGF), eosinophil-CSF (E-CSF), hematopoietic cell growth factor (HCGF), burst-promoting activity (BPA)	5q23-q31	152 AA, 15 kDa
IL-4	B-cell stimulating factor 1 (BSF-1)	5q31	Globular structure with a hydrophobic nucleus, 129 AA, 15 kDa
IL-5	Eosinophil differentiation factor/colony stimulation factor (EDF/E-CSF), B-cell growth factor II (BCGFII), B-cell differentiation factor for IgM (BCDFµ), T-cell replacing factor (TRF)	5q23-q31	Disulfide-bound homodimer, 115 AA, 13 kDa
IL-6	Interferon-β$_2$, B-cell stimulating factor 2 (BSF-2), plasmacytoma growth factor, hepatocyte differentiation factor (HSF), monocyte granulocyte inducer type 2 (MGI-2)	7p21-p14	183 AA, 26 kDa
IL-7	Lymphopoietin 1 (LP-1), pre-B-cell growth factor	8q21-q13	152 AA, 20–28 kDa

EC = Endothelial cells, IL = interleukin, kDa = kilodalton, BM = bone marrow

Source	Target cells	Biological activity	Receptor
Monocytes, macrophages, DC, astrocytes, NK cells, B cells, EC, fibroblasts	T cells, B cells, endothelial cells, organs: hepatocytes, bone	Activation of lymphocytes and macrophages, increases cell adhesion, fever, weight loss, hypotension, acute-phase reaction	Type I receptor: CD121a, 80 kDa, 3 immunoglobulin-like domains. Type II receptor: CD121b, 60 kDa, 3 immunoglobulin-like domains; soluble receptor can bind IL-1β
T cells	T cells, NK cells, B cells, monocytes, macrophages, oligodendrocytes	Proliferation and differentiation of T and B cells, activation of monocytes	Three chains: α chain (p55), TAC, CD25; β chain (p75), CD122; γ chain (p64), common γ chain together with IL-4R, IL-7R, IL-9R, IL-13R, and IL-15R; α/γ or β/γ heterodimers form receptors of intermediate affinity; α/β/γ heterotrimers form high-affinity receptors
Activ. T cells, mast cells, eosinophil granulocytes	All bone marrow precursor cells	Growth factor for bone marrow precursor cells, B cells, monocytes	Two subunits: IL3Rα (CD123) and a β chain form a high-affinity IL-3 receptor. The β chain is shared with IL-5R and GM-CSFR
Mast cells, T cells, bone marrow stromal cells	T cells, B cells, monocytes, endothelial cells, fibroblasts	Isotype switch by B cells, secretion of IgG4 (IgG1) and IgE by B cells	Two chains: α chain = p140 (CD124), high-affinity binding of IL-4; γ chain (p64), common γ chain; increases the affinity for IL-4
Mast cells, T cells, eosinophil granulocytes	Eosinophil granulocytes	Induces eosinophil differentiation, B-cell growth and differentiation (in mice only)	Two chains: α chain = (CD125) low-affinity binding of IL-5; β chain = shared with IL-3R and GM-CSFR
T cells, B cells, macrophages, bone marrow stromal cells, fibroblasts, EC	B cells, plasmacytes, T cells, hepatocytes, bone marrow cells	B cell growth and differentiation, T cell proliferation, acute-phase reaction	Two chains α chain = (CD126) low-affinity binding of IL-6; β chain (gp130) associated with α chain/IL-6 complex
BM cells, thymic stromal cells, splenic cells	T cells, B cells	Proliferation and maturation of T- and B-cell progenitor cells	Two chains: α chain = (CD127), binding of IL-7; γ chain: shared with IL-4R, IL-9R, IL-13R and IL-15R

(**Table 9:** Most Important Cytokines in Immunology, continued)

Cytokine	Other designations	Gene locus	Structure
IL-8	*See chemokines*		
IL-9	P40, mast cell growth-enhancing activity, T-cell growth factor III	5q31.1	126 AA, 32–39 kDa
IL-10	Cytokine synthesis inhibitory factor (CSIF)	1	160 AA, 35–40 kDa
IL-11	Adipogenesis inhibitory factor	19q13.3-13.4	179 AA, 23 kDa
IL-12	Natural killer cell stimulatory factor (NKSF), cytotoxic lymphocyte maturation factor (CLMF)	?	Heterodimer with two chains (p35 and p40), 196 AA/306 AA and 30–33 kDa/35–44 kDa, respectively
IL-13	P600	5q31	112 AA, 9/17 kDa
IL-14	High molecular weight B-cell growth factor (HMW-BCGF)	?	483 AA, 60 kDa
IL-15	T-cell growth factor	4q31	Similarity with interleukin-2, 114 AA, 14 kDa
IL-16	Lymphocyte chemoattractant factor (LCF)	?	130 AA, 40 kDa (precursor: 632 AA)

Source	Target cells	Biological activity	Receptor
T_H2 cells	Hodgkin's cells, T cells, mast cells, megakaryocytes, erythrocyte precursor cells	Increases the proliferation of T cells and basophils	IL-9 receptor can associate with the common γ chain
T_H0 and T_H2 cells, activ. CD4$^+$ and CD8$^+$ T cells, monocytes, macrophages, DC	B cells, thymocytes, T_H1 cells, monocytes, NK cells	Activation and proliferation of B cells, thymocytes, mast cells	One chain, homology to IFN-γ and IFN-$\alpha\beta$ receptor
Fibroblasts, BM stromal cells	Hematopoietic precursor cells, plasmacytoma cells, adipocytes	Growth factor for hematopoietic precursor cells, inhibition of adipocytes	
DC, monocytes, macrophages, B cells	T cells, NK cells	IFN-γ production in T cells and NK cells; activation and differentiation of T_H1 T cells	One large receptor; structurally similar to the G-CSF receptor
Activ. T cells	B cells, monocytes	B cell proliferation and differentiation, IgE secretion	?
T cells, B cells	Activ. B cells	Stimulates the proliferation of activ. B cells, inhibits immunoglobulin synthesis	One single receptor type
Peripheral mononuclear cells (PBMC), placenta, skeletal muscles, kidney, lung, heart	T cells, lymphokine-activated killer cells	T-cell growth factor	Two receptor chains: β chain and γ chain, shared with IL-2 receptor; one variable α chain
CD8$^+$ T cells	Eosinophil granulocytes, CD4$^+$ T cells, monocytes	Chemotaxis	?

(**Table 9:** Most Important Cytokines in Immunology, continued)

Cytokine	Other designations	Gene locus	Structure
IL-17	Cytotoxic T-lymphocyte-associated antigen (CTLA-8)	?	132 AA, 20 kDa
IL-18	Interferon-γ-inducing factor (IGIF)	?	157 AA, 18 kDa, similar to IL-1β
IL-19 (IL-10 homolog)		1q32.2	
IL-20 (IL-10 homolog)		1q32.2	17.6 kDA, 152 AA
IL-21 (closely related to IL-2 and IL-15)			
IL-22 (IL-10 homolog)	T-cell-derived inducible factor (IL-TIF)	12q15	16.8 kD, 147 AAA
IL-23		12q13.13	
IL-24 (IL-10 homolog)	Melanoma differentiation-associated gene 7 (MDA-7); mob-5, IL-17F	1q32	23 kDa
IL-25 (member of the IL-17 family)	SF20		
IL-26 (IL-10 homolog)	AK155	12q15	

Source	Target cells	Biological activity	Receptor
CD4+ T cells	Stromal cells, fibroblasts	Proinflammatory effect like that of TNF and lymphotoxin	No homology to other receptors
Kupffer cells, keratinocytes, osteoclasts	T cells, NK cells	Induction of IFN-γ	One part of the receptor is shared with IL-1 receptor
	Monocytes	Production of IL-6, TNF-α; induces apoptosis and reactive oxygen species	
Keratinocytes	Keratinocytes (autocrine factor), monocytes	Plays a role in epidermal function and psoriasis, induces proliferation	
	T cells, NK cells, B cells	T-cell co-stimulation, NK cell expansion, B-cell proliferation, and immunoglobulin production	IL-21R and shares common cytokine receptor γ chain with IL-2, 4, 7, 9, and 15
T cells		Induction of acute phase reactants in liver and pancreas	IL-22R, IL-10Rβ
Activ. dendritic cells	Memory T cells	Secretion of IL-17	IL-23R, IL-12Rβ1; heterodimers composed of IL-12p40 subunit and novel subunit related to IL-12p35, termed p19
Growth-arrested and terminally differentiated melanoma cells, activ. monocytes and T cells		Tumor suppressor gene, stimulates T-cell growth and inhibits angiogenesis, induces endothelial cells to produce IL-2, TGF-β, and MCP-1	IL-22R1/IL-20R2; IL20R1/IL-20R2
Bone marrow stroma cells		Promotes a T$_H$2-like response	Thymic shared antigen-1 (TSA-1)
T cells			

(**Table 9:** Most Important Cytokines in Immunology, continued)

Cytokine	Other designations	Gene locus	Structure
IFN-α	Interferon-α, type I interferon, leuko-cyte interferon, buffy coat interferon	9	α-Interferons are a family of proteins with at least 24 genes, interferon-α1: 166 AA, 16–27 kDa, interferon-α2: 172 AA, ? kDa
IFN-β	Interferon-β, type I interferon, fibroblast interferon	9p22	166 AA, 20 kDa
IFN-γ	Interferon-γ, immune interferon or type II interferon, T-cell interferon	12q24.1	143 AA, 40–70 kDa, monomers of 20–25 kDa form dimers or multimers
TNF-α	Tumor necrosis factor, cachectin, necrosin, hemorrhagic factor, macrophage cytotoxin	6p21.3	157 AA, 52 kDa (primarily from 17.4 kDa units)
TNF-β	Tumor necrosis factor, lymphotoxin, cytotoxin	6p21	35% homology to TNF-α, 171 AA, 25 kDa
TGF-α	Transforming growth factor-α, sarcoma growth factor	2	50 AA, 6 kDa, high degree of homology to IgF
TGF-β	Transforming growth factor-β, differ-entiation inhibiting factor	19q13 1q41 14q24	Three related proteins, TGF-βI, -II, and -III, all with 112 AA and 25 kDa
EGF	Epidermal growth factor, β-urogastron	4, q25	Proteolytic cleavage product of a membrane protein, 53 AA, 6 kDa
G-CSF	Granulocyte colony-stimulating factor	17, q21-22	17 AA, 21 kDa

Source	Target cells	Biological activity	Receptor
Lymphocytes, monocytes, macrophages	Most cells in the body	Interferon-α induces viral resistance, inhibits cell proliferation, and regulates class I MHC expression	At least 2 different receptors, one of which binds with interferon-α and interferon-β. Homologies to interferon-γ and IL-10 receptor
Fibroblasts and epithelial cells	Virtually all cells of the body	Similar to interferon-α	Common receptor shared with interferon-α
CD8$^+$ and CD4$^+$ T cells, NK cells	Hematopoietic cells, epithelial and endothelial cells, numerous tumor cells	Activation, growth and differentiation of T and B cells, macrophages, NK cells, EC-enhanced antiviral effect of IFN-α and IFN-β	Two chains, one (CD119) with high-affinity binding of IFN-γ; β chain: accessory chain for signal transduction
Activ. monocytes and macrophages, DC, B lymphocytes, T cells, fibroblasts	Virtually all cells of the body	Proinflammatory cytokines, growth factor, and differentiation factor for many cells. Cytotoxic for many transformed cells	Type I receptor (CD120A), Type II receptor (CD120B). Both bind TNF-α and TNF-β; soluble receptors detectable in serum and urine
Activ. T and B cells	Virtually all cells of the body	Growth and differentiation of numerous cells	Receptor shared with TNF-α
Monocytes, keratinocytes, various tissues	Virtually all cells of the body	Growth and differentiation of numerous cells	Receptor shared with EGF (known as c-erbB)
Virtually all nuclear cells, many tumor cells	Virtually all cells of the body	Inhibition of cell growth, "tissue modeling"	Three receptors of variable activity
All ectodermal cells, monocytes, renal cells, glands	Virtually all cells of the body	Epithelial cell growth, wound healing	Receptor shared with TGF-α
Macrophages, fibroblasts, endothelial cells, BM stromal cells	Granulocytes and myeloid precursor cells, EC, thrombocytes and precursor cells	Growth, differentiation and activation factor for granulocytes and myeloid precursor cells; proliferation and migration of endothelial cells	Two receptor forms having differences in their intracytoplasmic segments

Appendix

(**Table 9:** Most Important Cytokines in Immunology, continued)

Cytokine	Other designations	Gene locus	Structure
GM-CSF	Granulocyte/macrophage colony-stimulating factor, CSF-α	5, q21q32	127 AA, 22 kDa
M-CSF	Macrophage colony-stimulating factor, CSF-I	5, q33.1	224, 406, 522 AA, 45–90 kDa; homodimer structure, 3 mRNA species exist
SCF	Stem cell factor, mast cell growth factor, kit ligand (KL), steel factor (SLF)	12, q22-24	Proteolytic cleavage product of transmembranous proteins, 222 AA and 248 AA, 36 kDa
Flt3L	fms-like-tyrosine kinase 3, flk-2 (fetal liver kinase-2)	19q13.3-13.3	235 AA
EPO	Erythropoietin	7pter-q22	166 AA, 36 kDa
TPO	Thrombopoietin	3q27	322 AA, 60 kDa

Chemokines

The name "chemokines" derives from chemotactic cytokines belonging to a superfamily of smallproinflammatory activation-inducible molecules that promote chemotaxis (migration) of different cell types. They have a molecular weight of 8–10 kDa and show a high degree of homology; they all have a number of conserved cystein residues. Two large families are defined: the **4q chemokines** are encoded for by genes on closely related loci called SCYB (small inducible cytokine subfamily member B) on chromosome 4q12-21. The chemokines of this family have two cysteine residues (C) separated by a single amino acid (X), so they are called **CXC chemokines**.

▶

Source	Target cells	Biological activity	Receptor
T cells, macrophages, fibroblasts, endothelial cells	Granulocytes, monocytes, precursor cells, EC, fibroblasts, Langerhans cells, dendritic cells	Growth factor for hematopoietic precursor cells, differentiation and activation factor for granulocytes and monocytes, growth factor for EC	Two chains: an α chain (CD116) of low-affinity binding and a β chain (shared with IL-3 and IL-5 receptors) bind with an α chain to form a high-affinity receptor
Lymphocytes, monocytes, fibroblasts, epithelial and endothelial cells	Macrophages and precursor cells	Growth, differentiation and activation of macrophages and precursor cells	M-CSF (CD115) is coded by the c-*fms* proto-oncogene
Stromal cells, brain, liver, kidney, lung, fibroblasts, ovocytes	Virtually all hematopoietic precursor cells except B cells	Growth factor for hematopoietic cells	The proto-oncogene c-kit is the receptor for SCF (CD117)
T-cell lines	Hematopoietic precursor cells	Stem cell mobilization in the peripheral blood, ex vivo expansion of stem cells, ex vivo and in vivo expansion of DC, in vitro antitumor activity	Flt3R, 993 AA, 5 immunoglobulin-like extracellular domains
Liver, kidney	Erythroid precursor cells, endothelial cells	Differentiation and growth factor for erythrocyte precursor and blood vessels	One chain, 484 AA
Liver, kidney, skeletal muscles	Megakaryocytes	Differentiation and growth factor for megakaryocytes	One α chain; the β chain is shared with IL-3, IL-5, and GM-CSF receptors

This is in contrast to the second large family, the **17q chemokines**, which have the first two cystein residues adjacent (**CC chemokines**) and are encoded on chromosome 17q11-32 (the SCYA locus). Other chemokines are characterized by the presence of a single disulfide bridge and a cytoplasmic C terminus that is needed for signaling (**C chemokines**), while some are characterized by the presence of three amino acid residues between the two cystein residues (**CX$_3$C chemokine** or **fractalkine**). Only a few members of these two groups have been identified so far.

(Table 9: Most Important Cytokines in Immunology, continued)

Systematic name	Most frequent name	Other designations	Gene locus, gene symbol
CXC Chemokines: Two Cysteine (C) Molecules are Divided by Another Amino Acid (X)			
CXCL1	GROα	Growth-related oncogene α (GROα), melanoma growth stimulatory activity α (MGSAα), neutrophil-activating peptide-3 (NAP-3)	4q12-q13, small inducible cytokine sub-family member B1 (SCYB1)
CXCL2	GROβ	Growth-related oncogene β (GROβ), melanoma growth stimulatory activity β (MGSAβ), macrophage inflammatory protein-2-α (MIP-2-α)	4q12-q13, SCYB2
CXCL3	GROγ	Growth-related oncogene γ (GROγ), melanoma growth stimulatory activity γ (MGSAγ), macrophage inflammatory protein-2-β (MIP-2-β)	4q12-q13, SCYB3
CXCL4	PF4	Platelet factor-4 (PF4), Oncostatin A	4q12-q13, SCYB4
CXCL5	ENA-78	Epithelial cell-derived neutrophil attractant-78 (ENA-78)	4q12-q13, SCYB5
CXCL6	GCP-2	Granulocyte chemotactic peptide-2 (GCP-2), LPS-induced CXC (LIX)	4q12-q13, SCYB6
CXCL7	NAP-2	Neutrophil-activating protein-2 (NAP-2), connective tissue activating protein-3 (CTAP-3), low affinity platelet factor-4 (LA-PF4), platelet basic protein (PBP), β-thromboglobulin	4q12-q13, SCYB7

Structure	Source	Target cells	Biological activity	Receptor
73 AA, 7.9 kDa	Activ. mono-cytes, fibro-blasts, endothelial cells, epithelial cells, synovial cells	Neutrophils, endothelial cells	Neutrophil chemotaxis and degranulation; growth of fibroblasts, melanoma, and oligodendrocyte pre-cursor cells	CXCR2 > CXCR1
73 AA, 7.9 kDa	Activ. mono-cytes, fibro-blasts, endothelial cells, epithelial cells, synovial cells	Neutrophils, endothelial cells	Neutrophil chemotaxis and degranulation; growth of fibroblasts, melanoma, and oligodendrocyte pre-cursor cells	CXCR2
73 AA, 7.9 kDa	Activ. mono-cytes, fibro-blasts, endothelial cells, epithelial cells, synovial cells	Neutrophils, endothelial cells	Neutrophil chemotaxis and degranulation; growth of fibroblasts, melanoma, and oligodendrocyte pre-cursor cells	CXCR2
70 AA, 7.8 kDa	Megakaryocytes and platelets, mast cells, en-dothelial cells of umbilical veins	Monocytes, neutrophils	Chemotaxis of monocytes, activation and degranula-tion of neutrophils, inhi-bits angiogenesis	Unknown (chondroitin-sulfate pro-teoglycan of neutrophils)
78 AA, 8.4 kDa	Epithelial cells	Neutrophils	Chemotaxis and activation of neutrophils	CXCR2
75 AA, 8 kDa	Fibroblasts, epithelial cells	Neutrophils	Chemotaxis of neutrophils	CXCR1, CXCR2
69–85 AA, 6–7.5 kDa (different trun-cated forms derived from a precursor: leukocyte-de-rived growth factor (LDGF). Deletion of 2 AA from NAP-2 gives origin to throm-bocidin-1)	Macrophages, platelets, epithelial cells, endothelial cells	Monocytes, neutrophils, fibroblasts	Chemotaxis of fibroblasts, neutrophils, and mono-cytes; mitogenic for fibro-blasts; releases hyaluronic acid, glycosaminoglycans, plasminogen activator, and PGE2; histamine re-lease by basophils	CXCR2

Appendix

(Table 9: Most Important Cytokines in Immunology, continued)

Systematic name	Most frequent name	Other designations	Gene locus, gene symbol
CXCL8	IL-8	Neutrophil attractant/activating protein-1 (NAP-1), neutrophil-activating factor (NAF), leukocyte adhesion inhibitor (LAI), granulocyte chemotactic protein (GCP), endothelial cell neutrophil-activating peptide (ENAP-β)	4q12-q13, SCYB8
CXCL9	Mig	Monokine induced by IFN-γ (mig), cytokine responsive gene-10 (CRG-10)	4q21.21, SCYB9
CXCL10	IP-10	Interferon-inducible protein-10 or immune protein-10 (IP-10), cytokine responsive gene-2 (CRG-2)	4q21.21, SCYB10
CXCL11	I-TAC	Interferon-inducible T-cell α chemoattractant (I-TAC), interferon-γ-inducible protein-9 (IP-9)	4q21.21, SCYB11
CXCL12	SDF-1α/β	Stromal cell-derived factor-1 (SDF-1), pre-B-cell growth stimulating factor (PBSF)	10q11.1, SCYB12
CXCL13	BLC/BCA-1	B-lymphocyte chemoattractant (BLC), B-cell attracting chemokine-1 (BCA-1), Angie	4q21, SCYB13
CXCL14	BRAK	CXC chemokine in breast and kidney (BRAK), B-cell and monocyte-activating chemokine (BMAC), bolekine	5q31, SCYB14

Structure	Source	Target cells	Biological activity	Receptor
72 AA, 8 kDa, processed from a larger precursor of 99 AA. Longer and shorter forms exist	Activ. endothelial cells and monocytes, fibroblasts, keratinocytes, melanocytes, hepatocytes, chondrocytes, and a number of tumor cell lines	All immune cells, erythrocytes, endothelial cells, some epithelial cells	Chemotaxis of all migratory immune cells, activation of neutrophils, inhibits histamine release by basophils, IgE production by B cells, promotes angiogenesis	CXCR1, CXCR2
103 AA, 11.7 kDa	Macrophages, neutrophils, endothelial cells, tumor cells, upon IFN-γ stimulation	Activ. bronchial epithelium	Chemotaxis of monocytes, modulates cell growth and activation during inflammation	CXCR3
98 AA	Lymphocytes, monocytes, activ. keratinocytes, endothelial cells, neutrophils	Lymphocytes, monocytes, neutrophils, endothelial cells	Regulates the growth of immature hematopoietic progenitor cells, inhibits angiogenesis, induces proliferation of mesangial cells	CXCR3
73 AA, 8.3 kDa	Activ. astrocytes, activ. monocytes	IL-2-activated T cells	Potent chemoattractant for IL-2-activated T cells	CXCR3
89 and 93 AA (4 additional AA in SDF-1β), 32 kDa	Ubiquitous expression (not on blood cells)	Mainly lymphocytes and monocytes	Chemotaxis of mononuclear cells including BM progenitor cells	CXCR4, pre-B-cell-derived chemokine receptor (PB-CRK)
109 AA, 13.2 kDA, SWIB13	Follicles of the spleen, lymph nodes, Peyer's patches	Cells expressing Burkitt lymphoma receptor-1 (blr-1)	Activates and promotes chemotaxis of B lymphocytes	CXCR5, blr-1
88 AA	Ubiquitously expressed in normal tissue, produced by fibroblasts, keratinocytes, lamina propria cells	Activ. monocytes	Selectively attracts activ. monocytes in inflamed tissues	Unknown

(Table 9: Most Important Cytokines in Immunology, continued)

Systematic name	Most frequent name	Other designations	Gene locus, gene symbol
CXCL15 (so far identified only in mice)	Weird chemokine (WECHE)	Lungkine	Murine chr. 5.51.5, SCYB15
C Chemokines			
XCL1	Lymphotactin (Ltn, Lptn)	Single C motif-1α (SCM-1α), activation induced T-Cell derived and chemokine related (ATAC)	1q23
XCL2	SCM-1β	Single C motif-1β (SCM-1β)	1q23
CX₃C Chemokines			
CX3CL1	Fractalkine (FK, FKN)		16q13
CC Chemokines			
CCL1	I-309	P500, TCA-3 (murine homologue of I-309)	17q11.2, SCYA1
CCL2	MCP-1/MCAF	Monocyte chemoattractant protein-1 (MCP-1), monocyte chemoattractant and activating factor (MCAF), glioma cell-derived chemotactic factor (GDCF), tumor necrosis factor-stimulated gene sequence-8	17q11.2-q21.1, JE gene at SCYA2
CCL3	MIP-1-α/LD78α	Macrophage inflammatory protein-1-α (MIP-1-α), G0/G1 switch gene (GOS-19)	17q11.2, SCYA3

Structure	Source	Target cells	Biological activity	Receptor
17 kDa	Highly expressed in murine lung, fetal liver, yolk sac	Murine BM cells	Inhibits the growth of hematopoietic erythroid precursor cells, promotes migration of bone marrow cells	
93 AA, 2 different structural conformations	Activ. pro-T cells, thymocytes, CD8+ T cells	T cells, NK cells, B cells, neutrophils	Chemotactic factor for lymphocytes, NK cells, and neutrophils	XCR1
Only 2 AA differ from XCL1	Similar to XCL1?	Similar to XCL1?	Similar to XCL1?	XCR1
397 AA, a chemokine-like domain placed atop a mucin stalk and a transmembrane domain	Endothelial cells, epithelial cells, neurons	Monocytes, T cells, NK cells	Membrane-bound fractalkine induces binding and adhesion of CX3CR1-positive cells. Soluble fractalkine induces activation and migration of CX3CR1-positive cells	CX3CR1
72 AA, 15–16 kDa	Activ. T lymphocytes	Monocytes	Chemotaxis and activation of monocytes	CCR8
76 AA, 6–7 kDa unglycosylated, up to 30 kDa glycosylated	Monocytes and macrophages, fibroblasts, endothelial cells, keratinocytes, smooth muscle cells, astrocytes, and various tumor cells lines	Monocytes, T cells, basophil, and eosinophil granulocytes	Chemotaxis on monocytes, activating effect on monocytes and basophils (induces histamine release)	CCR2
69 AA, 7.8 kDa	Monocytes and macrophages (upon stimulation with bacterial endotoxins), memory T cells (upon activation)	Granulocytes, T cells, hematopoietic precursor cells	Inhibits hematopoiesis, induces T-cell migration, enhances adherence of monocytes to endothelial cells	CCR1, CCR5

(**Table 9:** Most Important Cytokines in Immunology, continued)

Systematic name	Most frequent name	Other designations	Gene locus, gene symbol
CCL4	MIP-1-β	Immune activation gene-2 (ACT-2), macrophage inflammatory protein-1-β (MIP-1-β)	17q11.2, SCYA4
CCL5	RANTES	**R**egulated upon **a**ctivation, **n**ormal **T**-cell **e**xpressed, and **s**ecreted (RANTES), small inducible secreted chemokine-delta (SIS-delta), eosinophil chemotactic polipeptide-1 (EoCP-1)	17q11.2, SCYA5
CCL6 (only murine)		C10, macrophage inflammatory protein-related protein-1 (MRP-1)	Unknown, SCYA6
CCL7	MCP-3	Monocyte chemoattractant protein-3 (MCP-3), mast cell activation-related chemokine (MARC), NC28	17q11.2 (close to the erbB2 locus), SCYA7
CCL8	MCP-2	Monocyte chemoattractant protein-2 (MCP-2)	17q11.2, SCYA8
CCL9 (only murine)	Unknown	Macrophage inflammatory protein-1-γ (MIP-1-γ), CCF18	Murine chromosome 11, SCYA9
CCL10 (only murine)	Unknown	Eventually related to human CCL15?	SCYA10
CCL11	Eotaxin		17q21.1-17q21.2, SCYA11
CCL12	Murine MCP-5	Monocyte chemotactic protein-5 (MCP-5)	Murine chromosome 11, SCYA12

Structure	Source	Target cells	Biological activity	Receptor
Highly homologous to MIP-1-α	Monocytes and macrophages (upon stimulation with bacterial endotoxins), memory T cells (upon activation)	Granulocytes, T cells, hemato-poietic pre-cursor cells	Promotes growth of hematopoietic precursor cells, activation of killer cells, induces adhesion of T cells to endothelial cells	CCR5
8 kDa	T cells (induced by TNF-α and IL-1α)	T cells, eosino-phils, baso-phils, mono-cytes, synovial fibroblasts	Recruits cells to inflam-matory sites, induces release of granules by eosinophils, promotes activation of killer cells	CCR1, CCR3, CCR5
Homologue to MIP-1-δ?	Hematopoietic cells, fibroblasts	Monocytes, T cells	Involved in monocyte and macrophage migra-tion upon injury	Unknown
97 AA, 8–18 kDa	Epithelial and endothelial cells, blood mono-nuclear cells upon activation	Monocytes, T cells, eosi-nophil gran-ulocytes	Chemotaxis of monocytes, eosinophils; induces protease secretion by macrophages	CCR1, CCR2, CCR3, CCR10?
76 AA, 8–18 kDa	Fibroblasts, endothelial cells, epithelial cells, blood mono-nuclear cells	Monocytes, T cells, eosinophil granulocytes	Chemotaxis of monocytes	CCR1, CCR2B, CCR5
100 AA	Murine macro-phages	Hematopoi-etic cells in the bone marrow, T cells	Suppression of colony for-mation in stimulated bone marrow, induces calcium release in neutrophils, acti-vates and recruits T cells	Unknown
				Unknown
97 AA	Epithelial cells, macrophages, T cells, fibro-blasts	Eosinophils	Chemotaxis of eosino-phils, activation and calcium release	CCR3
82 AA, 9.3 kDa	Lymph nodes, strongly upregu-lated in activ. monocytes	Monocytes, macro-phages	Strong chemoattractant for monocytes, macro-phages	CCR2

(Table 9: Most Important Cytokines in Immunology, continued)

Systematic name	Most frequent name	Other designations	Gene locus, gene symbol
CCL13	MCP-4	Monocyte chemotactic protein-4 (MCP-4)	17q11.2, SCYA13
CCL14	HCC-1	Hemofiltrate CC chemokine-1 (HCC-1), macrophage colony inhibitory factor (M-CIF)	17q11.2, SCYA14
CCL15	MIP-1-δ	Macrophage inflammatory protein-5 (MIP-5), hemofiltrate CC-chemokine-2 (HCC-2), NCC-3, leukotactin-1	17q11.2, SCYA15
CCL16	LEC	Liver-expressed chemokine (LEC), monotactin-1, new CC chemokine-4 (NCC-4), hemofiltrate CC-chemokine-4 (HCC-4)	17q11.2, SCYA16
CCL17	TARC	Thymus and activation-regulated cytokine (TARC), ABCD-2	16q13, SCYA17
CCL18	DC-CK1	Pulmonary and activation-regulated chemokine (PARC), alternative activated macrophage associated CC-chemokine (AMAC-1), dendritic cell-derived chemokine-1 (DC-CK1)	17q11.2, SCYA18
CCL19	MIP-3-β/ELC	EBI-1-ligand chemokine (ELC), exodus-3	9p13, SCYA19

Structure	Source	Target cells	Biological activity	Receptor
75 AA	Epithelial and endothelial cells (upon TNF-α and IL-1 stimulation), macrophages	Monocytes, T cells	Potent chemoattractant for monocytes and T lymphocytes.	CCR2, CCR3
74 AA, 8.6 kDa	Spleen, liver, skeletal and heart muscle, gut, and bone marrow; present as soluble protein in the blood	Monocytes, myeloid progenitors	Weakly chemotactic on monocytes, induction of proliferation on CD34$^+$ myeloid cells, inhibits colony formation induced by M-CSF	CCR1
92 AA, 6 conserved cystein residues instead of 4, similarity to murine C10	Leukocytes in liver, intestine, lung	Monocytes, immature DC, T and B cells, eosinophils	Attracts monocytes, DC, lymphocytes, eosinophils; inhibits colony formation by progenitor cells	CCR1, CCR3
100 AA, 11.2 kDa, a 120 AA propeptide exists	Hepatocytes, activ. monocytes (upregulation by IL-10), some NK cells, $\gamma\delta$ T cells	Monocytes, lymphocytes, DC	Promotes cell adhesion, recruits antigen presenting cells to transfected tumor cells	CCR1, CCR2, CCR5, CCR8
94 AA, 8 kDa	Thymocytes, IL-13-activated macrophages, bronchial epithelial cells, keratinocytes	T cells	Attracts predominantly T_H2-differentiated T cells	CCR4, CCR8
69 AA, 7.8 kDa	DC in germinal centers and T-cell areas of lymph nodes, alveolar macrophages, activ. monocytes	Resting T cells	Chemoattractant for T cells to antigen presentation sites	Unknown
98 AA	Thymus, lymph nodes, macrophages	T cells, B cells	Chemoattractant for CD34$^+$ cells, activ. T and B cells	CCR7

Appendix

Tables

(**Table 9:** Most Important Cytokines in Immunology, continued)

Systematic name	Most frequent name	Other designations	Gene locus, gene symbol
CCL20	MIP-3-α/LARC	Liver and activation regulated chemokine (LARC), exodus-1	2q33-q37, SCYA20
CCL21	6Ckine/SLC	Chemokine with 6 cysteines (6Ckine), secondary lymphoid-tissue chemokine (SLC), exodus-2	9p13, SCYA21
CCL22	MDC	Macrophage-derived chemokine (MDC), stimulated T-cell chemo-attractant protein-1 (STCP-1), DC/B-CK	16q13, SCYA22
CCL23	MPIF-1	Myeloid progenitor inhibitory factor-1 (MPIF-1), chemokine-β-8	17q11.2, SCYA23
CCL24	MPIF-2/eotaxin-2	Myeloid progenitor inhibitory factor-2 (MPIF-2), chemokine-β-6	7q11.23, SCYA24
CCL25	TECK	Thymus-expressed chemokine (TECK)	19p13.2, SCYA25
CCL26	Eotaxin-3	Macrophage inflammatory protein-4-α (MIP-4-α), thymic stroma chemokine-1 (TSC-1)	7q11.23, SCYA26
CCL27	CTACK/ILC	Cutaneous T-cell-attracting chemokine (CTACK), IL-11Rα-locus chemokine (ILC), ALP, skinkine, eskine, MILC	9p13, SCYA27
CCL28	MEC	Mucosa-associated epithelial chemokine (MEC)	5, SCYA28

Structure	Source	Target cells	Biological activity	Receptor
96 AA	Liver, fibroblasts, LPS-stimulated leukocytes	Immature DC, T cells	Chemoattractant for lymphocytes, weak chemoattractant for granulocytes	CCR6
111 AA, has a 30 AA carboxy-terminal domain with 2 additional cystein residues	High endothelial venules of lymphoid organs, lymphatic endothelium of different organs	Thymocytes, activ. T cells	Induces adhesion and migration of T cells, particularly naive T cells	CCR7
69 AA, 8.1 kDa	Macrophages, DC, B cells	Activ. T lymphocytes and monocytes	Recruitment of activ. T cells for interaction with antigen-presenting cells	CCR4
99 AA	Variety of tissues	Monocytes, DC, resting T cells	Chemoattractant for monocytes, DC, resting T cells, osteoclast precursors; inhibition of colony formation by myeloid precursors	CCR1
93 AA, 10.6 kDa	Activ. monocytes	Resting T cells, eosinophils, basophils, hematopoietic precursor cells	Chemotaxis of resting T cells, eosinophils, and basophils; release of histamine and leukotriene; inhibition of colony formation in stem cells	CCR3
127 AA	Thymic DC, small intestine epithelial cells	Intestinal intra-epithelial lymphocytes	Chemotattractant for IgA-secreting cells	CCR9
71 AA	Endothelial cells, epithelial cells of different tissues	Eosinophils	Activation of fibroblasts and eosinophils, chemotaxis of eosinophils and basophils	CCR3
95 AA, 10.9 kDa	Keratinocytes	Memory T cells	Selectively attracts skin-associated T cells	CCR10
108 AA, 12.3 kDa	Epithelial cells (particularly mucosa)	Resting CD4 and CD8 T cells, eosinophils	Attracts resting T cells, eosinophils	CCR10, CCR3

Appendix

Glossary

Affinity maturation	The increase in average antibody affinity that occurs during a secondary immune response.
Affinity	Measure of binding strength between an antigenic determinant (epitope) and a binding site on an antibody (paratope).
Agretope	The region of an antigen or antigen fragment that interacts with an MHC molecule.
Allele	Alternative form of a particular gene locus within a given species.
Allergy	Originally defined as the altered reaction state that occurs upon secondary contact with an antigen; today an allergy is generally considered to be a type I or type IV hypersensitivity reaction.
Allogeneic	Allogeneic variation denotes the genetic differences between members of the same species.
Allotype	Protein product of an allele recognized as an antigen by another member of the same species.
Anaphylatoxins	Complement peptides (C3a and C5a) that induce the degranulation of mast cells and the contraction of smooth muscles.
Anaphylaxis	Antigen-specific, primarily IgE-mediated immune response associated with vasodilatation and contraction of smooth muscles (and of the bronchi); the outcome may be fatal.
Antibody (Ab)	Molecule formed in response to contact with an antigen and which can specifically bind to that antigen.
Antigen (Ag)	Any substance that can trigger a specific immune response or react with components of an already ongoing immune response (e.g., cross-react with antibodies). The main substances that act as antigens are proteins and other substances with high molecular weights. Some low-molecular-weight substances that cannot trigger an immune response alone are able to trigger an immune response by binding to endogenous proteins (hapten–carrier complex), thus rendering them full-fledged antigens.
Antigen processing	The transformation of an antigen to a form recognizable by lymphocytes.
Antigen-presenting cell (APC)	Cells such as macrophages, dendritic cells, Langerhans cells that express antigens, e.g., from microorganisms bound to their surface, and present them along with MHC products to T lymphocytes. This process of making the antigens "palatable" is essential for an effective immune response.
Apoptosis	Programmed cell death (suicide).

Atopia	The clinical manifestations of type I hypersensitivity, including eczema, asthma, and rhinitis.
Autologous	Originating from the same individual.
Avidity	The functional binding potential of an antibody to its antigen; dependent on the affinity between epitopes and paratopes as well as the valences of antibody and antigen.
Bursa of Fabricius	Lymphoepithelioid organ on the cloaca of birds; site of B-cell maturation in birds.
C1–C9	Components of the classical and lytic complement pathways of the complement system which mediate inflammatory reactions, the opsonization of particles, and the lysis of cell membranes.
Carrier	An immunogenic molecule (or part of a molecule) recognized by T cells during an immune response.
CD	See **cluster of differentiation**.
CDR	See **complementarity-determining region**.
Cell cycle	Process of cell division, which can be divided into four phases: G_1, S, G_2 and M. DNA is copied during the S phase, whereas cell division occurs in the M phase (mitosis phase).
Cell line	Cells that can be bred in vitro in a defined cell culture. Cell lines usually contain several individual cell clones.
CFU	See **colony-forming unit**.
Chemokinesis	Increased (nondirectional) migration activity of cells.
Chemotaxis	Directional movement of cells along a concentration gradient of certain chemotactic factors.
Chimerism	The presence of cells from genetically different individuals in a given individual.
Clone	A family of cells or organisms with an identical genetic configuration.
Cluster of differentiation (CD)	Internationally standardized nomenclature for antigens on cell surfaces. Cell populations can be differentiated using monoclonal antibodies directed against these antigenic determinants.
Colony-forming unit (CFU)	Term for bone marrow stem cells that become mature blood cells after further differentiation.
Colony-stimulating factor (CSF)	(Growth factors). Polypeptides produced, for example, by T lymphocytes that stimulate the proliferation and differentiation of hematopoietic stem cells.

Appendix

Complementarity-determining region (CDR)	Hypervariable region of antibodies or T-cell receptors. Contact with the antigen is established via the CDR.
Conjugate	Reagent formed by the covalent binding of two molecules, e.g., fluorescein bound to an immune molecule.
Cytokine	Common name for soluble molecules that mediate cell–cell interactions.
Dendritic cells	Antigen-presenting cells that occur in the skin as Langerhans' cells, in the lymph nodes as follicular or interdigitating cells, and in the blood and lymph as veiled cells.
Desetope	Part of the MHC molecule that binds with an antigen or processed antigen.
Effector cells	Functional designation for lymphocytes and phagocytes that exert the actual end effects of an immune response.
Enhancement	Extension of the survival time of a transplant by antibodies that attach to and mask alloantigens of the donor tissue.
Epitope	An individual determinant of an antigen to which the paratope of the antibody binds.
Exon	A protein-coding gene segment.
Framework regions	Portions of the V regions of antibodies that lie between the hypervariable regions.
Genome	The entire genetic material of a cell.
Haplotype	A set of genetic determinants on a single chromosome.
Hapten	A small molecule that can assume the function of an epitope but cannot evoke an antibody response without assistance.
Heterologous	Belonging to another species.
Heteronuclear RNA (hnRNA)	The fraction of a nuclear RNA molecule containing the primary DNA transcript before it is processed for formation of messenger RNA.
High responder	Pertains to a specific antigen of an individual (or cultured breed) that responds with a strong immune response.
Histocompatibility	The property of transplant acceptance among different individuals.
Homologous	Belonging to the same species.
Hybridoma	In vitro hybridized lines from two cell types (usually lymphocytes), one of which originates from a tumor.

Idiotope	A single antigenic determinant on the variable domain of an antibody.
Idiotype	The overall set of an antibody's idiotopes that also have antigenic properties. Anti-idiotypic antibodies that are identical to the epitope of the original antigen can therefore be generated.
Immune complex	Product of an antigen–antibody reaction; it may also contain components of the complement system.
Interferons (IFNs)	Interferons are synthesized by a number of different cell types, especially T lymphocytes. They play an important role in the "nonspecific" defense against viral infections and are involved in the lysis of infected cells, thereby inducing the interruption of viral replication.
Interleukins (ILs)	Group of molecules that transmit signals between cells of the immune system. More than 17 interleukins have been characterized so far. Larger amounts can be manufactured by genetic engineering. Consequently, the therapeutic use of interleukins is now feasible.
Intron	Gene segment between two exons that does not code a protein.
Isologous	Characterized by an identical genetic constitution.
Isotype	Of the several possible variants of specific proteins or peptides, the variants anchored isotypically in the genome are identical with all individuals of a species (e.g., immunoglobulin classes)
Kinins	A group of vasoactive mediator substances released when tissue is damaged.
Ligand	A molecule that can mediate a binding or a linkage.
Linkage disequilibrium	Linkage disequilibrium exists if the coincidence of two genes in a population is more frequent than would be expected based on the product of their individual gene frequencies.
Locus	The position of a specific gene on a chromosome.
Low responder	An individual or animal breed with weak reactivity to one or more defined antigens.
Lymphokine-activated killer cells (LAK cells)	Upon incubation with interleukins, lymphoid precursor cells can differentiate into mature effector cells with a high cytotoxic potential, e.g., against tumor cells.
β_2-Microglobulin	Polypeptide constituent of class I molecules (light chain).
Migration-inhibition factor (MIF)	Peptides released by lymphocytes that limit the migration of macrophages.
Mitogen	Substance that induces the transformation and division of cells (mainly lymphocytes).

Appendix

303

Mononuclear phagocytic system (MPS)	The concept of the MPS as a morphological and functional unit has replaced the former term, "reticuloendothelial system" (RES). This cytogenetically uniform cell complex can differentiate into promonocytes, histiocytes, Kupffer cells (stellate cells), pulmonary alveolar macrophages, sinus endothelial cells of the spleen, lymph node macrophages, sinus endothelial cells of the bone marrow, peritoneal macrophages, or osteoclasts.
Opsonization	Phagocytosis of an antigen is facilitated by the deposition of opsonins on the antigen (e.g., antibody and C3b).
Paratope	That part of an antibody molecule by which contact with the antigenic determinant (epitope) is established.
Pathogen	Disease-causing organism
Pinocytosis	Process by which fluids or very small particles are incorporated into a cell.
Pokeweed mitogen (PWM)	Lectins of *Phytolacca americana*. In experimental immunology, this mitogen is used for stimulation of lymphocytes and macrophages.
Primary response	Initial immune response (cellular or humoral) after the first exposure to a specific antigen.
Priming	The initial sensitization of a cell to a specific antigen.
Pseudoalleles	Tandem variants of a gene that occupy nonhomologous positions on the chromosome (e.g., C4).
Pseudogenes	Genes that have structures homologous to those of other genes but are not expressed.
Secondary response	The immune response to the second exposure and each subsequent exposure to a specific antigen.
Secretory component (SC)	Constituent of secretory IgA. It facilitates the transport of the immunoglobulin through the intestinal epithelium and protects it from proteolytic degradation by enzymes.
Somatic mutation	Rearrangement of antibody genes occurs during B-cell maturation, resulting in the development of a wide range of antibody specificities.
Syngeneic	Animals of inbred strains are syngeneic if all of their autosomal pairs are identical.
T-helper cell	Human T-helper (T_H) lymphocytes bear antigen markers of the CD4 subclass. They play a central role in the initiation and maintenance of immune responses. They recognize an antigen only if it occurs in conjunction with a class II MHC molecule.
Tolerance	State of specific immunologic unresponsiveness.

Regulatory T cell (T_R)	A regulatory T cell (T_R) is a suppressor T cell that has a regulatory effect on the course of humoral and cell-mediated immune responses. Hence, T_R cells play an important role in the avoidance of allergic reactions and autoimmune diseases.
Xenogeneic	Pertaining to antigenic differences between different species.

Appendix

Further Reading

Textbooks

Abbas AK, Lichtman AH. *Basic Immunology: Functions and Disorders of the Immune System*. Philadelphia: W.B. Saunders Co, 2001.

Abbas AK, Lichtman AH. *Cellular and Molecular Immunology*. 5th ed. Philadelphia: Saunders, 2003.

George AJT, Urch CE, eds. *Diagnostic and Therapeutic Antibodies*. Totowa, NJ: Humana Press, 2000.

Janeway CA, Travers P, Walport M, Shlomchik M. *Immunobiology*. 5th ed. Edinburgh: Churchill Livingstone, 2001.

Kaufmann SHE, Sher A, Ahmed R, eds. *Immunology of Infectious Diseases*. Washington, DC: ASM Press, 2002.

Paul WE, ed. *Fundamental Immunology*. 4th ed. Philadelphia: Lippincott-Raven, 1999.

Roitt I, Brostoff J, Male D, eds. *Immunology*. 6th ed. Edinburgh; New York: Mosby, 2001.

Sell S, Max EE. *Immunology, Immunopathology, and Immunity*. 6th ed. Washington, DC: ASM Press, 2001.

Reference works

Barclay AN, Brown MH, Law SKA, et al. *The Leukocyte Antigen Factsbook*. 2nd ed. San Diego: Academic Press, 1997.

Delves PJ, Roitt IM, eds. *Encyclopedia of Immunology*. 2nd ed. San Diego: Academic Press, 1998.

Fitzgerald KA, O'Neill LAJ, Gearing AJH. *The Cytokine Factsbook*. 2nd ed. San Diego: Academic Press, 2001.

Periodicals

Advances in Immunology. Annual. San Diego: Academic Press. ISSN: 0065-2776.

Annual Review of Immunology. Palo Alto, CA: Annual Reviews. ISSN: 0732-0582.

Arthritis and Rheumatism. Monthly. New York: John Wiley Sons. ISSN: 0004-3591.

Current Opinion in Immunology. Bimonthly. London: Current Biology. ISSN: 0952-7915.

Current Opinion in Rheumatology. Bimonthly. Philadelphia: Lippincott Williams Wilkins. ISSN: 1040-8711.

Immunity. Monthly. Cambridge, MA: Cell Press. ISSN: 1074-7613.

Journal of Immunology. Semimonthly. Bethesda, MD: Amer Assoc Immunologists. ISSN: 0022-1767.

Trends in Immunology. Monthly. Oxford: Elsevier Sci. ISSN: 1471-4906.

Illustration credits

The illustration on page 47B was adapted from Bjorkman PJ, Saper MA, Samraoui B, et al. The foreign antigen binding site and T cell recognition regions of class I histocompatibility antigens. *Nature* 329 (October 1987): 512–18.

Illustration A.1 on page 159 was taken from Koolman J, Röhm KH. *Taschenatlas der Biochemie.* Stuttgart: Thieme, 1998.

Index

Note: page numbers in *italics* refer to illustrations